THE GENETICS OF MALE INFERTILITY

THE GENETICS
OF MALE INFERTILITY

Edited by

DOUGLAS T. CARRELL, PhD

Departments of Surgery (Urology),
Obstetrics and Gynecology, and Physiology
University of Utah School of Medicine
Salt Lake City, UT

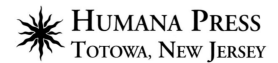

HUMANA PRESS
TOTOWA, NEW JERSEY

This publication is printed on acid-free paper. ∞
ANSI Z39.48-1984 (American Standards Institute)

Permanence of Paper for Printed Library Materials.
Cover illustration: Fig. 1 from Chapter 5, "Physiological and Proteomic Approaches to Understanding Human Sperm Function: Prefertilization Events" by Sarah J. Conner, Linda Lefièvre, Jackson Kirkman-Brown, Gisela S. M. Machado-Oliveira, Frank Michelangeli, Stephen J. Publicover, and Christopher L. R. Barratt, Fig 3. from Chapter 7, "The Immunocytogenetics of Human Male Meiosis: A Progress Report" by Daniel Topping, Petrice Brown, and Terry Hassold, and Figs. 1 and 2 from Chapter 8, "The Clinical Relevance of Sperm Aneuploidy", by Renee H. Martin.

Production Editor: Jennifer Hackworth

Cover design by Patricia F. Cleary

For additional copies, pricing for bulk purchases, and/or information about other Humana titles, contact Humana at the above address or at any of the following numbers: Tel.: 973-256-1699; Fax: 973-256-8341; E-mail: orders@humanapr.com; or visit our Website: www.humanapress.com

Printed in Singapore. 10 9 8 7 6 5 4 3 2 1
1-59745-176-2 (e-book)

Library of Congress Cataloging-in-Publication Data

The genetics of male infertility / edited by Douglas T. Carrell.
    p. ; cm.
  Includes bibliographical references and index.
  ISBN 1-58829-863-9 (alk. paper)
  1. Infertility, Male--Genetic aspects--Congresses. 2.
Spermatogenesis--Genetic aspects--Congresses. I. Carrell, Douglas T.
  [DNLM: 1. Infertility, Male--genetics--Congresses. 2. Genetic
Techniques--Congresses. WJ 709 G3287 2007]
  RC889.G46 2007
  616.6'921042--dc22   2006015411

PREFACE

Male infertility is a common and severe health problem. Infertility not only affects one's ability to have children, but also has emotional, psychological, family, and societal effects. Despite the prevalence and significance of this health problem, resources and attention have not been sufficiently focused on this important issue.

Approximately 7% of men suffer from infertility, and the incidence may be increasing. Of those affected, roughly 40% have idiopathic infertility. It is likely that the majority of those patients have genetic abnormalities that are the cause of their infertility. However, it is important to remember that there are genetic ramifications for essentially all infertile male patients. For example, it is likely that there are genetic predispositions to pathologies such as varicoceles, and environmental factors almost certainly modulate the underlying condition. The understanding of the genes involved in spermatogenesis, sperm maturation, and normal sperm function is key, but we must also focus on better methods of accelerating advances into meaningful clinical diagnostic tests and therapies.

During the past 20 years, significant improvements in technology have advanced the treatment of male infertility. The primary advance has been intracytoplasmic sperm injection (ICSI) in conjunction with in vitro fertilization. Although this technological leap has allowed thousands of men to father a child who otherwise would have been unable to do so, the scientific study of the causes of male infertility has not kept pace. In fact, the clinical application of ICSI proceeded without sufficient scientific study of its safety to the offspring, or the future genetic ramifications.

We currently stand at a point in history in which new tools are available to evaluate genetic diseases. The completion of the Human Genome Project has ushered in an era of unprecedented momentum and ability to tackle the complex issues in the genetics of male infertility. New tools include in vitro methodologies, *in silico* technologies, and new model organisms. Together these advances portend great possibilities.

In January 2006, an international symposium was held at the University of Utah Campus in Salt Lake City to address the genetic causes of male infertility and the translation of the knowledge to the clinical realm. Twenty-one researchers and clinicians, and an international audience of experts in the field, reviewed the study of the genetics of male infertility, the tools available in the laboratory and clinic, the current state of knowledge, and the future of research and translation into clinical diagnostics and treatments. This book is the result of the symposium. The book is intended as a review of our current understanding of genetic causes of male infertility, a guide to evidence-based clinical applications, and a preview of future possibilities.

Douglas T. Carrell, PhD

CONTENTS

CONTRIBUTORS

ALEXANDER I. AGOULNIK, PhD, *Department of Obstetrics and Gynecology, Baylor College of Medicine, Houston, TX*

VINCENT W. AOKI, PhD, *Seattle Reproductive Medicine, Seattle, WA, and University of Utah School of Medicine, Department of Surgery (Urology), Salt Lake City, UT*

LESLIE AYENSU-COKER, MD, *Department of Obstetrics and Gynecology, Baylor College of Medicine, Houston, TX*

MARCO A. AZARO, PhD, *Department of Molecular Genetics, Microbiology and Immunology, University of Medicine and Dentistry of New Jersey, Robert Wood Johnson Medical School, Piscataway, NJ*

CHRISTOPHER L. R. BARRATT, PhD, *Reproductive Biology and Genetics Group, Division of Reproductive and Child Health, University of Birmingham, Edgbaston, Birmingham, UK*

COLIN BISHOP, PhD, *Department of Obstetrics and Gynecology, Baylor College of Medicine, Houston, TX*

DAVIDE BIZZARO, PhD, *Institute of Biology and Genetics, University of Ancona, Ancona, Italy*

PETRICE BROWN, MS, *School of Molecular Biosciences, Washington State University, Pullman, WA, and Department of Genetics, Case Western Reserve University, Cleveland, OH*

DOUGLAS T. CARRELL, PhD, *University of Utah School of Medicine, Department of Surgery (Urology), Obstetrics and Gynecology, and Physiology, Salt Lake City, UT*

SANDRA CHANTOT-BASTARAUD, MD, *Reproduction, Fertility and Populations, Institut Pasteur and Service d'Histologie, Biologie de la Reproduction et Cytogenetique, Hopital Tenon, Paris, France*

NYAM-OSOR CHIMGE, PhD, *Department of Molecular Genetics, Microbiology and Immunology, University of Medicine and Dentistry of New Jersey, Robert Wood Johnson Medical School, Piscataway, NJ*

YI CHU, MS, *Department of Molecular Genetics, Microbiology and Immunology, University of Medicine and Dentistry of New Jersey, Robert Wood Johnson Medical School, Piscataway, NJ*

SARAH J. CONNER, PhD, *Reproductive Biology and Genetics Group,
Division of Reproductive and Child Health, University
of Birmingham, Edgbaston, Birmingham, UK and Assisted
Conception Unit, Birmingham Women's Hospital, Birmingham, UK*

GAIL A. CORNWALL, PhD, *Department of Cell Biology and Biochemistry,
Texas Tech University Health Sciences Center, Lubbock, TX*

DAVID CRAM, PhD, *Monash IVF, Monash Institute of Medical Research,
Monash University, Clayton, Melbourne, Victoria, Australia*

XIANGFENG CUI, BS, *Department of Molecular Genetics, Microbiology
and Immunology, University of Medicine and Dentistry of New
Jersey, Robert Wood Johnson Medical School, Piscataway, NJ*

CHRISTINA J. DECOSTE, PhD, *Department of Molecular Biology,
Princeton University, Princeton, NJ*

CHRISTOPHER DE JONGE, PhD, *HCLD, Reproductive Medicine Center,
University of Minnesota, Minneapolis, MN*

DAVID M. DE KRETSER, MD, *Andrology Australia, Monash Institute
of Medical Research, Monash University, Clayton, Melbourne,
Victoria, Australia*

DAVID J. DIX, PhD, *National Center for Computational Toxicology,
Office of Research and Development, U.S. Environmental
Protection Agency, Durham, NC*

BRAHIM EL HOUATE, MSc, *Reproduction, Fertility and Populations,
Institut Pasteur, Paris, France*

SHU FENG, PhD, *Department of Obstetrics and Gynecology, Baylor
College of Medicine, Houston, TX*

MARK S. FOX, PhD, *Program in Human Embryonic Stem Cell Biology,
University of California San Francisco, San Francisco, CA*

RICHENG GAO, MS, *Department of Molecular Genetics, Microbiology
and Immunology, University of Medicine and Dentistry of New
Jersey, Robert Wood Johnson Medical School, Piscataway, NJ*

FRANCESCA K. E. GORDON, BS, *Molecular and Cellular Biology,
Baylor College of Medicine, Houston, TX*

DANIELLE M. GREENAWALT, PhD, *Department of Molecular Genetics,
Microbiology and Immunology, University of Medicine
and Dentistry of New Jersey, Robert Wood Johnson Medical
School, Piscataway, NJ*

TERRY HASSOLD, PhD, *School of Molecular Biosciences, Washington
State University, Pullman, WA*

NORMAN B. HECHT, PhD, *Center for Research on Reproduction
and Women's Health, University of Pennsylvania School
of Medicine, Philadelphia, PA*

GUOHONG HU, PhD, *Department of Molecular Genetics, Microbiology and Immunology, University of Medicine and Dentistry of New Jersey, Robert Wood Johnson Medical School, Piscataway, NJ*

CLAIRE KENNEDY, PhD, *Monash Institute of Medical Research, Monash University, Clayton, Melbourne, Victoria, Australia*

JACKSON KIRKMAN-BROWN, PhD, *Reproductive Biology and Genetics Group, Division of Reproductive and Child Health, University of Birmingham, Edgbaston, and Assisted Conception Unit, Birmingham Women's Hospital, Birmingham, UK*

NOORA KOTAJA, PhD, *Institut de Génétique et de Biologie Moléculaire et Cellulaire, Illkirch–Strasbourg, France*

STEPHEN A. KRAWETZ, PhD, *Department of Obstetrics and Gynecology, Center for Molecular Medicine and Genetics, Institute for Scientific Computing, Wayne State University School of Medicine, Detroit, MI*

CSILLA KRAUSZ, MD, PhD, *Andrology Unit, Department of Clinical Physiopathology, University of Florence, Florence, Italy*

DOLORES J. LAMB, PhD, *Molecular and Cellular Biology and Scott Department of Urology, Baylor College of Medicine, Houston, TX*

LINDA LEFIÈVRE, PhD, *Reproductive Biology and Genetics Group, Division of Reproductive and Child Health, University of Birmingham, Edgbaston, Birmingham, UK*

HONGHUA LI, PhD, *Department of Molecular Genetics, Microbiology and Immunology, University of Medicine and Dentistry of New Jersey, Robert Wood Johnson Medical School, Piscataway, NJ*

JAMES Y. LI, BS, *Department of Computer Science, University of Maryland, Baltimore County, Baltimore, MD*

YI-NAN LIN, MSc, *Departments of Pathology and Molecular and Cellular Biology, Baylor College of Medicine, Houston, TX*

YONG LIN, PhD, *Department of Biometrics, University of Medicine and Dentistry of New Jersey, Robert Wood Johnson Medical School, Piscataway, NJ*

ZHENWU LIN, PhD, *Department of Cellular and Molecular Physiology, Milton S. Hershey Medical Center, Pennsylvania State University College of Medicine, Hershey, PA*

MINJIE LUO, PhD, *Department of Molecular Genetics, Microbiology and Immunology, University of Medicine and Dentistry of New Jersey, Robert Wood Johnson Medical School, Piscataway, NJ*

MICHAEL LYNCH, PhD, *Prince Henry's Institute, Clayton, Melbourne, Victoria, Australia*

GISELA S. M. MACHADO-OLIVEIRA, BsC, *School of Biosciences, University of Birmingham, Edgbaston, Birmingham, UK*

JACQUELINE MANDELBAUM, MD, PhD, *Reproduction, Fertility and Populations, Institut Pasteur and Service d'histologie, biologie de la reproduction et cytogenetique, Hopital Tenon, Paris, France*

GIAN C. MANICARDI, PhD, *Department of Animal Biology, University of Modena and Reggio Emilia, Modena, Italy*

RENEE H. MARTIN, PhD, FCCMG, *Department of Medical Genetics, University of Calgary, Calgary, Alberta, Canada*

MARTIN M. MATZUK, MD, PhD, *Departments of Pathology, Molecular and Cellular Biology and Molecular and Human Genetics, Baylor College of Medicine, Houston, TX*

KEN MCELREAVEY, PhD, *Reproduction, Fertility and Populations, Institut Pasteur, Paris, France*

ROBERT I. MCLACHLAN, MD, PhD, *Prince Henry's Institute, Clayton, Melbourne, Victoria, Australia*

GISELA S. M. MICHADO-OLIVEIRA, BSc, *School of Biosciences, University of Birmingham, Edgbaston, Birmingham, UK*

FRANK MICHELANGELI, PhD, *School of Biosciences, University of Birmingham, Edgbaston, Birmingham, UK*

DURGA PRASAD MISHRA, PhD, *Department of Pharmacology, Gillespie Neuroscience, University of California, Irvine, Irvine, CA*

MOIRA K. O'BRYAN, PhD, *Monash Institute of Medical Research, Monash University, Clayton, Melbourne, Victoria, Australia*

MARTTI PARVINEN, MD, PhD, *Department of Anatomy, University of Turku, Turku, Finland*

ADRIAN E. PLATTS, BSc, *Department of Obstetrics and Gynecology, Wayne State University School of Medicine, Detroit, MI*

SREEMANTA PRAMANIK, PhD, *Department of Molecular Genetics, Microbiology and Immunology, University of Medicine and Dentistry of New Jersey, Robert Wood Johnson Medical School, Piscataway, NJ*

STEPHEN J. PUBLICOVER, PhD, *School of Biosciences, University of Birmingham, Edgbaston, Birmingham, UK*

CELIA RAVEL, MD, *Reproduction, Fertility and Populations, Institut Pasteur and Service d'histologie, biologie de la reproduction et cytogenetique, Hopital Tenon, Paris, France*

ANNE REILLY, BScHons, *Monash Institute of Medical Research, Monash University, Clayton, Melbourne, Victoria, Australia*

RENEE A. REIJO PERA, PhD, *Program in Human Embryonic Stem Cell Biology, University of California San Francisco, San Francisco, CA*

JAN ROHOZINSKI, PhD, *Department of Obstetrics and Gynecology, Baylor College of Medicine, Houston, TX*

ANGSHUMOY ROY, MBBS, *Departments of Pathology and Molecular and Human Genetics, Baylor College of Medicine, Houston, TX*

DENNY SAKKAS, PhD, *Department of Obstetrics, Gynecology and Reproductive Sciences, Yale University School of Medicine, New Haven, CT*

PAOLO SASSONE-CORSI, PhD, *Department of Pharmacology, Gillespie Neuroscience, University of California, Irvine, Irvine, CA*

PETER N. SCHLEGEL, MD, *Department of Urology, New York Presbyterian Hospital, Weill Medical College of Cornell University, New York, NY*

LI SHEN, MS, *Department of Molecular Genetics, Microbiology and Immunology, University of Medicine and Dentistry of New Jersey, Robert Wood Johnson Medical School, Piscataway, NJ*

WEICHUNG J. SHIH, PhD, *Department of Biometrics, University of Medicine and Dentistry of New Jersey, Robert Wood Johnson Medical School, Piscataway, NJ*

JEAN-PIERRE SIFFROI, MD, PhD, *Service d'Histologie, Biologie de la Reproduction et Cytogenetique, Hopital Tenon, Paris, France*

IRINA V. TERESHCHENKO, MD, PhD, *Department of Molecular Genetics, Microbiology and Immunology, University of Medicine and Dentistry of New Jersey, Robert Wood Johnson Medical School, Piscataway, NJ*

DANIEL TOPPING, MD, *School of Molecular Biosciences, Washington State University, Pullman, WA*

HANS H. VON HORSTEN, PhD, *Department of Cell Biology and Biochemistry, Texas Tech University Health Sciences Center, Lubbock, TX*

HUI-YUN WANG, MD, PhD, *Department of Molecular Genetics, Microbiology and Immunology, University of Medicine and Dentistry of New Jersey, Robert Wood Johnson Medical School, Piscataway, NJ*

QIFENG YANG, MD, PhD, *Department of Molecular Genetics, Microbiology and Immunology, University of Medicine and Dentistry of New Jersey, Robert Wood Johnson Medical School, Piscataway, NJ*

I

METHODS AND TOOLS FOR THE STUDY OF THE GENETICS OF MALE INFERTILITY

1

The Genetics of Male Infertility in the Era of Genomics

Tools for Progress

Douglas T. Carrell, PhD

Summary

The histories of progress in the fields of genetics and andrology are rich and include many breakthroughs. The era of genomics, initiated with the completion of the Human Genome Project, is upon us and offers many new tools for better understanding the genetics of male infertility. Genomic breakthroughs give us a better understanding of structural components of DNA, new types of genetic polymorphisms, regulation of gene expression, and the identity of genes involved in male infertility. The advances we have seen in genomics are key to facilitating some of the studies needed to gain a better understanding of the genetics of infertility, but researchers in this field can better maximize resources and tools through focused collaboration on studies of major issues.

Key Words: Male infertility; genomics; medical resequencing; consortium; gene; spermatogenesis; Human Genome Project.

1. GENETICS AND ANDROLOGY: COLLABORATION BETWEEN TWO FIELDS

With the recent passing of the 50th anniversary of the publication of Watson and Crick's elucidation of the structure of DNA, much attention has been focused on the rich history of the field of genetics. From the identification of DNA as the molecule responsible for heredity in 1944 to the completion of the Hapmap Project last year, the history of genetics is marked by regular advances in techniques and understanding that have fueled the hope of future therapies to alleviate suffering and provide a higher quality of life. Although those hopes have not been realized as quickly as desired and often predicted, recent breakthroughs, largely accelerated by the Human Genome Project (HGP), have raised

From: *The Genetics of Male Infertility*
Edited by: D.T. Carrell © Humana Press Inc., Totowa, NJ

expectations higher than ever before. It is clear that we are currently in an era of genomics, an era in which advances in genetic tools are shaping the methods and capabilities available to treat disease.

Although the term *andrology* was sporadically used as far back as 150 yr ago, the use of the term to denote the study of male reproduction and infertility was coined and commonly accepted in 1951, 2 yr before the elucidation of the structure of DNA *(1)*. Since that time, the evaluation and treatment of male infertility have evolved from simple techniques to evaluate sperm characteristics to a better understanding of underlying endocrinology to today's common use of intracytoplasmic sperm injection, chromatin evaluation, and sperm function assays, and the initiation of candidate gene evaluation. The interaction of genetics and andrology has been continual and productive throughout the past, bringing breakthroughs such as the identification of sexual differentiation abnormalities, Y-chromosome microdeletions, and DNA nicks and breaks. However, with the completion of the HGP and our entrance into the era of genomics, it is clear that many of the major concerns facing those studying male infertility will likely be solved using the techniques and tools the field of genomics is producing.

The era of genomics does not have a start date, however, it is clear that the genomics movement gained great momentum in 1990 with the planning of the HGP, and was officially ushered in by the initial publication of the sequence of the human genome in 2001 *(2–4)*. The HGP has spawned other major initiatives, such as the Hapmap Project, which is described in Section 3, and the Encyclopedia of DNA Elements project, a study that aims to identify all control mechanisms involved in a representative sample (~1%) of the genome *(5)*. Major consortia have been formed to study these and other big-issue questions, such as the role of the environment in gene function and the genetics of cancer. It is apparent that the progress made in genomics is largely a result of unprecedented collaboration of various specialties (sequencing, bioinformatics, statisticians, classical genetics, etc.) and this model of collaboration could benefit most areas of biomedical research.

Major questions in the study of male infertility include: What are the genes involved in normal spermatogenesis, sperm maturation, and sperm function? Can we identify what polymorphisms or mutations result in infertility, and if so, how can we screen and treat patients better? What are the regulators of normal gene expression during spermatogenesis? What role does abnormal meiotic recombination and segregation play in male infertility? What effect does abnormal DNA nicks and breaks have on embryogenesis? What is the role of abnormal protamines in infertility and does it relate to imprinting or epigenetic defects? What is the role of the environment, diet, and other factors in the variation of the degree of pathology seen in different individuals (i.e., varicoceles, smoking effects, etc.)? These and many other important questions will largely be addressed through genetic studies. Proteomics, physiology, endocrinology, and other fields of study will assist in the quest, but it is likely that many of the large leaps made in the study of male infertility will be largely because of genetic advances, lessons learned, and the technologies developed from the HGP. Therefore, it is important to remember not only the advances spurred through the genomics revolution, but also the significant and unique collaborative efforts used in the process.

2. THE CONTRIBUTION OF THE HGP

The HGP was initiated with great hope that the sequencing of the human genome would yield tremendous advances in the understanding of gene function and the etiology of human diseases *(6)*. However, it is likely that, at this time, many of the major breakthroughs of the HGP are in the basic understanding of the human genome. Foremost is the identification of 20,000–25,000 genes, a number much lower than previously predicted *(2,7)*. Previous studies have estimated that at least 2000 genes may be involved in normal spermatogenesis, a strikingly high percentage of the total complement of human genes *(8)*.

Although the number of genes in the human genome is smaller than expected, the diversity of gene products is larger. It is estimated that as many as 35–60% of genes undergo alternative splicing, which increases the diversity of the proteome and the complexity of regulatory and functional mechanisms. Additionally, the data indicate a surprisingly narrow range in the number of genes found in a comparison of humans and other animals.

Another basic finding from the HGP that highlights the increased diversity of products of the genome is the common transcription of non-protein-coding RNA. Some of these RNAs may simply be the result of alternative 5′ start sites during transcription, or may they may be involved in regulatory mechanisms, but it is obvious now that nonprotein-coding RNAs are essential to normal cellular function. More than 800 human micro-RNA "genes" have been identified and appear to be essential to normal development and metabolism *(9)*. The micro-RNAs are apparently an essential regulator of gene expression and very relevant to sperm function *(10)*. The mechanisms and functions of micro-RNAs are a current area of major research, and addressed in Chapters 3 and 4.

In addition to a better understanding of the diversity of the genome and its messenger RNA products, genomic advances have improved our understanding of several structural components of the genome. One such discovery is the presence of ultraconserved elements (UCEs;

ref. *11*). UCEs are sequences of at least 200 bp with complete homology between the human, mouse, and rat sequences. Thus far, 481 human UCEs have been identified. Their function has not been entirely worked out; however, it appears that they contain enhancer elements *(6,12)*. Given their evolutionary conservation, it seems likely that the UCEs play a vital role in gene expression regulation.

Another finding is that the genome contains "gene deserts," which are regions of 3 megabases or more that are devoid of genes *(3)*. The regions do not appear to be a result of the normal statistical distribution of the genes, which raises interesting questions as to their function. At this point, the only possible function of these regions is the possible identification of enhancers for lateral genes *(13)*. Nobrega et al. *(14)* have experimentally removed two such deserts in mice, with no apparent effect. Additionally, there is at times a clustering of functionally related genes of nonrelated origin *(15)*. It would appear that an evolutionary advantage might sometimes be found in the clustering of functionally related genes into "neighborhoods," with obvious implications for coordinated expression regulation.

Studies have found that the genome is polymorphic in a structural sense on a much larger scale than previously thought *(16)*. Using comparative microarray technology, large differences in copy number variation were shown, and it was suggested that large-scale DNA variations of up to several hundred kilobases were responsible. Several studies have since shown that these deletions and other changes are relatively common and more than 1000 such polymorphisms have been identified *(16–19)*. The studies that identified these polymorphisms used different assays and had small overlaps, indicating that the ideal assays to identify the polymorphisms are not yet known, and that there may be many more polymorphisms to be found *(20)*. This exciting find is likely to have profound implications in many areas, including a better understanding of polymorphic phenotypes, including infertility.

3. THE IDENTIFICATION AND EVALUATION OF CANDIDATE MALE INFERTILITY GENES

The great promise of the HGP is in the identification and evaluation of candidate genes in patients. Previous estimates have predicted that about 10% of the genes in the human genome may be related to spermatogenesis and fertility *(8)*. Those estimates are based largely on animal studies, with human data recently beginning to significantly add to the pool. Table 1 is a current list of genes known to affect male fertility.

Table 1
Genes That Cause Male Infertility When Targeted

Gene symbol	Gene name	Reproductive phenotype
ADAM1a	A disintegrin and metallopeptidase domain 1a	Asthenospermia, penetration defect
ADAM2	A disintegrin and metallopeptidase domain 2	Sperm–egg fusion defect
ADAM3	A disintegrin and metallopeptidase domain 3; cyritestin	Sperm–zona fusion defect
AKAP4	A kinase (PRKA) anchor protein 4	Abnormal tail morphology, asthenospermia
Acr	Acrosin	Sperm are not capable of binding and penetrating the zona pellucida
Acvr2	Activin receptor-type IIA	Small testes, delayed fertility
ACOX	Acyl-Coenzyme A oxidase 1, palmitoyl	Leydig cell hypoplasia, small testes, abnormal spermatogenesis
ADFP	Adipose differentiation -related protein	Male infertility
Arl4	ADP-ribosylation factor-like 4	Significantly reduced testicular weights and sperm counts
AFF1	AF4/FMR2 family, member 1	Male subfertility (decreased litter size)
AFF4	AF4/FMR2 family, member 4	Enlarged seminal gland, small testis, azoospermia, arrest of spermatogenesis, abnormal epididymis morphology
Man2a2	α-mannosidase IIx	Defect in adherence of spermatogenic cells to Sertoli cells; germ cells prematurely released from the testis
Amhr2	AMH receptor	Abnormal semal differentiation
Npepps	Aminopeptidase puromycin-sensitive	Asthenospermia, abnormal tubules

(Continued)

Table 1 *(Continued)*

Gene symbol	Gene name	Reproductive phenotype
Ar; tfm	Androgen receptor; testicular feminization	Feminized external genitalia; hypogonadal; cryptorchidism with a block in spermatogenesis
ACE	Angiotensin I-converting enzyme; peptidyl-dipeptidase A 1	Presumed penetration defect; normal testicular histology, concentration, sperm morphology
Ace	Angiotesin-converting enzyme	Compromised ability of sperm to fertilize ova
AE2	Anion exchanger 2	Disrupted spermiogenesis, complete absence of spermatozoa in tubules
Amh	Anti-Mullerian hormone	Uteri development in males causes obstruction and secondary infertility
Apob	Apolipoprotein B	Decreased sperm count, motility, survival time, and ability to fertilize ova
Apaf1	Apoptotic protease-activating factor 1	Spermatogonial degeneration
Atm	Ataxia Telangiectasia	Germ cells degenerate; disruptions evident in meiosis I
Atxn7	Ataxin 7	Reduced fertility at 16 wk of age
AGTPbp1	ATP/GTP-binding protein 1	Oligospermia, teratospermia, asthenospermia
Atp2b4	ATPase, Ca^{++} transporting, plasma membrane 4	Infertile
Atp8b3	ATPase, class I, type 8B, member 3	Impaired sperm–egg interaction, reduced zona pellucida-induced acrosome reaction
Bbs2	Bardet-Biedl syndrome 2 homolog (human)	Sperm lack flagella
Bbs4	Bardet-Biedl syndrome 4 homolog (human)	Flagella are absent throughout the seminiferous tubules, even on cells with condensed sperm heads
BSG	Basigin	Azoospermia, arrest at meiosis I

(Continued)

Table 1 *(Continued)*

Gene symbol	Gene name	Reproductive phenotype
Bsg	Basign	Block in spermatogenesis at metaphase I
Bax	Bc12-associated X protein	Premeiotic arrest of spermatogenesis
Bc16	B-cell leukemia/ lymphoma 16	Apoptosis in metaphase I spermatocytes
Bclw; *Bc12l2;* *Bc12-like 2*	BCL2-like 2 protein apoptosis regulator *BCL-W*	Late meiotic arrest with loss of germ cells
	β 1-4-galactosyl-transferase	Male infertility; defects in sperm–egg interaction
Btrc	β-transducin repeat-containing protein	Meiotic arrest with multiple errors
bs	Blind-sterile	Small testis, oligospermia
Bmp4	Bone morphogentic protein 4	Absent primordial germ cell (PGC) population; defect in PGC development
Bmp8a	Bone morphogentic protein 8a	Degeneration of germ cells and epididymis
Bmp8b	Bone morphogentic protein 8b	Reduced or absent PGCs (developmental defect); postnatal germ cell defects and spermatocyte apoptosis
Bdnf	Brain-derived neurotrophic factor	Reduced male fertility
Brca1	Breast cancer 1	Spermatogenic arrest
BUB1B	Budding uninhibited by benzimidazoles 1 homolog β	Oligzoospermia
Camk4	Calcium/calmodulin-dependent protein kinase IV	Impaired chromatin packaging during spermiogenesis
Clgn	Calmegin	Defect in sperm-zona pellucida binding
	Cα(2)/Prkaca	cAMP-dependent protein kinase catalytic subunit 2 Males infertile, motility and fertilization affected
Crem	cAMP-responsive element modulator	Defective spermiogenesis with aberrant postmeiotic gene expression
Csnk2a2	Casein kinase IIa 1	Globozoospermia (no acrosomal cap)

(Continued)

Table 1 *(Continued)*

Gene symbol	Gene name	Reproductive phenotype
Catsper1	Cation channel of sperm 1	Asthenospermia, normal count and testis weight
Catsper2	Cation channel of sperm 2	Capacitation defect
Cnot7	CCR4-NOT transcription complex, subunit 7	Abnormal testis morphology, testis hypoplasia
Cd59b	CD59b antigen	Teratozoospermia, oligozoospermia, asthenozoospermia
Cks2	CDC28 protein kinase regulatory subunit 2	Male and female germ cells arrest at anaphase I
Cenpb	Centromere protein B	Hypogonadal and have low sperm counts
Cldn11; Osp-11	Claudin 11	No tight junctions between Sertoli cells
Csf1	Colony-stimulating factor (macrophage)	Reduced testosterone
Gja1; C43	Connexin 43	Small ovaries and testes; decreased numbers of germ cells from E11.5
Ros1	c-ros protoncogene	Sperm motility defects
Crsp	Cryptorchidism with white spotting, deletion region	Azoospermia
Cut11; CDP/Cux	Cut-like 1	Severely reduced fertility
Ccna1	Cyclin A1	Block in spermatogenesis before the first meiotic division
Ccnd2	Cyclin D2	Fertile with decreased testis size
p27Kip1; Cdkn1b	Cyclin-dependent inhibitor 1b	Fertile with testicular hyperplasia
p57kip2; Cdkn1c	Cyclin-dependent inhibitor 1c	Surviving mice show sexual immaturity
p18Ink4c; Cdkn2c	Cyclin-dependent inhibitor 2c	Leydig cell hyperplasia and reduced testosterone production
p19ink4d; Cdkn2d	Cyclin-dependent inhibitor 2d	Testicular atrophy and germ cell apoptosis
Ccne1	Cyclin E1	Testicular hypoplasia
Ccne2	Cyclin E2	Testicular hypoplasia

(Continued)

Table 1 *(Continued)*

Gene symbol	Gene name	Reproductive phenotype
Cdkn2d	Cyclin-dependent kinase inhibitor 2D (p19, inhibits CDK4)	Increased germ cell apoptosis, small testis
Adam3	Cyritesin	Altered sperm protein expression and adhesion defects during fertilization
CYP17	Cytochrome P450 17α-hydroxylase/ 17,20-lyase	Abnormal morphology, reduced motility, sexual behavior
Cyp11a	Cytochrome P450, 11a, cholesterol side-chain cleavage	Males feminized with female external genitalia, underdeveloped sex organs; gonads degenerate
Cyp19	Cytochrome P450, 19, aromatase	Early spermatogonial arrest, Leydig cell hyperplasia, and defects in sexual behavior
Cpeb	Cytoplasmic polyadeny-lation element-binding protein	Disrupted germ cell differentiation and meiosis I synaptonemal complex formation
Tial1	Cytotoxic granule-associated RNA-binding protein-like 1	PGCs lost by E13.5
Dax1 (Nr0b1)	Orphan nuclear receptor	Progressive degeneration of the germinal epithelium
Ddx4	DEAD (Asp-Glu-Ala-Asp) box polypeptide 3, Y-linked (DBY) Symbol-DDX3Y, AZFa region; VASA homolog	Defective proliferation/ differentiation of PGCs
Dazl	Deleted in azoospermia-like	Reduced germ cells; differentiation failure and degeneration of germ cells
Dhh	Desert hedgehog	Complete absence of mature sperm; defects in Sertoli-to-Leydig cell signaling
Dmc1h	Disrupted meiotic cDNA 1 homolog	Defects in chromosome synapsis in meiosis
	DNA polymerase λ	Asthenozoospermia

(Continued)

Table 1 *(Continued)*

Gene symbol	Gene name	Reproductive phenotype
Dnaja1	DnaJ (Hsp40) homolog, subfamily A, member 1	Small testis, tubal degeneration
Dms	Dominant male sterility	Testicular degeneration, azoospermia
Dspd	Dominant spermiogenesis defect	Teratozoospermia, oligozoospermia
Dmrt1	Doublesex and Mab-3-related transcription factor 1	Defects in postnatal testes differentiation; disorganized seminiferous tubules and absence of germ cells
Spo11	DPO11 homolog	Defects in meiosis
Cnahc1	dynein heavy chair 7	Defects in sperm flaggelar motility
Ube2b	E2B ubiquitin-conjugating enzyme; HR6B	Alterations in sperm chromatin structure, an incomplete meiotic arrest, abnormal sperm morphology
Egr1; NGFI-A	Early growth response 1	Lack of LH
Egr4	Early growth response 4	Germ cells undergo apoptosis during pachytene stage
Esgd12d	Early spermiogenesis defective 12d	Some epididymal sperm present, asthenozoospermia, teratozoospermia
Elk1	ELK1, member of ETS oncogene family	Asthenozoospermia
Emk	Elkl motif kinase	Infertile
Emx2	Empty spiracles homolog 2	Defective development of gonads and urogenita tracts
Esr1	Estrogen receptor (ER)α	Develop disruptions of the seminiferous epithelium because of abnormal epididymal function, no ejaculations
Esr2	ERβ	Fertile, but develop prostate hyperplasia
Etv4	Ets variant gene 4 (E1A enhancer-binding protein, E1AF)	Severe oligozoospermia
Etv5	Ets variant gene 5	Early testicular degeneration
Fanc	Fanconi anemia complementation group A	Hypogonadism, reduced fertility

Table 1 *(Continued)*

Gene symbol	Gene name	Reproductive phenotype
Fancc	Fanconi anemia complementation group C	Hypogonadism, compromised gametogenesis
Fancg	Fanconi anemia complementation group G	Hypogonadism, compromised gametogenesis
Adam2	Fertilin β	Altered sperm protein expression and adhesion defects during fertilization
Fgf9	Fibroblast growth factor 9	XY male-to-female sex reversal; phenotype ranges from testicular hypoplasia to complete sex reversal
Fkbp6	FK506-binding protein 6	Absence of normal pachytene spematocytes
Fmr1	Fragile-X mental retardation syndrome 1 homolog	Macroorchidism
Fishb	FSH hormone β-subunit	Decreased testis size
Fshr	FSH receptor	Decreased testis size
Gpr 106	G protein-coupled receptor 106	Crsp males homozygous for trans gene integration exhibit a high intra-abdominal position of the testes, complete sterility
Gpr64	G protein-coupled receptor 64	Enlarged testis, azoospermia
Gcl	Germ cell-less homolog (Drosophila)	Asthenozoospermia, teratozoospermia (giant heads with multiple tails), oligozoospermia
Gdnf	Glial cell line-derived neurotrophic factor	Depletion of stem cell reserves; spermatogonia differentiate
GAPDS	Glyceraldehyde 3-phosphate dehydrogenase-*S*	Severely decreased sperm motility
Cga	Glycoprotein hormone α-subunit	Hypogonadal because of FSH and LH deficiency
GRTH/ Ddx25	Gonadotropin-regulated testicular RNA helicase	Arrest of spermiogenesis, elongation failure
iPLA(2)β	Group VIA phospholipase A2	Reduced motility, impaired fertilization, unable to fertilize

(Continued)

Table 1 *(Continued)*

Gene symbol	Gene name	Reproductive phenotype
Gdf7	Growth differentiation factor-7	Defects in seminal vesicle development
Ghrhr	Growth hormone-releasing hormone receptor	Idiopathic
Gdi1	Guanosine diphosphate dissociation ihibitor 1; Rho GDI α	Impaired spermatogenesis, vaculolar degeneration in males
HSFY	Heat shock factor Y	Deleted in individual with idiopathic azoospermia
Hsp70-2	Heat shock protein 70-2	Meiosis defects and germ cell apoptosis
Hfe2	Hemochromatosis type 2 (juvenile; human homolog)	Sterility
Tcf1	Hepatocyte nuclear factor (HNF-1α) transcription factor 1	Vestigial vas deferens, seminal vesicles and prostate, impaired spermatogenesis, no mating behavior
Hmga1	High mobility group AT-hook 1	Abnormal Sertoli cells, abnormal epididymis morphology
Hmgb2	High mobility group box 2	Sertoli and germ cell degeneration and immotile spermatozoa
H3f3a	Histone 3.3A	Reduced copulatory activity and fewer matings result in pregnancy
H2afx	Histone H2A family, member X	Pachytene stage arrest in spermatogenesis; defects in chromosome segregation and MLH1 foci formation
Hrb	HIV-1 Rev-binding protein	Round-headed spermatozoa lack an acrosome (Globozoospermia)
Hoxa10	Homeobox A10	Variable infertility; cryptorchidism
Hoxa11	Homeobox A11	Males have malformed vas deferens and undescended testes
HOOK1	Hook homolog 1	Teratozoospermia and decapitation
HE6/ GPR64	Human epididymal protein 6	Dysregulation of efferent ductule fluid reabsorbtion, stasis of spematozoa within the ducts

(Continued)

Table 1 *(Continued)*

Gene symbol	Gene name	Reproductive phenotype
BclX; *Bcl2l*	Hypomorph	PGCs are lost by E15.5
Inha	Inhibin a	Granulosa/Sertoli tumors, gonadotropin hormone-dependent
Inpp5b	Inositol polyphosphate-5-phosphatase	Sperm have reduced motility and reduced ability to fertilize eggs; defects in fertilin β processing
Igf1	Insulin-like growth factor 1	Hypogonadal and infertile; disrupted spermatogenesis and vestigial ductal system, defects in mating behavior
Insl3	Insulin-like hormone 3	Bilateral cryptorchidism results in abnormal spermatogenesis
Izumo1	Izumo sperm–egg fusion 1	Normal zona penetration, abnormal oolema binding
JunD; *Jund1*	Jun D proto-oncogene	Anomalous hormone levels and sperm structural defects
Klhl10	Kelch-like 10 (Drosophila)	Sertoli cell only
Kitl	Kit ligand	Defect in PGC migration/survival
Kit	Kit receptor	White spotting null mutation causes PGC defects
Ggtp	λ-Glutamyl transpeptidase	Hypogonadal and infertile; phenotype corrected by feeding mice *N*-acetylcysteine
LGR8 *(GREAT)*	Leucine-rich repeat-containing G protein-coupled receptor	Intra-abdominal cryptorchidism and sterility
Lep; *ob/ob*	Leptin	Obese and infertile with hypogonadotrophic hypogonadism
Lepr; *db/db*	Leptin receptor	Obese and infertile with hypogonadotrophic hypogonadism
Lgr7	Leucine-rich repeat-containing G protein-coupled receptor	Spermatic apoptosis at meiotic stage 12
Lipe; *HSL*	Lipase, hormone-sensitive	Multiple abnormalities in spermatogenesis
Lhcgr	LH receptor	Underdeveloped sex organs and infertility; spermatogenesis

(Continued)

Table 1 *(Continued)*

Gene symbol	Gene name	Reproductive phenotype
		arrested at round spermatid stage
Smad5; Madh5	MAD homolog 5	Developing embryos lose PGCs
Smad; Madh1	MAS homolog 1	Developing embryos lose PGCs
Mell1	Mel-transforming oncogene-like 1	Decreased fertilization and embryogenesis
Mitf	Microphthalmia-associated transcription factor	Reduced male fertility
Morc	Microrchidia	Early arrest in meiosis and germ cell apoptosis
Mtap7; E-MAP-115	Microtubule-associated protein	Abnormal microtubules in germ cells and Sertoli cells
Mlh3	MutL homolog 3 (*E. coli*)	Increased sperm aneuploidy, increased arrest at pachytene
Mlh1	MutL homolog 1	Meiotic arrest and genomic instability
Msh4	MutS homolog 4	Prophase I meiotic defects apparent at the zygotene/pachytene stage; germ cells lost within a few days postpartum
Msh5	MutS homolog 5	Zygotene/pachytene meiotic defects with aberrant chromosome synapsis and apoptosis
Myhl1; A-myb	Myeloblastosis oncogene-like 1	Germ cell meiotic arrest at the pachytene stage
NKCC1; Slc12a2	Na(+) –K(+) –2Cl(–) cotransporter; solute carrier family 12, member 2	Low spermatid counts and compromised sperm transport
Nkd1	Naked cuticle 1 homolog (Drosophila)	Oligozoospermia
Nanos2	Nanos homolog 2 (Drosophila)	Azoospermia
Nanos3	Nanos homolog 3 (Drosophila)	Increased germ cell apoptosis, no germ cells were detected in the testes by E15.5

(Continued)

Table 1 *(Continued)*

Gene symbol	Gene name	Reproductive phenotype
Neurl	Neuralized-like homolog (Drosophila)	Asthenozoospermia, missing sperm heads
Nxph1	Neurexophilin 1	Infertility appears to be an artifact of homologous recombination
Nhlh2	Neuronal helix–loop–helix 2	Infertile and hypogonadal
NIR	Neuronal insulin receptor	Hypothalamic hypogonadism; impaired spermatogenesis
Nkx3-1	NK-3 transcription factor, locus 1 (Drosophila)	Accessory gland deformation
Nmp4	Nuclear matrix protein 4	Abnormal seminiferous tubule morphology, decreased spermatocytes
Nr5a1	Nuclear receptor subfamily 5, group A, member 1	Prostate hypoplasia, seminal gland hypoplasia, germ cell depletion
Ncoa1; SRC1	Nuclear receptor co-activator; steroid receptor coactivator-1	Decreased responsiveness to steroid hormones in testes and prostate
Nr0b1	Nuclear receptor subfamily 0, group B, member 1	Early testicular degeneration
Nr2c2	Nuclear receptor subfamily 2, group C, member 2	Oligozoospermia, cells arrest in meiotic prophase stage/pachytene spermatocyte stage resulting in an increase in the ratio of stage X to stage XII tubules
Nr5a1; SF-1	Nuclear receptor subfamily 5, group A, member 1; steroidogenic factor-1	Gonadal agenesis in both sexes
Ovo	Ovo protein (Drosophila melanogaster homolog)	Reduced fertility and underdeveloped genitalia
P2rx1	P2X1 receptor	Oligospermia and defective vas deferens contraction
Wip1	p53-induced phosphatase	Runting and testicular atrophy
PLCdelta4	Phospholipase C δ 4	Sperm fail to activate eggs, no calcium transients
Pi3k	Phosphatidylinositol 3′-kinase	Defects in proliferation and increased apoptosis of spermatogonia

(Continued)

Table 1 *(Continued)*

Gene symbol	Gene name	Reproductive phenotype
Piga	Phosphatidylinositol glycan, class A	Abnormal testes, epididymis and seminal vesicles
Pss2/ Ptdss2	Phosphatidylserine synthase 2	Reduced testis weigth, some infertile males
Styx	Phosphoserine/threonine/ tyrosine interaction protein	Defects in round and elongating spermatid development
mili/piwil2	Piwi-like homolog 2	Spermatogenesis arrested in early prophase I
Pafah1b1	Platelet-activating factor acetylhydrolase, isoform 1b, β1 subunit	Azoospermia, abnormal testicular morphology
Nectin-2/ Pvrl2	Poliovirus receptor-related 2	Abnormal morphology, males are sterile
TPAP/ Papolb	Polymerase β (testis-specific)	Sperm arrest during spermiogenesis
Pea3	Polyomavirus enhancer activator 3	Normal mating behavior, but males do not set plugs or release sperm
Pms2	Postmeiotic segregation increase 2	Abnormal chromosome synapsis in meiosis
Doppel/ Prnd	Prion protein dublet	Reduced counts, motility and morphology
Adamts2	Procollagen *N*-proteinase	Defects in spermatogenesis; marked decrease in sperm within testes tubules
Prlr	Prolactin receptor	Variability in infertiity and subfertility
Prm1	Protamine 1	Protamine haploinsufficiency; abnormal spermatogenesis
Prm2	Protamine 2	Protamine haploinsufficiency; abnormal spermatogenesis
PN-1	Protease inhibitor protease nexin-1; serpine2	Abnormal seminal vesicle morphology and altered semen protein composition
Ppp1cc	Protein kinase A, catalytic subunit λ	Defects in spermiogenesis
P2rx1	Purinergic receptor P2X, ligand-gated ion channel 1	Impaired neurogenic vas deferens contraction, azoospermia
CatSper	Putative sperm cation channel	Defects in motility and fertilization

(Continued)

Table 1 *(Continued)*

Gene symbol	Gene name	Reproductive phenotype
Rsn/ CLIP-170	Reed-Steinberg cell-expressed intermediate filament-associated protein	Abnormal head morphology
Rara	Retinoic acid receptor α	Complete arrest and degeneration or germ cell depletion
Rarg	Retinoic acid receptor λ	Squamous metaplasia of the seminal vesicles and prostate
Rxrb	Retinoid X receptors	Germ cell maturation defects and tubular degeneration
RNF17	Ring finger protein 17	Component of granuales, arrest as round spermatids
Sept4	Septin 4	Mice sterile because of defective motility, tail morphology
Serac1	Serine active site containing 1	Male sterility
Serpina5	Serine proteinase inhibitor A 5; protein C inhibitor	Sertoli cell destruction
SH2-B	SH2-B homolog	Small testes and reduced sperm count
NHEt	Sodium hydrogen exchanger-testis	Normal morphology and count, but severely reduced motility
sAC	Soluble adenylyl cyclase	Total loss of forward motility
SLC19A2	Solute carrier family 19 (thiamine transporter), member 2	Germ cells arrest as primary spermatocytes
Sp4	Sp4 *trans*-acting transcription factor	Defects in reproductive behavior
PF20/ Spag16	Sperm-associated antigen 16	Significant loss of sperm cells at round spermatid stage, disorganized axoneme structure
SMCP	Sperm mitochondria-associated cysteine-rich protein	Reduced motility, impaired fertilization
SMCP	Sperm mitochondrion-associated cysteine-rich protein	Defects in sperm motility and migration into the oviduct; defects in fertilization
	Sperm-1	Defect in haploid sperm function

(Continued)

Table 1 *(Continued)*

Gene symbol	Gene name	Reproductive phenotype
Spnr	Spermatid perinuclear RNA-binding protein	Defects in seminiferous epithelium and spermatogenesis
Sycp1	Synaptonemal complex protein 1	Ensures formation of crossovers, spermatocytes arrest in pachynema
Sycp3	Synaptonemal complex protein 3	Defects in chromosome synapsis during meiosis; germ cell apoptosis
Tlp;TRF2	TATA-binding protein-like protein	Postmeiotic spermiogenesis block (defective acrosome formation in early stage spermatids)
TLF	TBP-like factor	Complete arrest of spermiogenesis at round spermatid stage
Tektin-t	Tektin-t	Abnormal morphology, bent tails, reduced motility
Tert	Telomerase reverse transcriptase	Progressive infertility
PC4; Pcsk4	Testicular germ cell protease	Sperm have impaired fertilizaiton ability
Tenr	Testis nuclear RNA binding protein	Infertile males with reduced sperm count, motility, and morphology
SSTK	Testis-specific serine kinase	Profound impairment of motility and morphology
Theg; Kisimo	THEG homolog isoform 2	Abnormal elongated spermatids; asthenospermia
Tnp1	Transition protein 1	Abnormal chromosome condensation, sperm motility
Tnp2	Transition protein 2	Abnormal chromosome condensation
Fus1	Translocated in liposarcoma; TLS	Defects in spermatocyte chromosome pairing
Utp14b	U3 small nucleolar ribonucleoprotein, homolog B	Type A spermatogonia fail to differentiate
UTP14c	U3 small nucleolar ribonucleoprotein, homolog C	In frame stop codon identified in infertile males
Siah1a	Ubiquitin protein ligase seven in absentia 1A	Block in spermatogenesis and germ cell apoptosis; failure to complete transition to telophase

(Continued)

Table 1 *(Continued)*

Gene symbol	Gene name	Reproductive phenotype
		of meiosis I
Ube3a	Ubiquitin proteinligase E3A; E6-AP ubiquitin protein ligase	Testicular hypoplasia, defects in spermatogenesis and prostate gland development
USP26	Ubiquitin-specific protease 26	Mutations identified in infertile males
USP9Y; DFFRY	Ubiquitin-specific protease 9; AZFa region	Azoospermia
Ube2b	Ubiquitin-conjugating enzyme E2B, RAD6 homology	Increased apoptosis of primary spermatocytes, infertile males
HR23B; Rad23b	Ubiquitin-like DNA repair gene	Most knockouts die during development or shortly after birth; surviving mice have multiple abnormalities and male sterility
Vdr	Vitamin D receptor	Defects in estrogen biosynthesis, elevated serum gonadotropins
VDAC3	Voltage-dependent anion channel 3	Normal counts, abnormal axonemes, loss of a single microtubule doublet
Vdac3	Voltage-dependent anion channel type 3	Immotile sperm; axonemal defects with sperm maturation
Wt1	Wilms tumor homolog	Gonadal agenesis
Wnt7a	Wingless-type MMTV integration site family member 7A	Do not have Mullerian duct regression
MSY2/ YBX2	Y box protein 2	Spermatogenesis disrupted in postmeiotic null germ cells with misshapen spermatids, no sperm in epididymis
Synj2	Ynaptojanin 2	Male sterility
Zfp148	Zinc finger protein 148	Required for development of fetal germ cells
Zfx	Zinc finger protein X-linked	Reduced germ cell numbers; males have reduced sperm, but are fertile
Dax1 (Nr0b1)	Orphan nuclear receptor	Progressive degeneration of the germinal epithelium

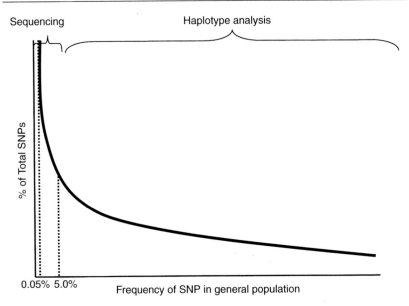

Fig. 1. A plot of the relationship between gene variants and overall polymorphisms. It is expected that many disease causing variants are found in low frequency and will likely require gene sequency studies to identify relevant polymorphisms. On the other hand, common variants can be evaluated using linkage disequilibrium studies, such as haplotype analysis.

The list has been updated from an original listing of both male and female infertility genes by Matzuk and Lamb 4 yr ago *(21)*. Since that time, the number of "male infertility genes" identified has more than doubled.

The strategy used to identify and analyze novel candidate genes in infertile men will be largely dependent on information available about the gene from animal studies, the resources of the laboratory, and the frequency of the variants (polymorphism/mutation) that cause the altered phenotype. Figure 1 demonstrates the hypothetical distribution of gene variants causing disease in relation to the overall frequency of polymorphisms. Common variants, those seen in more than 5% of the population, lend themselves to be analyzed differently than rare variants. Many common diseases may be caused by common variants/ polygenic effects (the common disease/common variant hypothesis) such as is expected for heart disease and other common diseases. These types of common diseases may be more easily studied through classical linkage disequilibrium studies and using haplotypes analysis. Alternatively, many diseases are caused by rare (<5% frequency) or very rare (<0.05% frequency) variants. These variants cannot be as easily identified through linkage disequilibrium, rather will·likely necessitate large-scale medical resequencing studies. The causes of male infertility are likely many, and it is possible that numerous strategies will be used to identify and analyze relevant gene defects. Therefore, it is incumbent that new techniques be monitored and analyzed for their potential assistance.

Last year the International Hapmap Consortium released the first draft of the human hapmap *(22)*. The hapmap sequenced more than 1 million single-nucleotide polymorphisms (SNPs) in 269 individuals from four ethnic populations. One SNP was evaluated for approximately every 3 Kb of the genome, and eventually SNPs will be evaluated for every 1 Kb. The usefulness of the hapmap in identifying disease-causing genes is that nearby SNPs generally remain associated with the target SNP because of linkage disequilibrium. Therefore, rather than genotyping each SNP in the genome, targeted SNPs can be evaluated in patients and controls to evaluate haplotypes associated with a given phenotype, which can then be narrowed and further analyzed to identify disease causing polymorphisms *(23)*. Although this technique will undoubtedly be a great tool in identifying some disease-related polymorphisms, drug discovery, and other areas, it is uncertain how beneficial it will be in aiding the study of male infertility. However, it is apparent that such studies must be undertaken in the near future.

Because many causes of infertility are likely caused by rare functional variants not suitable for analysis using hapmap data, identification and analysis of those genes will be continue to be dependent on direct genotyping, or medical resequencing. Medical resequencing has already been performed on a number of candidate genes, largely identified by animal transgenic and knockout studies in which the targeted genes resulted in altered spermatogenesis without other severe phenotypic effects *(24)*. Medical resequencing has been used to identify polymorphisms in several genes affecting male fertility, including the estrogen receptor gene, protamine genes, transition nuclear protein genes, and genes related to globozoospermia *(25–28)*.

Because gene sequencing is key to future studies, advances in this area are of importance. The Sanger method of gene sequencing remains the gold standard for the evaluation of candidate genes in study populations. However, some reports highlight the potential of alternative strategies to more cheaply perform large screens. Current sequencing has been estimated to cost approx $1 per 1000 bases (sequencing costs only), or roughly $3.1 million per human genome *(5)*. The long-term prediction of the eventual ability to sequence a genome for $1000 highlights the predicted advances in improved sequencing capabilities. Whether the ideal sequencing technology will ultimately rely on modifications to the currently used Sanger technique, such as the application of microfluidic technology to improve injection and separation times, or new sequencing techniques will replace the Sanger method remains to be seen *(29)*. Several alternative sequencing techniques have been proposed and are yet to be refined to the point of practical application *(30)*. Additionally, some new techniques allow the pooling of study samples to identify low-variance polymorphisms and mutations, which could potentially reduce costs dramatically *(31)*.

4. THE FUTURE OF THE STUDY OF THE GENETICS OF MALE INFERTILITY

In 2003, Francis Collins wrote a perceptive evaluation of the future of genomics research *(4)*. Collins related the future to the building of a house, and proposed three levels of future development, all resting on the foundation of the HGP. The first level, genomics to biology, is dependent on three key needs: the development of a comprehensive catalog of all components encoded by the genome, the determination of how those components function in an integrated manner to maintain normal cellular functions, and the need to understand how genomes change. The second level, genomics to health, is dependent on the identification of gene pathways with a role in disease and a determination of how they interact with environmental factors, the development of genome-based diagnostic methods and evaluation of drug response, and the development of translational therapeutic advances. The third and final level, genomics to society, relies on the analysis of genomics, societal factors, and health, and the use of such data to define policy options and ethical guidelines. Six pillars relevant to each of the levels was proposed: resources; technology development; computational biology; training; ethical, legal, and social implications; and education.

Although an understanding of the genetics of male infertility rests on the foundation of areas other than just genomics, this model is of benefit in the development of a vision of the future of the study of the genetic causes and treatments of male infertility. In our field, the three levels are similar to those identified by Collins, and dependent on the same needs and approaches. For example, on the biological level an understanding of not only fertility-related genes is needed, but, as mentioned earlier, we also need to understand the role of micro-RNA, enhancers, promoters, and other regulators. The level of health is dependent on improved assays and treatments, including a stronger regard to the safety of the offspring.

Last, society will benefit by improved safety, lower costs, and broader coverage of assistance to those needing treatment.

Although each of the six pillars proposed by Collins are relevant to our field, focus should be made on three key areas. First, the prudent use of limited resources. With the lack of sufficient funding to assure completion of all relevant areas of study, prioritization and collaboration are key. Identification of a major goal, such as genotyping relevant candidate genes in a large population of well-characterized patients with an equally suitable control group would be an obvious undertaking for a collaborative consortium of researchers. This goal highlights a major area of need for most studies: quality DNA and tissue from patients and controls. Although most laboratories have small repositories of tissue available, pools are usually inadequate for large-scale studies that will be needed. Even more critical, phenotyping is usually inconsistent and incomplete. Last, many studies lack proper controls, both in quantity, diversity, and quality (phenotyping). The establishment of a funded collaborative research tissue repository with community sharing would greatly facilitate studies.

Education is needed on all levels, including interaction between basic scientists and clinicians. Progress is being made in this area as seen by this book and the underlying International Symposium on the Genetics of Male Infertility. However, more is needed. Proper clinical techniques and interpretation of assay results are lacking on the level of the clinician, the patient, and in the decisions society makes regarding health care; these problems can only be solved through education.

The third pillar that we must be especially cognizant of is technology development. Advances are made using proper techniques and utilizing new technologies to their fullest. In addition to equipment and procedures, the proper use of technology includes the use of other model organisms, sometimes more efficient for studies. Examples would be the exciting possibilities for a better understanding of the interaction of proteins with messenger RNA to regulate translation, a regulatory mechanism key to spermatogenesis, which can now be better studied using techniques such as the yeast three-hybrid system and the ability to use RNAi techniques in vivo to better understand protein function *(32,33)*. An example of technological advances involving other species, which can be exploited in the study of male infertility, is the use of the drosophila catalog of more than 2000 induced mutations related to male infertility *(34)*. Most medical and scientific meetings and symposia that deal directly with the diagnosis and treatment of male infertility deal very little with technology. Future meetings must emphasize technology more, so those with a broad spectrum of backgrounds can more fully utilize available tools.

5. CONCLUSIONS

Genomics has brought many tools beneficial to the future study of male infertility. It is clear that the HGP and Hapmap Project could not have been completed without major collaboration and pooling of resources. The study of male infertility greatly benefits from the altruistic collaborative spirit of those pioneers, and will continue to progress using traditional approaches. However, it is clear that the concept of major collaborative efforts in the banking of study tissues, the careful and thorough phenotyping of controls and study subjects, the consistent and careful physiological evaluation of samples, and the genotyping of large study groups and controls are ideas that may hasten the breakthroughs needed to better understand the genetics of male infertility.

REFERENCES

1. Schirren C. History of the term "Andrology". Andrologia 2005;37:143–144.
2. International Human Genome Sequencing Consortium. Initial sequencing and analysis of the human genome. Nature 2001;409:860–921.
3. Venter JC, Adams MD, Myers EW, et al. The sequence of the human genome. Science 2001;291:1304–1351.
4. Collins FS, Green ED, Guttmacher AE, Guyer MS. A vision for the future of genomics research. Nature 2003;422:835–847.
5. Guttmacher AE, Collins FS. Realizing the promise of genomics in biomedical research. JAMA 2006;294:1399–1402.
6. Little PF. Structure and function of the human genome. Genome Res 2005;5: 1759–1766.
7. International Human Genome Sequencing Consortium. Finishing the euchromatic sequence of the human genome. Nature 2004;431:931–945.
8. Hargreave TB. Genetic basis of male infertility. Br Med Bull 2000;56:650–671.
9. Leaman D, Chen PY, Fak J, et al. Antisense-mediated depletion reveals essential and specific functions of microRNAs in drosophila development. Cell 2005;121: 1097–1108.
10. Miller D, Ostermeier GC, Krawetz SA. The controversy, potential and roles of spermatozoal RNA. Trends Mol Med 2005;11:56–63.
11. Bejerano G, Pheasant M, Makunin I, et al. Ultraconserved elements in the human genome. Science 2004;304:1321–1325.
12. Poulin F, Nobrega MA, Plajzer-Frick I, et al. In vivo characterization of a vertebrate ultraconserved enhancer. Genomics 2005;85:774–781.
13. De la Calle-Mustienes E, Feijoo CG, Manzanares M, et al. A functional survey of the enhancer activity of conserved non-coding sequences from vertebrate Iroquois cluster gene deserts. Genome Res 2005;15:1061–1072.
14. Norbrega MA, Zhu Y, Plajzer-Frick I, Afzal V, Rubin EM. Megabase deletions of gene deserts result in viable mice. Nature 2004;431:988–993.
15. Yamashita T, Honda M, Takatori H, Nishino R, Hoshino N, Kaneko S. Genome-wide transcriptome mapping analysis identifies organ-specific gene epression patterns along human chromosomes. Genomics 2004;84:867–875.
16. Tuzun E, Sharp AJ, Bailey JA, et al. Fine-scale structural variation of the human genome. Nat Genet 2005;36:949–951.

17. Hinds DA, Kloek AP, Frazer KA. Common deletions and SNPs are in linkage disequilibrium in the human genome. Nat Genet 2006;38:82–85.
18. McCarroll SA, Hadnott TN, Perry GH, et al. The International Hapmap Consortium. Nat Genet 2006;38:86–92.
19. Conrad DF, Andrews TD, Carter NP, Hurles ME, Pritchard JK. A high-resolution survey of deleti polymorphisms in the human genome. Nat Genet 2006;38:75–81.
20. Eichler EE. Widening the spectrum of human genetic variation. Nat Genet 2006;38:9–11.
21. Matzuk MM, Lamb DJ. Genetic dissection of mammalian fertility pathways. Nat Cell Biol 2002;4:s41–s49.
22. International HapMap Consortium. A haplotype map of the human genome. Nature 2005;437:1299–1320.
23. Gibbs R. Deeper into the genome. Nature 2005;437:1233–1234.
24. Christensen GL, Carrell DT. Animal models of genetic causes of male infertility. Asian J Androl 2002;4:213–219.
25. Guarducci E, Nuti F, Becherini L, et al. Estrogen receptor α promoter polymorphism: stronger estrogen action is coupled with lower sperm count. Hum Reprod 2006;21;994–1001.
26. Iguchi N, Yang S, Lamb DJ, Hecht NB. A protamine SNP: one genetic cause of male infertility. J Med Genet 2005;43;382–384.
27. Miyagawa Y, Nishimura H, Tsujimura A, et al. Single nucleotide polymorphisms and mutation analysis of the TNP1 and TNP2 genes of fertile and infertile human male populations. J Androl 2005;26:779–786.
28. Christensen GL, Ivanov IP, Atkins JF, Campbell B, Carrell DT. Identification of polymorphisms in the Hrb, GOPC, and Csnk2a2 genes in two men with globozoospermia. J Androl 2006;27:11–15.
29. KanCW, Fredlake CP, Doherty EAS, Barron AE. DNA sequencing and genotyping in miniaturized electrophoresis systems. Electrophoresis 2004;25:3564–3588.
30. Metzker ML. Emerging technologies in DNA sequencing. Genome Res 2005;15:1767–1776.
31. Li-Sucholeiki XC, Tomita-Mitchell A, Arnold K, et al. Detection and frequency estimation of rare variants in pools of genomic DNA from large populations using mutational spectrometry. Mut Res 2005;570:267–280.
32. Bernstein DS, Buter N, Stumpf C, Wickens M. Analyzing mRNA–protein complexes using a yeast three-hybrid system. Ethods 2002;26:123–141.
33. Prawitt D, Brixel L, Spangenberg C, et al. RNAi knock-down mice: an emerging technology for post-genomic functional genetics. Cytogenet Genome Res 2004;105:412–421.
34. Wakimoto BT, Lindsley DL, Herrera C. Toward a comprehensive genetic analysis of male fertility in drosophila melanogaster. Genetics 2004;167:207–216.

2 The Use of cDNA Libraries to Demonstrate a Linkage Between Transcription and Translation in Male Germ Cells

Norman B. Hecht, PhD

Summary

cDNA libraries have played a prominent role in developing the extensive database of gene expression in germ cells and somatic cells of the mammalian testis. Differential screening of cDNA libraries has allowed investigators to determine the temporal up- and downregulation of many genes. This chapter discusses how suppressive subtraction hybridization and cDNA sequencing have been used to define populations of messenger RNAs (mRNAs) that selectively bind, or do not bind, to the germ cell-specific Y-box protein, MSY2. MSY2 is an abundant DNA/RNA-binding protein that in vitro binds to all mRNAs, but shows selective binding to a subset of male germ cell mRNAs in cells. This specificity is regulated by MSY2 binding to a conserved sequence in gene promoters, which facilitates MSY2 binding to the transcripts from these promoters in the nucleus and coordinates the transport, storage, and translational suppression of these mRNAs in the cytoplasm.

Key Words: DNA/RNA-binding proteins; spermatogenesis; germ cells; transcription; translation; mRNA storage.

1. INTRODUCTION

The differentiation of male germ cells from diploid spermatogonia to haploid spermatozoa requires the precise temporal expression of a large number of genes. Based on the National Center for Biotechnology Information Mouse Unigene database, gene profiling, and analyses of testicular cDNA libraries, nearly 20,000 different sequence clusters have been identified *(1–4)*. Because many of the sequence clusters are

From: *The Genetics of Male Infertility*
Edited by: D.T. Carrell © Humana Press Inc., Totowa, NJ

derived from short expressed sequence tag sequences, and because splice variants are common in germ cells, the exact number of messenger RNAs (mRNAs) expressed in the diverse cell types of the mammalian testis is unknown. However, estimates that at least 3000 of these sequence clusters are expressed in the germ cells appear reasonable.

This chapter aims to first present a historical description of how cDNA libraries have been used to develop and build our current database of gene expression during spermatogenesis, and then discuss how cDNA libraries can be used to answer relevant current questions. Many different investigators have contributed to our understanding of testicular gene expression and in defining the cellular expression patterns of their favorite proteins using cDNA cloning procedures. Because of space limitations, I apologize in advance for my inability to cite the research of many important contributors.

2. HISTORICAL BACKGROUND

In the beginning, investigators isolated testis RNA and prepared cDNA libraries in vectors such as pBR322, λ gt10, and λ gt11. These libraries were usually screened with DNA or RNA probes, often designed from known sequences of genes expressed in other tissues or extrapolated from gene sequences from related species. cDNA protein expression libraries in vectors such as λ gt11 were an improvement and provided a means to isolate cDNAs encoding proteins or specific domains of proteins by allowing individual colonies of cDNAs to be screened with monoclonal or polyclonal antibodies. These approaches helped to characterize the temporal expression of many testicular proteins. Moreover, they also identified numerous germ cell-specific proteins whose isoforms are expressed in somatic cells.

Defining the cellular sites of expression of the testis-expressed proteins has proven both exciting and frustrating, largely because of the large number of different somatic and germ cells in the adult testis. Before the isolation of individual populations of male germ cells became a routine procedure in laboratories, researchers utilized the differentiating prepuberal testis as a means to relate protein expression and cell type(s). In the first wave of spermatogenesis, meiotic cells such as pachytene spermatocytes are present in testes of 17-d-old mice and spermiogenesis initiates with round spermatids in the testes of 22-d-old mice. However, analyzing changes in gene expression during this first prepuberal wave of differentiation had limitations in defining cell type expression because it only allowed cellular correlations to be made. With the development of testicular cell dissociation and cell separation procedures, such as unit gravity sedimentation *(5)* and centrifugal elutriation *(6)*, researchers in reproduction gained a powerful new means to better define temporal (cell type) expression patterns of specific proteins, often using testis cDNAs as probes.

3. DIFFERENTIAL SCREENING OF cDNA LIBRARIES

The utilization of testicular cell dissociation and separation and differential cDNA library screening made it possible to critically test hypotheses, such as whether haploid gene expression occurred in the mammalian testis. Autoradiographic studies had demonstrated a large amount of RNA synthesis occurs during meiosis and hinted at low levels of postmeiotic RNA synthesis in mammals *(7)*. To determine whether the RNAs transcribed during spermiogenesis were just a continued "leakage" of meiotic transcripts or represented additional and perhaps a novel distinct population of postmeiotic transcripts, an adult testis cDNA library was differentially screened with probes derived from cytoplasmic poly(A)+ RNA prepared from isolated populations of meiotic pachytene spermatocytes or postmeiotic round spermatids *(8)*. A number of cDNA clones were identified that hybridized more strongly with the round spermatid cDNAs than pachytene spermatocyte cDNAs. These cDNAs did not hybridize with cytoplasmic poly(A)+ from testes of 17-d-old mice, total RNA from cultured Sertoli cells, adult liver or brain, nonpolyadenylated mRNA from adult testis, or mouse mitochondrial DNA, suggesting selective expression in the haploid germ cells. Sequencing some of the cDNAs identified protamine 1 and 2 and transition protein 1, three genes now known to be first and solely expressed in spermatids. Differential cDNA screens were also successfully used with mRNAs isolated from mice carrying the sex-reversed and testicular-feminization mutations to identify mRNAs expressed during spermiogenesis *(9)*.

4. APPLICATIONS OF cDNA LIBRARY SCREENING

In a larger screening effort, Nishimune and colleagues utilized stepwise subtraction hybridization to identify mouse genes whose transcription is upregulated during spermiogenesis *(10)*. They prepared a cDNA library from adult mouse testis (35-d-old mice) and subtracted it from a cDNA library from prepuberal mouse testis (17-d-old mice). The testes of 17-d-old mice contain spermatogonia and spermatocytes as well as the somatic Leydig, myoid, and Sertoli cells, but lack significant numbers of postmeiotic haploid cell types. Of the approx 30% cDNA clones that were found to be expressing more intensely in the adult testes, the clones were grouped into three categories. Type 1 cDNA clones were not expressed in the prepuberal testes, type 2 cDNA clones showed an increased expression in the adult testis, and type 3 cDNA clones often detected multiple mRNAs with one size mRNA being present in equal amounts in prepuberal and adult testes and one being predominantly found in adult testis. The detection of mRNAs with different sizes in postmeiotic male germ cells compared with somatic cell types is common and often reflects the use of novel promoters and/or truncation of transcripts in round spermatids (reviewed in refs. *1* and *11*). The stepwise subtraction hybridization of Fujii et al. *(10)* was highly successful, identifying 153 mouse genes whose expression is upregulated during spermiogenesis. Eighty appear to be highly specific to the testis and upon sequencing many encoded novel uncharacterized genes. The stepwise subtraction hybridization methodology can be valuable for both defining temporal expression as well as for gene discovery. Subsequent detailed analyses of cDNAs isolated in this screen helped to identify and provide valuable insight into the expression timing of a number of novel testicular mRNAs encoding proteins such as Hils 1, Hanp 1, Tektin-t, t-actin 1 and 2, and Haprin (reviewed in ref. *12*).

Differential screening of cDNA libraries can be a valuable tool to identify molecular targets of proteins. For instance, cells that rely heavily on posttranscriptional regulation express many different RNA-binding proteins. To define the functions of these RNA-binding proteins, it is useful to determine their RNA target molecules. We have used suppressive subtractive hybridization (SSH) to understand how a very abundant male and female germ cell-specific DNA/RNA-binding protein, MSY2, selects which mRNAs it binds and have found it marks specific transcripts for transport in the nucleus and then helps stabilize them in the cytoplasm *(13)*.

MSY2 is a member of a widely expressed and highly conserved (bacteria to humans) family of nucleic acid-binding proteins. Y-box proteins serve as coactivators of transcription in the nucleus recognizing the DNA motif, CTGATTGGC/TC/TAA *(14)*. In the cytoplasm, they stabilize/store/suppress the translation of specific mRNAs. Y-box proteins are expressed in both somatic cells and germ cells in vertebrates. One member of this family, MSY2, is a 360 amino acid mouse protein encoded by a single-copy gene, which is solely expressed in meiotic and postmeiotic cells of the mouse *(15)*. It is an abundant protein, constituting about 0.7% of total protein in male germ cells *(16)* and 2% of total protein in oocytes *(17,18)*. Gene targeting of MSY2 has confirmed it is solely expressed in germ cells and demonstrated it is essential for male and female fertility *(16)*. Contrin, its highly conserved human ortholog, is also expressed in meiotic and postmeiotic germ cells *(19)*. Based on its abundance in germ cells *(16)* and from in vitro binding assays that indicate sequence-independent RNA-binding of MSY2, we wondered how germ cells manage to selectively synthesize certain proteins while avoiding random translational inactivation of all their mRNAs by MSY2. Suppressive subtractive hybridization and cDNA cloning gave us the answer by identifying the in vivo mRNA targets and non-targets of MSY2.

Using an affinity-purified antibody to recombinant *MSY2*, immuno-precipitation followed by SSH were used to fractionate MSY2-bound and -nonbound mRNAs. cDNA inserts from randomly chosen clones of the *MSY2*-bound subtracted cDNA library (MSY2-bound) and a non-bound (polysomal) mRNA cDNA library were amplified and sequenced to confirm the differential screening. Genes not expressed in germ cells, such as clusterin, which is expressed in Sertoli cells in the testis, served as valuable controls for binding specificity. A total of 98 clones (48 clones encoding *MSY2*-bound mRNAs and 50 clones of *MSY2*-nonbound mRNAs) were analyzed. Quantitative real time reverse transcriptase-polymerase chain reaction confirmed that the immuno-precipitation and cloning successfully differentiated between two distinct populations of mRNAs.

Using cluster analyses to identify related functions of the bound and non-bound mRNAs, many of the *MSY2*-bound mRNAs were shown to be gamete-specific transcripts expressed in meiotic and postmeiotic cells. Moreover, many of the *MSY2*-bound mRNAs were translationally delayed and specifically critical for male gamete development. In contrast, many nonbound mRNAs were involved in constitutive cellular processes such as cell growth and general metabolism and were translated immediately upon transcription.

Although SSH produced two distinct populations of *MSY2*-bound or -nonbound mRNAs, the molecular mechanism whereby MSY2 recognized specific mRNAs, but not others, was unknown. Analyses of sequence and secondary structures of the mRNA populations failed to detect obvious differences between the bound and non-bound mRNA populations. However, many of the *MSY2*-bound mRNAs contained Y-box sequences in the promoters of their genes, whereas nonbound mRNAs often were transcribed from promoters lacking Y-boxes. To test for a possible linkage between transcription and translation, we compared whether exogenous green fluorescent protein (GFP) transcripts from transgenic mice fractionated in the *MSY2*-bound or -nonbound populations when they were transcribed from promoters containing or lacking the Y-box sequence *(13)*. When GFP was expressed from SP-10 promoters containing or lacking the *MSY2* DNA-binding sequence, GFP mRNAs were either bound or not bound by MSY2, respectively. These experiments demonstrated selective marking by MSY2 of specific mRNAs transcribed from promoters containing Y-box sequences. Chromatin immunoprecipitation assays confirmed that the promoters of this population of mRNAs were preferentially bound by MSY2 (13). Thus, our use of cDNA libraries and SSH allowed us to dissect a mechanism whereby nuclear events associated with transcription were linked to selective mRNA storage and translational regulation in the cytoplasm of male germ cells.

5. cDNA SCREENING BY COMPUTER

The field of reproductive biology is fortunate to have attracted scientists such as M. Eddy, M. Griswold, J. McCarrey, M. Primig, and their colleagues who are willing to prepare and readily share their valuable databases. Through their efforts they have made available to the scientific community detailed expression profiling analyses *(2–4)* and valuable cDNA libraries prepared against many different types of highly purified testicular germ cells (6-d primitive type A spermatogonia, type A spermatogonia, type B spermatogonia, 18-d pre-leptotene spermatocytes, 18-d leptotene and zygotene spermatocytes, spermatocytes, and round spermatids) and from 20-d Sertoli cells and the mouse embryonal carinoma cell line F9 (www.ncbi.nlm.nih.gov/UniGene/library.cgi). With such resources, it is now possible to clone unknown novel genes and define their temporal expression pattern without leaving one's office.

6. CONCLUSION

In summary, cDNA libraries have been instrumental in establishing the extensive databases of gene expression during spermatogenesis. Early efforts at cDNA screening were labor intensive, whereas current technologies provide a rapid means or *in silico* gene identification. Such approaches will greatly enhance our abilities to define the molecular bases of many human male infertilities as well as provide valuable insights for the control of mammalian fertility.

REFERENCES

1. Eddy EM. Male germ cell gene expression. Recent Prog Horm Res 2002;57:103–128.
2. Shima JE, McLean DJ, McCarrey JR, Griswold MD. The murine testicular transcriptome: characterizing gene expression in the testis during the progression of spermatogenesis. Biol Reprod 2004;71:319–330.

3. Schlecht U, Demougin P, Koch R, et al. Expression profiling of mammalian male meiosis and gametogenesis identifies novel candidate genes for roles in the regulation of fertility. Mol Biol Cell 2004;15:1031–1043.

4. Wrobel G, Primig M. Mammalian male germ cells are fertile ground for expression profiling of sexual reproduction. Reproduction 2005;129:1–7.

5. Romrell LJ, Bellve AR, Fawcett DW. Separation of mouse spermatogenic cells by sedimentation velocity. A morphological characterization. Dev Biol 1976;49: 119–131.

6. Grabske RJ, Lake S, Gledhill BL, Meistrich ML. Centrifugal elutriation: separation of spermatogenic cells on the basis of sedimentation velocity. J Cell Physiol 1975;86:177–189.

7. Monesi V, Geremia R, D'Agosino A, Boitani C. Biochemistry of male germ cell differentiation in mammals: RNA synthesis in meiotic and postmeiotic cells. Curr Top Dev Biol 1978;12:11–36.

8. Kleene KC, Distel RJ, Hecht NB. cDNA clones encoding poly (A) RNAs which first appear at detectable levels in haploid phases of spermatogenesis in the mouse. Dev Biol 1983;98:455–464.

9. Dudley K, Potter J, Lyon MF, Willison KR. Analysis of male sterile mutations in the mouse using haploid stage expressed cDNA probes. Nucleic Acids Res 1984;25:4281–4293.

10. Fujii T, Tamura K, Masai K, Tanaka H, Nishimune Y, Nojima H. Use of stepwise subtraction to comprehensively isolate mouse genes whose transcription is up-regulated during spermiogenesis. EMBO Rep 2002;3:367–372.

11. Hecht NB. Molecular mechanisms of male germ cell differentiation. BioEssays 1998;20:555–561.

12. Tanaka H, Baba T. Gene expression in spermiogenesis. Cell Mol Life Sci 2005;62:344–354.

13. Yang J, Medvedev S, Reddi PP, Schultz RM, Hecht NB. The DNA/RNA-binding protein MSY2 marks specific transcripts for cytoplasmic storage in mouse male germ cells. Proc Natl Acad Sci USA 2005;102:1513–1518.

14. Yiu GK, Hecht NB. Novel testis-specific protein-DNA interactions activate transcription of the mouse protamine 2 gene during spermatogenesis. J Biol Chem 1997;272:26,926–29,933.

15. Gu W, Tekur S, Reinbold R, et al. Mammalian male and female germ cells express a germ cell-specific Y-Box protein, MSY2. Biol Reprod 1998;59:1266–1274.

16. Yang Y, Medvedev S, Yu J, et al. Absence of the DNA/RNA-binding protein MSY2 results in male and female infertility. Proc Nat Acad Sci USA 2005;102: 5755–5760.

17. Yu J, Hecht NB, Schultz RM. Expression of MSY2, a germ cell-specific Y-box protein in the female mouse. Biol Reprod 2001;65:1260–1270.

18. Yu J, Hecht NB, Schultz RM. RNA-binding properties and translation repression in vitro by germ cell-specific MSY2 protein. Biol Reprod 2002;67:1093–1098.

19. Tekur S, Pawlak A, Guellaen G, Hecht NB. Contrin, the human homologue of a germ-cell Y-box-binding protein: cloning, expression, and chromosomal localization. J Androl 1999;20:135–144.

3

Considerations When Using Array Technologies for Male Factor Assessment

Adrian E. Platts, BSC,
David J. Dix, PhD,
and Stephen A. Krawetz, PhD

Summary

Expression profiles from sets of genes are currently being explored as candidate diagnostics to assess male fertility status and as surrogate makers of paternal toxicological exposure. In this chapter, we describe considerations for their design when using microarrays to create a clinical diagnostic tool. Two commercially available oligonucleotide-based platforms were compared. The results are then referenced against an expressed sequence tag data set and a cDNA array. The concordance between the different platforms for genes indicated as present with high confidence and absent with high confidence when provided with the same pool of RNA is presented. Based on these data, the capacity for this technology to develop into a robust diagnostic for male factor fertility is discussed.

Key Words: Microarray; sperm mRNA; expressed sequence tags; EST; cDNA.

1. INTRODUCTION

Two methods have principally been adopted for high-throughput transcriptome analysis. These are the transcript sequencing approaches that include serial analysis of gene expression (SAGE) and expressed sequence tag (EST) library sequencing and hybridization-based microarray approaches *(1–4)*. Familiarity and cost have led many investigators to adopt the microarray technology. Inherently, the array approach assumes that the informative transcripts in a given tissue have been characterized. This assumption may require further evaluation in light of recent data from high-resolution transcript mapping *(5)*. Conversely, the EST or SAGE strategies are independent of *a priori* assumptions regarding the

From: *The Genetics of Male Infertility*
Edited by: D.T. Carrell © Humana Press Inc., Totowa, NJ

presence or absence of transcripts. This approach can have a higher discovery rate, but the statistical confidence of the resulting analysis is dependent on the level of the sequencing or depth of coverage that the tags provide. SAGE is likely to remain a discovery tool for the time being, not generally suited to the clinical setting. This reflects the cost constraints imposed by the technology.

Various microarray platforms holding the promise of designer-based medicine *(6–9)* are beginning to be adopted as clinical diagnostics *(10–15)*. Implementation of array technologies in the clinical setting will need to be considered with careful reference to cross-platform and biological reproducibility of the results *(16)*. Some comparative studies have been undertaken *(17,18)*, but have tended not to address whether a robust set of platform-independent probes can be identified. In this chapter, we examine the high-confidence data from two commercially available oligonuceotide microarray platforms to define the human testis transcriptome. This is compared to a cDNA microarray platform and as a function of the EST data available from the National Center for Biotechnology Information (NCBI) dbEST repository *(19)*.

2. PLATFORMS

The advent of a variety of high-throughput technologies that are accessible to many laboratories has spawned an interest in developing diagnostics based on these technologies. One of the foci of our laboratories is to develop DNA microarrays for characterizing sperm RNA content and assessing the genetic and environmental basis of male fertility status *(20–22)*. Several strategies have been implemented to address this task of creating a diagnostics tool. They include both *in silico* and wet-bench approaches. For example, *in silico* tools have been built to combine public data from numerous projects. This has been made possible by the research community primarily adopting two standards: first, a uniform means to describe a microarray experiment and data (i.e., the minimum information about a microarray experiment; refs. *23* and *24*) and second, extensible markup language (XML) protocols describing how high-throughput data can be represented (e.g., microarray and gene expression markup language [MAGE-ML]; ref. *25*). With these standards in place, a range of databases have been constructed to warehouse microarray data. These include subject area-specific repositories, such as the mammalianreproductive genetics (MRG) database (http://mrg.genetics.washington.edu/), and super-repositories, such as the NCBI Gene Expression Omnibus *(26)* and European Molecular Biology Laboratory-European Bioinformatics Institute

ArrayExpress *(27)* projects, that archive data from all high-throughput platforms. Parallel databases derived from transcript sequencing, such as the NCBI dbEST, complement these assets. These harbor a wealth of information that have enabled data mining and various meta-analyses. However, caution must be exercised, because the primary data represent a variety of perspectives that were each tailored to address the initial primary research goal.

Although the *in silico* avenue will provide a guide *(28)*, wet-bench laboratory analysis is required to develop and put a clinical diagnostic into practice. The platforms discussed in this chapter reflect some of the technologies that may soon be considered or have even entered the pipeline towards clinical application, including the Illumina Sentrix® 6: Human Whole Genome BeadChip array *(29)* and the Affymetrix Human U133+2 GeneChip® array *(30)*. Both assess a wide distribution of transcripts, many of which overlap between the platforms. The Illumina BeadChip interrogates 47,300 segments using a series of 50 basepair (bp) probes. A subset of 23,259 was mapped directly through GenBank to known gene transcripts. In comparison, the Affymetrix Human U133+2 array interrogates 54,613 segments using a series of 25 bp probesets of which 41,282 were mapped to known gene transcripts representing 38,572 distinct genes.

3. EXPERIMENTAL CONSIDERATIONS AND ANALYTICAL PROCEDURES

Many excellent texts have already been devoted to the various statistical aspects of analyzing microarray-based experiments *(31–33)*. Approaches and array technologies continue to evolve. A host of tools are being made available online, where they are frequently updated. Their URLs are best found by searching the Internet, or where this fails by using www.archive.org to identify deprecated tools. Similarly, when seeking the most recent statistical perspectives, a search of PubMed for microarray analysis provides a good starting point.

Table 1 lists some of the most frequently cited primary analysis software tools that are commercially or freely available. These include GeneSpring *(34)*, which provides a generic turnkey analysis solution with limited data mining capabilities; the oligonucleotide centric DChip *(35)*; and others, such as BeadStudio, that is array platform- and manufacturer-specific.

3.1. Experimental Design

Most microarray studies are comparative rather than absolute and are designed as time series, dose–response, or disease state comparisons.

Table 1
Examples of Microarray Analysis Software Suites
With Their Literature Citation Frequency

Analysis suite	Citations[a]	Platform specificity
TIGR suite (www.tigr.org)	1890	Primarily aimed at cDNA platforms
GeneSpring (Silicon Genetics)	1440	All platforms
Imagene	938	Generic one- and two-color arrays
Bioconductor/R	690	All platforms
DChip (www.dchip.org)	546	Primarily oligonucleotide, although import is possible for other platforms
GCOS/MAS5 (Affymetrix)	513	Affymetrix array analysis software tools
BeadStudio	1	Illumina Sentrix® BeadChip analysis software

[a]As of January 1, 2006.

They do not seek to quantify a gene's expression in absolute terms, but rather demonstrate whether a significant change in the level of the transcript has occurred between states. This may be assessed relative to a single comparator (e.g., an initial time point or a "normal" state or between different states).

The design of these differential experiments generally reflects the question being addressed and the technological solution adopted. Multichannel platforms are capable of simultaneously measuring two states. The test condition can thus be associated with one channel, whereas the second channel can be dedicated to a control that is common among all arrays. This approach permits the relative expression from all experiments to be evaluated with one intermediate array at most. Alternatively, when a single-channel platform is employed, a second array provides a control for each condition. The cost can prove prohibitive when multiple conditions are explored. A compromise of cross-referencing the samples, by comparing sample 1 to sample 2, sample 2 to sample 3, and so on, is frequently employed.

Whether exploring differential or absolute expression, the underlying biological differences between the conditions tested are only one source that contributes to the differential signal. Sources of signal variance can arise through subject differences, sampling differences, or through the technical variance that is introduced by small differences in target preparation. There are many experimental designs that can be adopted to identify this variance. Selection of the appropriate design depends on a number of factors, including whether there is a need to identify all sources of variance or merely to characterize variance with respect to test variables and a subset of candidate nuisance elements. Factorial designs, typified by the Latin-square, are the most complete experimental designs. At least one array is devoted to each combination of parameters. This optimizes the potential to quantitatively link the nuisance and tested contributions to the measured outcomes through, for example, analysis of variance (ANOVA). Unfortunately, the Latin-square can prove cost-prohibitive for complex protocols. Consequently, several variables are usually clustered together to define groups of factors rather than individual factors.

The primary source of analytical discordance between differential analyses is encountered in the chip-normalization procedure *(36)*. This step is necessitated when sources of variation cannot be adequately addressed by the experimental design even when the same target is independently hybridized to an identical array. Slight differences in hybridization conditions, chip preparation, processing, and data capture lead to global differences between the two arrays. As shown in Fig. 1, these differences are usually observed as broad changes to the chip's envelope, i.e., the histogram of the signal from all of the chip's probes. In some cases, one chip might be brighter than the other, exhibiting a greater dynamic range of signal while having the same rank order of genes. Without compensation, some probes can exhibit substantially different signal levels between chips where no transcript differential is biologically present.

For many platforms, the initial chip normalization will be the median normalization. This simple adjustment globally factors the signal levels across a chip such that the median signals between chips are equalized. However, this approach is unable to compensate for changes in the shape of the envelope that leave the median signal unchanged. Hence, more advanced envelope-shaping normalizations such as invariant-set and percentile normalizations may be considered. Additional pre-analyses that model the signal and noise of the individual probes have become available to determine which probes are inherently noisy and which probes are stable. A range of models are available in Bioconductor *(37)* and GeneSpring, including the Robust Multichip Average (RMA) and the basepair-adjusted extension gcRMA. In comparison DChip *(35)* uses the model-based expression index approach. The relative merits of each have been compared *(38)*.

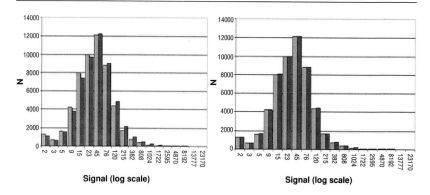

Fig. 1. Two histograms showing the distribution of signal intensity illustrating the signal envelope of two arrays before and after normalization. **(Left panel)** Before normalization signal intensities greater than 45 show a clear skew towards the darker bars. A similar skew is observed toward the lower signal intensity values less than 45 as illustrated by the lighter bars. **(Right panel)** After normalization, the level of hybridization between the arrays is similar.

The final stage of preanalysis typically identifies the genes that exhibit the largest quantifiable changes with respect to the test variables while determining which changes are likely significant and which likely result from stochastic processes. Approaches can be graphical and simple (like volcano plots, in which the fold log of the change in signal is plotted as a function of the log of significance or representations of the coefficient of variation [CV]). Alternatively approaches can be complex and graphically involved, like hierarchical clustering or principle component analyses. They are now routinely utilized to identify groups of genes that appear to be responding in a coordinated manner. Within each group regression, approaches that model the causes and outcomes of variance, such as ANOVA or multivariate ANOVA, are used to indicate whether a result is likely to be by chance alone. The decision of what to accept and what to reject is complex, given that an array can contain tens of thousands of probes. If a p value of 0.05 is adopted as the significance criteria for a 50,000-probe array, then in any given experiment 2500 genes could be reported by chance alone. This multiple comparison problem can be reconciled by the strict Bonferroni correction. However, this will reduce type I (false-positive) error, at the expense of a significant penalty to type II (false-negative) error. Other approaches are available to optimize the balance between type I and II errors. These include data-independent step-down procedures as well as data- and prior-based approaches, such as Storey's Q *(39)* value and the permutation-based Westfall and Young adjustment *(40)*.

4. ORIGINS OF DIFFERENCES BETWEEN PLATFORMS

Platforms exhibit different capacities to measure a broad range of signal. One or more probe sequences are available for hybridization for each gene detected on a given platform. The characteristics of each probe are determined by their corresponding sequence and system design. Thus, although a platform can be generally characterized, there are probes that differ from these general trends. Other innate factors brought about by the platform's design impact concordance among probes, including probe length, the data analysis strategy used to generate high-specificity probes, the distribution of probes with respect to translation initiation and termination signals, the number of times each probe is represented on the chip, the approach to measuring background signal and spurious hybridization, and the experimental technologies and protocols employed. Misannotation is inevitable, in these rapidly evolving platforms that incorporate tens of thousands of probes. This is usually reflective of genes that are not well understood or gene predictions. Generally, subjecting the probe sequences to another round of BLAST analysis will resolve this issue. This is particularly useful when comparing the results from older versions of arrays because genome builds and locations during their respective development are subject to change.

4.1. Platforms and Analytical Approach

A common reference standard of commercially available pooled testes RNA has been used to define amplification, hybridization, and image capture differences within two platforms and inclusivity and sensitivity characteristics between platforms. Data from each platform was analyzed based on our past experience with each platform. The specific approaches undertaken for this study were:

- Affymetrix. GeneChip images were processed with GCOS 1.1 (Affymetrix) and normalized relative to each other using DChip 2006 for invariant set normalization. Signal consistency was then assessed using the DChip model-based expression index approach in PM-MM mode.
- Illumina. The Illumina Sentrix array was imaged, validated, and then signal derived using the custom BeadStudio software.
- Platform-specific normalization within platforms containing duplicates. Only the probes corresponding to well characterized genes and well annotated within Genbank were compared between arrays.
- Rank invariant normalization between platforms. This approach was conducted using the National Institute of Aging online ANOVA system *(41)*.

4.2. Platform Performance in Limited Technical Replicates

Before assessing the extent to which platforms accord, it is useful to explore concordance within platforms. Because each platform has a preparation protocol that may bring about discordant results, reproducibility with respect to independent target preparation from the same biological specimen was assessed. These constitute technical replicates intended to incorporate elements of preparation protocol variance *(42)*, rather than simply technical repeats.

4.2.1. AFFYMETRIX U133+2 PLATFORM

Two samples of Clontech-pooled human testes RNA were independently amplified using the Ambion Message Amp™ amplification system according to the manufacturer's protocol. The RNA was hybridized to the arrays and the signal preprocessed as described. Affymetrix technologies report a signal value that is linearly related to RNA concentration across a broad range beyond which it becomes nonlinear *(43)*. The platform also uses signal stability across probe pairs relative to a mismatched background probe to deliver a "call" or confidence of detection. Assigning a confidence of detection above 0.96 (one-sided Wilcoxon rank sum divided by the signal discrimination score) leads to a P or present denotation, between 0.96 and 0.94, an M or marginal denotation, and below 0.94, an A or absent denotation. Because previous research has largely shown good cross-platform concordance only with the assignment of presence or absence *(44)*, it is useful to explore the extent to which the Affymetrix platform is concordant among technical replicates with respect to both signal and the assignment of presence or absence. This permits us to validate a set of clinical analysis parameters well-suited to the data from this platform.

As illustrated in Fig. 2A, the Affymetrix technical replicate signal values concord well. Signal-dependent variance that reduces signal correspondence among replicates is observed at lower signal intensity values. A least squares fit validates the data normalization approach, indicating a scaling M of 0.99 between chips and r^2 of 0.9895 [Log(I) r^2 0.9]. Analysis of the CV, with respect to signal, pinpoints signals below 100 units as the primary origin of spurious covariance. When assessed as a function of the signal being deemed present or absent, 89%, (i.e., 49,062/54,613) of probesets on the arrays were concordant between replicates. The remaining 11% were principally located in the lower quartile signals. Implementing a variable lower signal threshold cutoff yielded 95% presence–absence concordance, once the signals below 110 units were excluded from the analysis. This suggests a lower boundary of reliable, validated present signal of between 50 and 150 signal units. The lower bound is dependent on the user's preference for inclusivity or reproducibility.

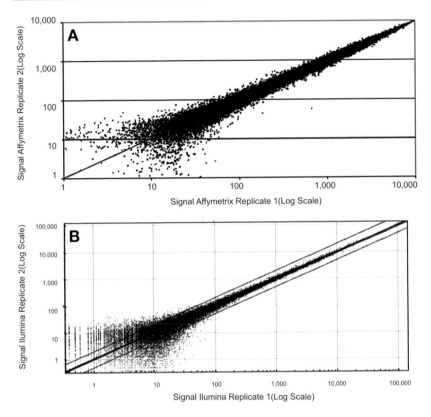

Fig. 2. Log_{10}–Log_{10} dot plot technical replicates illustrating excellent co-linearity and good signal correspondence above a threshold. **(A)** Affymetrix data. **(B)** Illumina data, after cubic-spline normalization. Normalization corrects for signal skew between replicates but introduces some noise below the lower signal threshold.

4.2.2. ILLUMINA SENTRIX 6: HUMAN WHOLE GENOME BEADCHIP PLATFORM

An additional sample of Clontech-pooled human testes RNA was independently amplified using the Ambion Message Amp amplification system. Signal from the Illumina Sentrix 6 BeadChip arrays was first validated for quality using the insuite array validation function and then further analyzed in the Illumina BeadStudio software suite. BeadStudio offers several options for array normalization. These include background, invariant set, and average normalizations. Although this normalization will not affect the confidence of a signal being assigned present or absent between platforms, it is key to attaining optimal signal concordance. Comparison of the various normalization strategies revealed little difference. Each did not substantially improve the signal correlation between the two arrays. However, spline normalization did correct a slight non-linearity at higher signal strengths to the linear relationship as shown in Fig. 2B. Signal intensity correlation determined by least squares fit generated r^2 0.9899 [log(I) r^2 0.988] with an M of 0.99 after normalization. The Pearson product moment of 0.994 indicates that 99% of the detected signal can be correlated between the replicates. Approximately 99% of the CoV was below 40 signal units and 80% below 25 signal units. Of the 47,300 probes on the platform, 28,455 were identified as definitely present ($p > 0.99$) or definitely absent ($p < 0.75$). These exhibited 100% concordance between experiments. The remaining 18,845 probes were of marginal intensity and not assigned as being present or absent and were not considered further. This reflects our conservative choice of $p < 0.75$ when assigning definitely absent. It contrasts the more inclusive value of $p < 0.94$ that is typically used when Affymetrix arrays are analyzed but marginally impacts the concordance of the assignment of presence or absence.

4.3. Comparing Oligonucleotide Platforms

Describing the Affymetrix and Illumina technologies jointly as only oligonucleotide platforms is a significant oversimplification. There exist a number of substantial differences between the technologies. The Affymetrix U133+2 platform has multiple probesets for some well-characterized genes, derived through the subclustering of EST data within 600 bp of the 3'-end of the transcript. Signal is measured through sets of 25-mer probes (probesets) aligned to a sequential region of the transcript with correction for nonspecific hybridization made relative to a parallel set of 1-bp centrally mismatched probes. This is key to the successful use of shorter oligonucleotide probes. By contrast, the Illumina Sentrix 6 platform uses longer 50-mer oligonucleotide-coated beads randomly dispersed across a very high-density array of pits with up to 60 identically coated oligonucleotide beads for each probe. This larger number of repeat measurements yields a very stable signal for each longer oligonucletide probe, lessening the need for probesets. Unlike the Illumina platform, the Affymetrix platform often queries a gene using several independent probesets that are offset from one another. This may have the advantage of simultaneously examining isoforms. Therefore, we can anticipate that only a subset of the Affymetrix probesets targeted to a gene will report the same biological behavior as the Illumina probe(s). Addressing this difference, albeit at the risk of biasing the assessment, can be achieved by either screening the Affymetrix probes for those that best correlate with the expression for that gene on the Illumina platform or by masking those reporters that are aligned to spatially distinct genomic locations. Of the 23,259 probes on the Sentrix Whole Genome GeneChip arrays that were

Table 2
Distribution of Known Transcripts Identified as Present

Platform	Cross-referenced probes	Total probes identified	Common transcripts identified	Total probes identified (%)
Affymetrix	25,635	9598	5265	37
Illumina	18,916	6837	5265	36

annotated relative to GenBank sequences, 18,916 could be matched through their Entrez Gene IDs to the Affymetrix arrays. These subsets of probes were normalized to each other using the National Institute of Aging normalization tool.

As shown in Table 2, 5265 unique platform-independent probesets (i.e., transcripts) were identified as common between the platforms. Both platforms possess a similar ability to detect probes (i.e., 37 and 36%, for the Affymetrix and Illumina platforms, respectively). The concordance of those genes defined as present is 77%. Although the platforms generally accord with respect to transcript identification, only 7% concordance is observed for the relative level of the signal. This can arise from at least two independent sources of interplatform discordance. On the one hand, the inherent differences in platform design (e.g., oligonucleotide length and probeset composition) could lead to different measurements even when the probes are assessing the same region. On the other hand, differences in the probe sequence may discern different isoforms leading to their independent measurement. These differences that arise from sequence selection may be assessed by restricting the probes included in the analysis. Restricting the data set to those probes that target sequences in closer proximity allows one to begin to identify the contribution of reporter location to platform concordance. The sequence alignments from the group of well annotated genes from each platform has already been undertaken by others and the results reported *(45)*. There is an evident leap in agreement to 21% when only the closest matching Affymetrix probeset is compared with its Illumina counterpart for each gene. Beyond this, the further thinning of the data sets to include only those probes targeted to within 200 bp or less of each other only reconciles 31% of the signal between the platforms, which is similar to the value obtained (27%) when the subsets of probesets that show a similar relative expression are compared. Accordingly, approx 60% of the interplatform signal variance may arise from causes beyond simple probe choice. This is consistent with the view that signal

Table 3
Number of Transcripts Sequenced in a Combined Testis Expressed
Sequence Tag Library That Were Also Detected Present
on Each of Three Microarray Platforms

Platform	Unigenes represented on the platform	Probes identified	Unigenes identified	Unigenes identified (%)	χ^2 Unigenes identified[a]
dbEST	11,784	52,000	11,784	100	
cDNA	6563	4226	2817	43	5 ($p < 0.05$)
Affymetrix	7468	12,306	6431	86	1411 ($p < 0.005$)
Illumina	7326	4887	4887	67	1648 ($p < 0.005$)

[a]The χ^2 statistical correlation of array platforms with the dbEST data set is given. The corresponding p value is parenthesized.

strength comparison among platforms is, at best, poorly correlated even when inclusivity is compromised.

5. DATA CONCORDANCE
WITH A REFERENCE TECHNOLOGY

Four EST libraries were aggregated from the NCBI dbEST totaling approx 52,000 sequence reads (libraries 18,517, 16,441, 18,476, 1752). These were combined to form a single external reference library of 11,784 distinct unigene clusters. Because many platforms, Affymetrix most notably, derive their hybridization sequences and calculate cross-hybridization resilience primarily from dbEST, it might be anticipated that a platform with probes so constructed would yield results in good agreement with dbEST. This has been reported for large SAGE projects (46). Table 3 illustrates the correlation between a gene being identified as present on the Affymetrix and Illumina oligonucleotide platforms together with a cDNA platform (2) alongside being identified in the combined dbEST library. The percentage of genes discovered by sequencing that are also discovered on the array platforms is informative. This suggests that the Affymetrix platform can identify a larger number of the transcripts present. The apparent enhanced performance of the Affymetrix platform may reflect the concurrent probesets that cover the same gene region, each being independently considered.

The ability to model the data can also be considered using the χ^2 statistic to inform on the level of agreement and disagreement and the significance of such agreement. As shown in Table 3, this analysis indicates that the cDNA platform does not model the EST data well. Both the Affymetrix and Illumina platforms concord to a greater extent with the EST data. However, the higher number of Affymetrix probe-sets directed toward the same gene region that increased its ability to identify a given probe reduces the corresponding χ^2 statistic when compared with the Illumina single multireiterated probe platform.

6. DISCUSSION

Previous studies reporting expression differences across platforms have drawn vastly different conclusions. Some have found the level and direction of differential expression to be somewhat concordant *(18,47–49)*. Others have found little in common between platforms in terms of their absolute signal *(50)*. Similarly, the microarray platforms tested did not strongly reflect the EST discovery frequency, a proxy value for expression level that is measured by EST sequence count per million averaged across the libraries. To an extent the differences and similarities reported are as much functions of the analytical pathway adopted *(51)* as they are functions of differences and similarities between the platforms themselves. Nevertheless, there is encouraging but not absolute agreement between the platforms when the presence or absence of a transcript is assessed relative to an external EST data set of known transcripts.

From the series of hybridizations conducted, the data suggests that the oligonucleotide platforms have excellent internal consistency. The exceptionally high signal and reproducibility of presence or absence assignment on the Illumina platform is statistically similar to that observed when real-time polymerase chain reaction techniques are employed. However, it is not possible to assert that one oligonucleotide platform outperforms another. Both are likely capable of drawing similar conclusions when given the task of identifying whether a broad set of genes are, as a group, expressed or silent. This directs us to explore larger and not smaller sets or individual genes when using these technologies. What is the number of transcripts that must be monitored to enable diagnosis? It has recently been shown by others *(13)* that as few as 70 probes can reliably inform on breast cancer prognosis. This may provide a lower bound, but it is not clear whether this would have sufficient power to distinguish among the various forms of male factor infertility.

Although still in its infancy *(10,14,21,52–54)*, the application of these technologies to assessing male factor fertility status holds considerable promise. Compared with the criteria currently in use that includes the well-accepted World Health Organization standards for normal semen analysis *(55)*, these new strategies may provide for the objective evaluation of male factor status. Analogous to a heterozygous CREM⁻ oligospermic individual, the ability of oligonucleotide-based micorarrays to convincingly discern differences among "normal" and CREM⁻ mouse testis transcripts has been demonstrated *(56)*. In our own laboratories, we have used microarrays to identify differences in testicular gene expression in mouse genetic models and human cases of infertility *(57)*, as well as from mice exposed to testicular toxicants resulting in infertility *(58,59)*. Although these are only a few examples of male factor infertility, it is reasonable to assume that the implementation of these arrays or other genomic technologies in the clinical setting will also enable the rapid identification and classification of what are currently cases of "idiopathic" infertility. This would constitute a significant advance for both our clinical and our basic understanding of this disease.

7. ABBREVIATIONS/TECHNICAL REFERENCES

ANOVA: analysis of variance (http://en.wikipedia.org/wiki/ANOVA).

CoV, coefficient of variation 100 × standard deviation/mean (http://en.wikipedia.org/wiki/Coefficient_of_variation).

dbEST, NCBI database of expressed sequence tags (http://www.ncbi.nlm.nih.gov/dbEST/).

EMBL-EBI, European Molecular Biology Laboratory-European Bioinformatics Institute (http://www.ebi.ac.uk/).

gcRMA, nucleotide (G/C) enrichment-adjusted robust multichip average (http://www.bioconductor.org/repository/devel/vignette/gcrma.pdf).

MAGE-ML, MicroArray Gene Expression-Markup Language (http://www.mged.org/Workgroups/MAGE/mage-ml.html).

MANOVA, multivariate ANOVA (http://en.wikipedia.org/wiki/MANOVA).

NCBI, National Center for Biotechnology Information (http://www.ncbi.nlm.nih.gov/).

Presence Significance on the Affymetrix Platform (http://www.affymetrix.com/support/technical/technotes/statistical_reference_guide.pdf).

Probe, an element, usually a sequence, that is printed onto an array to which a labeled target sequence in the sample can hybridize (note that *probe* and *target* are sometimes interchanged in the literature).

Probeset, a set of probes that investigate a near-sequential sequence of a gene. The signal from perfectly matched sequences is generally assessed relative to a 1-bp centrally mismatched sequence to determine the level of spurious hybridization.

RMA, robust multichip average (http://stat-www.berkeley.edu/users/bolstad/RMAExpress/RMAExpress.html).

Target, usually a mixture of labeled RNA, DNA, or protein elements from a tissue or other source that can hybridize to a probe.

XML, extensible markup language (http://www.xml.org/).

ACKNOWLEDGMENTS

The authors gratefully acknowledge the Michigan Economic Development Corporation and the Michigan Technology Tri-Corridor for the support of this program by grant 085P1000819 to SAK. This work was reviewed by the Environmental Protection Agency (EPA) and approved for publication but does not necessarily reflect official agency policy. Mention of trade names or commercial products does not constitute endorsement or recommendation by EPA for use.

REFERENCES

1. Carninci P, Kasukawa T, Katayama S, et al. The transcriptional landscape of the mammalian genome. Science 2005;309:1559–1563.
2. Ostermeier GC, Dix DJ, Krawetz SA. A bioinformatic strategy to rapidly characterize cDNA libraries. Bioinformatics 2002;18:949–952.
3. Shima JE, McLean DJ, McCarrey JR, Griswold MD. The murine testicular transcriptome: characterizing gene expression in the testis during the progression of spermatogenesis. Biol Reprod 2004;71:319–330.
4. Harbers M, Carninci P. Tag-based approaches for transcriptome research and genome annotation. Nat Methods 2005;2:495–502.
5. Cheng J, Kapranov P, Drenkow J, et al. Transcriptional maps of 10 human chromosomes at 5-nucleotide resolution. Science 2005;308:1149–1154.
6. Designer medicine works for asthmatics. Chem Ind 2000;19:623.
7. Designer medicine works for asthmatics. J Sci Ind Res 2001;60:172–173.
8. Collins FS, McKusick VA. Implications of the human genome project for medical science. JAMA 2001;285:540–544.
9. Dream R. Customized medicine—beyond designer drugs. Chem Eng Prog 2005;101:16–17.
10. Moldenhauer JS, Ostermeier GC, Johnson A, Diamond MP, Krawetz SA. Diagnosing male factor infertility using microarrays. J Androl 2003;24:783–789.
11. Martins RP, Krawetz SA. RNA in human sperm. Asian J Androl 2005; 7:115–120.
12. Cobb JP, Mindrinos MN, Miller-Graziano C, et al. Application of genome-wide expression analysis to human health and disease. Proc Natl Acad Sci USA 2005;102:4801–4806.
13. van't Veer LJ, Dai H, van de Vijver MJ, et al. Gene expression profiling predicts clinical outcome of breast cancer. Nature 2002;415:530–536.

14. Ostermeier GC, Goodrich RJ, Diamond MP, Dix DJ, Krawetz SA. Toward using stable spermatozoal RNAs for prognostic assessment of male factor fertility. Fertil Steril 2005;83:1687–1694.

15. Rockett JC, Burczynski ME, Fornace AJ, Herrmann PC, Krawetz SA, Dix DJ. Surrogate tissue analysis: monitoring toxicant exposure and health status of inaccessible tissues through the analysis of accessible tissues and cells. Toxicol Appl Pharmacol 2004;194:189–199.

16. Jarvinen AK, Hautaniemi S, Edgren H, et al. Are data from different gene expression microarray platforms comparable? Genomics 2004;83:1164–1168.

17. Zhu B, Ping G, Shinohara Y, Zhang Y, Baba Y. Comparison of gene expression measurements from cDNA and 60-mer oligonucleotide microarrays. Genomics 2005;85:657–665.

18. Yauk CL, Berndt ML, Williams A, Douglas GR. Comprehensive comparison of six microarray technologies. Nucleic Acids Res 2004;32:E124.

19. Boguski MS, Lowe TM, Tolstoshev CM. dbEST—database for "expressed sequence tags." Nat Genet 1993;4:332–333.

20. Miller D, Ostermeier GC, Krawetz SA. The controversy, potential and roles of spermatozoal RNA. Trends Mol Med 2005;11:156–163.

21. Ostermeier GC, Dix DJ, Miller D, Khatri P, Krawetz SA. Spermatozoal RNA profiles of normal fertile men. Lancet 2002;360:772–777.

22. Wykes SM, Miller D, Krawetz SA. Mammalian spermatozoal mRNAs: tools for the functional analysis of male gametes. J Submicrosc Cytol Pathol 2000;32:77–81.

23. Brazma A, Hingamp P, Quackenbush J, et al. Minimum information about a microarray experiment (MIAME)—toward standards for microarray data. Nat Genet 2001;29:365–371.

24. Stoeckert CJ, Jr, Causton HC, Ball CA. Microarray databases: standards and ontologies. Nat Genet 2002;32:469–473.

25. Spellman PT, Miller M, Stewart J, et al. Design and implementation of microarray gene expression markup language (MAGE-ML). Genome Biol 2002;3: RESEARCH0046.

26. Barrett T, Suzek TO, Troup DB, et al. NCBI GEO: mining millions of expression profiles—database and tools. Nucleic Acids Res 2005;33:D562–D566.

27. Parkinson H, Sarkans U, Shojatalab M, et al. ArrayExpress—a public repository for microarray gene expression data at the EBI. Nucleic Acids Res 2005;33: D553–D555.

28. Platts AE, Moldenhauer JS, Fayz B, Wang D, Borgaonkar DS, Krawetz SA. LARaLink 2.0: a comprehensive aid to basic and clinical cytogenetic research. Genet Test 2005;9:334–341.

29. Steemers FJ, Gunderson KL. Illumina, Inc. Pharmacogenomics 2005;6:777–782.

30. Affymetrix. Design and performance of the GeneChip® Human Genome U133 Plus 2.0 and Human Genome U133A 2.0 array. Technical Note 2003;701483:1–9.

31. Baldi P, Hatfield GW. DNA microarrays and gene expression: from experiments to data analysis and modeling. Cambridge University Press, Cambridge:2002;xvi, 213.

32. Speed TP. Statistical analysis of gene expression microarray data. Interdisciplinary statistics. Chapman & Hall/CRC, Boca Raton, FL; London:2003;xiii, 24, 222.

33. Drăghici S. Data analysis tools for DNA microarrays. Chapman & Hall/CRC, Boca Raton, FL; London:2003;xxv, 477.

34. Grewal A, Conway A. Tools for analyzing microarray expression data. Journal of Lab Automation 2000;5:62–64.

35. Li C, Wong WH. Model-based analysis of oligonucleotide arrays: expression index computation and outlier detection. Proc Natl Acad Sci USA 2001;98:31–36.

36. Xu L, Maresh GA, Giardina J, Pincus SH. Comparison of different microarray data analysis programs and description of a database for microarray data management. DNA Cell Biol 2004;23:643–651.
37. Fred Hutchinson Cancer Research Center. Bioconductor website. Available from: http://bioconductor.org/pub/. Accessed: 11/01/05.
38. Irizarry RA, Bolstad BM, Collin F, Cope LM, Hobbs B, Speed TP. Summaries of affymetrix GeneChip probe level data. Nucleic Acids Res 2003;31:e15.
39. Storey JD, Tibshirani R. Statistical significance for genomewide studies. Proc Natl Acad Sci USA 2003;100:9440–9445.
40. Zaykin DV, Young SS, Westfall PH. Using the false discovery rate approach in the genetic dissection of complex traits: a response to Weller et al. Genetics 2000;154: 1917–1918.
41. Sharov AA, Dudekula DB, Ko MS. A web-based tool for principal component and significance analysis of microarray data. Bioinformatics 2005;21:2548–2549.
42. Irizarry RA, Warren D, Spencer F, et al. Multiple-laboratory comparison of microarray platforms. Nat Methods 2005;2:345–350.
43. Chudin E, Walker R, Kosaka A, et al. Assessment of the relationship between signal intensities and transcript concentration for Affymetrix GeneChip arrays. Genome Biol 2002;3:RESEARCH0005.
44. Shippy R, Sendera TJ, Lockner R, et al. Performance evaluation of commercial short-oligonucleotide microarrays and the impact of noise in making cross-platform correlations. BMC Genomics 2004;5:61.
45. Barnes M, Freudenberg J, Thompson S, Aronow B, Pavlidis P. Experimental comparison and cross-validation of the Affymetrix and Illumina gene expression analysis platforms. Nucleic Acids Res 2005;33:5914–5923.
46. Kim HL. Comparison of oligonucleotide-microarray and serial analysis of gene expression (SAGE) in transcript profiling analysis of megakaryocytes derived from CD34+ cells. Exp Mol Med 2003;35:460–466.
47. Tan PK, Downey TJ, Spitznagel EL, Jr, et al. Evaluation of gene expression measurements from commercial microarray platforms. Nucleic Acids Res 2003;31: 5676–5684.
48. Larkin JE, Frank BC, Gavras H, Sultana R, Quackenbush J. Independence and reproducibility across microarray platforms. Nat Methods 2005;2:329–330.
49. Petersen D, Chandramouli GV, Geoghegan J, et al. Three microarray platforms: an analysis of their concordance in profiling gene expression. BMC Genomics 2005;6:63.
50. Mah N, Thelin A, Lu T, et al. A comparison of oligonucleotide and cDNA-based microarray systems. Physiol Genomics 2004;16:361–370.
51. Shi L, Tong W, Fang H, et al. Cross-platform comparability of microarray technology: intra-platform consistency and appropriate data analysis procedures are essential. BMC Bioinformatics 2005;6:S12.
52. Carreau S, Bourguiba S, Lambard S, Silandre D, Delalande C. The promoter(s) of the aromatase gene in male testicular cells. Reprod Biol 2004;4:23–34.
53. Lambard S, Galeraud-Denis I, Martin G, Levy R, Chocat A, Carreau S. Analysis and significance of mRNA in human ejaculated sperm from normozoospermic donors: relationship to sperm motility and capacitation. Mol Hum Reprod 2004;10:535–541.
54. Wang H, Zhou Z, Xu M, et al. A spermatogenesis-related gene expression profile in human spermatozoa and its potential clinical applications. J Mol Med 2004;82: 317–324.

55. Auger J, Eustache F, Ducot B, et al. Intra- and inter-individual variability in human sperm concentration, motility and vitality assessment during a workshop involving ten laboratories. Hum Reprod 2000;15:2360–2368.
56. Beissbarth T, Borisevich I, Horlein A, et al. Analysis of CREM-dependent gene expression during mouse spermatogenesis. Mol Cell Endocrinol 2003;212:29–39.
57. Rockett JC, Patrizio P, Schmid JE, Hecht NB, Dix DJ. Gene expression patterns associated with infertility in humans and rodent models. Mutat Res 2004;549: 225–240.
58. Rockett JC, Mapp FL, Garges JB, Luft JC, Mori C, Dix DJ. Effects of hyperthermia on spermatogenesis, apoptosis, gene expression, and fertility in adult male mice. Biol Reprod 2001;65:229–239.
59. Tully DB, Luft JC, Rockett JC, et al. Reproductive and genomic effects in testes from mice exposed to the water disinfectant byproduct bromochloroacetic acid. Reprod Toxicol 2005;19:353–366.

4 Microarray Analysis of a Large Number of Single-Nucleotide Polymorphisms in Individual Human Spermatozoa

Honghua Li, PhD, Xiangfeng Cui, BS, Danielle M. Greenawalt, PhD, Guohong Hu, PhD, Nyam-Osor Chimge, PhD, Sreemanta Pramanik, PhD, Minjie Luo, PhD, Hui-Yun Wang, MD, PhD, Irina V. Tereshchenko, MD, PhD, Marco A. Azaro, PhD, Yong Lin, PhD, Qifeng Yang, MD, PhD, James Y. Li, BS, Yi Chu, MS, Zhenwu Lin, PhD, Richeng Gao, MS, Li Shen, MS, Christina J. DeCoste, PhD, and Weichung J. Shih, PhD

Summary

Genetic studies in humans have been limited by various factors, including small family size and diploidy of the human genome. The ability to use individual spermatozoa as subjects has significantly facilitated these studies. However, because each sperm usually

From: *The Genetics of Male Infertility*
Edited by: D.T. Carrell © Humana Press Inc., Totowa, NJ

contains only one copy of the genome and the sensitivity of the available detection methods was low, single sperm could not be used for large-scale genetic analysis. After a series of enhancements, a high-throughput genotyping system has been developed. With this system, more than 1000 genetic markers consisting of single-nucleotide polymorphisms (SNPs) in a single sperm genome can be amplified to a detectable amount in a single tube. Sequences amplified from different polymorphic loci are then resolved by hybridizing these sequences to the corresponding probes spotted on a microarray. The allelic sequences of each SNP are then discriminated by the commonly used allele-specific single-base-extension assay with dideoxyribonucleotides labeled with different fluorescent dyes. Using single sperm cells as subjects, the highly sensitive and high-throughput multiplex genotyping system was used to analyze the physical structure of the human immunoglobulin heavy chain variable region that contains highly repetitive sequences and may not be easily analyzed with conventional methods. This system was also used to understand the contribution of meiotic recombination to haplotype structure formation in the human genome. The system may have various applications including study of genetic factors underlying male infertility.

Key Words: Single sperm; single-nucleotide polymorphisms; genetic analysis; high-throughput genotyping; microarray analysis.

1. INTRODUCTION

Genetic studies involve analysis of genetic material that are informative about the behavior of genetic markers. The resulting information can then be used for various purposes, such as determination of gene locations, recombination rates in given chromosomal regions, and parental origins of certain genetic variants. In mammals, including humans, individual gametes are ideal subjects for these studies because their genomes are simple and contain abundant information about the behavior of genetic markers. Unfortunately, because individual gametes are haploid and contain only one genome copy, genetic information in gametes is usually deduced by study of individual organisms that are the result of fusion of gametes from two sexes. Unlike other organisms in which the number of individuals with interesting phenotypes/genotypes can be expanded by breeding, in humans, individuals of interest for study have to be identified in the population, which involves an unusual amount of effort. The human families are so small that the conventional methods based on scoring the individuals with different phenotypes/genotypes from certain mating arrangements is not practical. Therefore, these analyses in humans usually require pedigree information from at least two generations *(1)*.

Like other higher organisms, the diploidy of the human genome also complicates genetic analysis. Spermatozoa (sperm) and oocytes are both gametes, ideal subjects for genetic analysis. Because these cells are haploid, when used for genetic studies the complications associated with diploid cells can be avoided. However, acquiring and using oocytes are practically much more difficult than using sperm and the number of oocytes from a donor is usually limited. In contrast, sperm cells are much easier to obtain. From each donor, a practically unlimited number of sperm can be obtained. If sperm can be used as subjects, genetic analysis may be performed by direct scoring and may not need pedigree information and complicated statistical analysis. A sufficient number of sperm may be collected from any voluntary doners or interest. However, because sperm are haploid, each sperm usually contains one genome copy, which cannot be analyzed by most available genotyping methods.

2. EFFORTS IN THE DETECTION OF GENETIC MARKERS IN INDIVIDUAL SPERM

The advent of DNA amplification technology, namely polymerase chain reaction (PCR) *(2,3)*, made it possible to detect DNA sequences from a very small amount of material. Detection of polymorphic sequences at single-nucleotide polymorphism (SNP) in single sperm loci enhanced the sensitivity to the high end *(4)*.

In the early stages, most single sperm were prepared by micromanipulation. The most commonly used method was the spread-scraping method. With this method, a small aliquot of the semen sample was first washed and suspended in 1% low-melting-point agarose to a concentration at which sperm can be well separated when a thin layer of the suspension is spread on a glass slide. Single sperm can then be picked up by scraping the areas of the thin layer containing well separated sperm with a fine needle *(5,6)*. Later, the manual method was replaced by flow cytometric separation *(7–9)*. Although it is very efficient, flow sorting of single sperm cells requires access to a flow cytometer and well-trained personnel. Correct alignment and sorting setup of the instrument to ensure single sperm delivered into wells of a microtiter plate at a high percentage can be time-consuming and rather challenging. Once the instrument is correctly aligned, a large number of single sperm can be rapidly sorted. Success in single sperm analysis also relied on the development of sperm lysis solutions that allows DNA to be released from sperm and is suitable for the subsequence PCR amplification of high efficiency *(10)*.

The earliest sperm typing method involved a two-round PCR protocol. In the first round, two to three polymorphic sequences were coamplified in a single tube. Small aliquots were then used to amplify individual sequences separately in different tubes. The amplified products were then analyzed by a method called allele-specific oligonucleotide hybridization. With this method, amplified sequences were immobilized onto nylon filters followed by hybridization with radioisotope-labeled probes *(11,12)*. For each SNP, two probes were designed. Each probe perfectly matched one of the allelic sequences but differed from the other by a single base. Under optimized conditions, each probe mainly hybridized to the perfectly matched template allowing allelic state of a sample at the SNP locus to be determined by analyzing the signal on X-ray films. Such a strategy allowed determination of genetic distance between two genetic markers, *parathyroid hormone*, and ^{G}g *hemoglobin* on chromosome 11 *(10)* for the first time utilizing single sperm analysis.

The genotyping system was later further simplified *(13)*. With the simplified method, the allelic sequences at each marker locus were amplified with a pair of allele-specific primers of different lengths. Each of these primers had its sequence perfectly matched to one of the two allelic sequences but mismatched the other at its 3′-end. Therefore, the primers were preferentially extended only when they annealed to the perfectly matched allelic templates. Because the resulting PCR products from the two alleles differed in length, they could be easily separated by gel electrophoresis. When the lengths of the PCR products from different loci were also taken into consideration, PCR products generated from the alleles of several SNP loci could be analyzed in the same gel lane. Using gel electrophoresis to separate sequences amplified from different loci and from different alleles of each locus not only simplified the experimental procedure, but was also nonradioactive. This method was used for simultaneously typing three loci in single sperm cells *(13)* and for several genetic linkage studies with single sperm *(14–16)*.

To increase the number of markers that can be detected from a single sperm, a whole genome amplification (WGA) procedure was developed in Norman Arnheim's laboratory. The method is called primer-extension preamplification (PEP) *(17)*. With PEP, the entire sperm genome is preamplified with 15mers consisting of degenerated sequences. Aliquots of the PEP product are then used for later PCR amplification with individual primer pairs. With the WGA procedure, single sperm samples could be genotyped with up to 12 markers *(17,18)*. WGA is a linear increasing process. The probability of amplifying any sequence in the genome to a minimum of 30 copies is not less than 0.78 *(17)*. Because of the poisson distribution, it is impossible to separate every individual copy of the amplified sequences into different tubes. Therefor, a WGA product may only be used for approx 25 PCR amplifications.

Table 1
Interacting Pairs as a Function of the Number of Primers

Number of primer pair(s)	Interacting pairs
1	3
2	10
3	21
4	36
5	55
10	210
20	820
30	1830
n	$n(1 + 2n)$

By using a single set of family-specific PCR primers, we were able to amplify more than 30 sequences in the human *immunoglobulin heavy chain* variable *(IGHV)* region from single sperm. Because the differences among the amplified sequences were minor, these sequences could be separated by denaturing gradient gel electrophoresis *(19–22)*. With this approach, we determined the organization of these sequences on individual chromosomes *(5,23,24)*.

As the demand for analyzing a large number of SNPs increases and high-throughput genotyping approaches become available, PCR amplification has becomes an expensive and rate-limiting step. However, increasing multiplex PCR capacity is limited by primer dimerization. Primer dimers are very deleterious during PCR not only because they possess perfect primer anchoring sequences, but also because they are usually much shorter than the amplicons and therefore amplify easily. PCR becomes difficult when more then three pairs of primers are multiplexed. As shown in Table 1, the number of interacting pairs increases exponentially when the number of primer pairs increases. For this reason, the capacity of multiplex PCR was once a bottleneck in high-throughput genotyping.

To address this issue, a three-round amplification protocol (Fig. 1) was developed in our laboratory *(25)*. With this protocol, multiplex amplification is limited to the early stage of PCR, and is converted into "singleplex" later by using primers with universal tails. Experimentally, the target sequence at each locus is first amplified with a regular primer and a primer with a 20-base "tail" (tail 1) at its 5′-end. This tail sequence is universal to one of the primers used for each SNP. Amplification with the tailed primers attaches tail 1 to all amplified sequences. In the second round, an aliquot of the first-round PCR product is reamplified. All tailed primers are replaced by only one

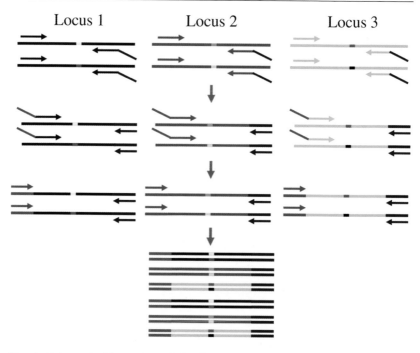

Fig. 1. Schematic illustration of the three-round multiplex amplification. Only three loci are shown. Regular primers, universal tails, and polymorphic sites are indicated as short arrowed lines, short diagonal lines attached to primers, and very short bars of different colors, respectively. *See* text in section 2 for more details.

primer that is identical to tail 1. The regular primer for each locus is then replaced by a primer containing another universal 5′-tail (tail 2). The second tailed primer is an internal (nested) primer with respect to the replaced regular primer to enhance the amplification specificity and yield. In the third round, only two primers identical to tails 1 and 2 are needed to amplify the target sequences to the detectable amounts. The number of PCR cycles in the first and second round is minimized so that amplification in the third round with only two primers significantly reduces primer–primer interaction. This protocol allowed us to amplify 26 loci simultaneously (Fig. 2; ref. 25), compared with approx 15 loci that could be amplified in a multiplex way in other publications (26,27) at that time.

By further optimizing PCR conditions including replacing the regular *Taq* DNA polymerase with a "hot-start" enzyme, the multiplex amplification protocol was simplified from three rounds to two rounds.

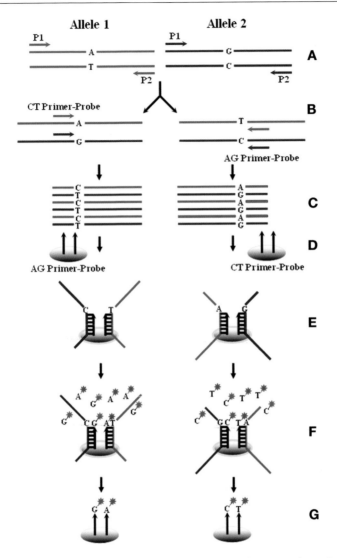

Fig. 2. Schematic illustration of the multiplex genotyping procedure. Only one polymorphism is shown. Primers and probes are shown as arrowed lines. Microarray spots are indicated as ellipsoids. **(A)** Amplification of the polymorphic sequence. Two alleles using the same set of primers, P1 and P2, are shown. **(B)** Generation of single-stranded DNA (ssDNA) by using the primer-probes in both directions in separate tubes. Only the two allelic template strands in each reaction are shown. **(C)** ssDNA generated from B. **(D)** Addition of the ssDNA to the respective microarrays containing probes in different directions. **(E)** ssDNA templates hybridized to their probes on the microarrays. **(F)** Labeling probes by incorporating fluorescently labeled ddNTPs. **(G)** Labeled probes on the microarray after washing off all other reagents. *See* text in section 2 for more details. (Adapted from ref. *36*.)

The procedure for the simplified protocol is generally the same as that for the first two rounds of the three-round PCR protocol described earlier. However, because the third round is not necessary, one primer (instead of two) with the universal tail is needed for each locus. With this protocol, 41 loci could be multiplexed in a single tube (Cui and Li, 1997, unpublished data).

More recently, the universal tail concept was applied to a few newly developed systems *(28–32)*. With these systems, universal sequences are attached to the amplicons by different approaches before PCR allowing more than 1000 SNP-containing sequences to be amplified in a single reaction. This advance has significantly facilitated high-throughput genotyping. The technique initially described by Yeakley et al. *(28)* has been commercialized by Illumina and used for completion of approx 65% of the International HapMap Project (www.hapmap.org). The technologies described by Hardenbol et al. and Kennedy et al. *(29,30)* have also been commercialized and used in large-scale genetic analyses *(33–35)*. However, attaching universal tails to the amplified sequences requires additional experimental steps in comparison with amplification with regular PCR primers, limiting the detection sensitivity. As a result, hundreds of nanograms to 2 μg of genomic DNA are required for each multiplex reaction. Some of these procedures also require pooling of individually amplified PCR products from multiple tubes, followed by column purification. Requirements of specialized probes and detection platforms and long oligonucleotides also limit the flexibility and cost-effectiveness of these systems.

3. DEVELOPMENT OF A HIGH-THROUGHPUT GENOTYPING SYSTEM WITH HIGH SENSITIVITY/DETECTION OF MORE THAN 1000 SNPs IN INDIVIDUAL SPERM CELLS

We have developed a simple genotyping system that requires a single round of multiplex PCR followed by a single step to generate single-stranded DNA (ssDNA) before genotype determination, with a sensitivity for detection of more than 1000 SNPs from a single sperm *(7,36)*. With our new system, instead of attaching universal tails, primers with no predictable productive interaction (i.e., lacking significant complementarity that might cause primer dimerization) are used. With these primers, all experimental effort toward minimizing and avoiding primer–primer interaction becomes unnecessary. A computer program was written to accomplish this task. The candidate sequence frames were first selected based on a user-defined melting temperature range within a sequence span flanking the polymorphic sites (usually 150 bp on each side). The qualified frames were then further selected based on the following criteria: (1) fewer than four consecutively complementary bases between the 3'-ends of any two frames; (2) fewer than eight but one consecutively complementary base between the 3'-ends of any two frames; (3) fewer than 10 consecutively complementary bases between the 3'-end of any frame and anywhere in all others; (4) fewer than 12 but 1 consecutively complementary base between the 3'-end of any frame and anywhere in all others; (5) complementary bases fewer than 75% anywhere between any two frames; and (6) fewer than 13 complementary bases between the 3'-end of any frame and any amplicon sequence. Results from our simulation study indicate that for 1200 or more SNPs selected from the National Center for Biotechnology Information dbSNP, primers could be designed for genotyping approx 90% of SNPs.

The high-throughput genotyping process is illustrated in Fig. 2. The polymorphic sequences of more than 1000 SNPs can be simultaneously amplified in a single tube with all primers (Fig. 2A). To generate ssDNA, a 1- to 2-μL aliquot of the amplified product is used as the template under the same conditions used in PCR. However, only one primer for each SNP is used. The primers used for ssDNA synthesis are designed in such a way that after annealing, their 3'-ends will be next to the polymorphic sites (Fig. 2B). Therefore, they could also be used as probes (primer-probes) on the microarray for genotyping (Fig. 2). For each SNP, two such primer-probes are designed in opposite directions so that they could be used as primers to generate ssDNA and as probes for genotyping in different directions. When used as primers, because they are internal (nested) with respect to primers used in multiplex PCR, the specificity and yield is increased for ssDNA production. The relative correspondence between these primer-probes and the regular primers is shown in Fig. 2. By hybridizing the resulting ssDNA to the probes arrayed onto a glass slide, sequences from different SNP loci are resolved (Fig. 2E).

To determine the allelic state of the sequences hybridized to their probes on the microarray, the commonly used single-base-extension assay *(37–41)* is used. As mentioned earlier, the 3'-ends of the primer-probes hybridizing to the ssDNA are immediately next to the polymorphic sites (Fig. 2E). Using ssDNA as a template, each probe is extended by a single ddNTP conjugated to a fluorescent chromophore (Cy3 or Cy5) in an allele-specific way. As a result, the allelic sequences of each SNP are labeled with different fluorescent colors (Fig. 2F). After labeling, everything but the labeled probes is washed off and the microarray is ready for scanning.

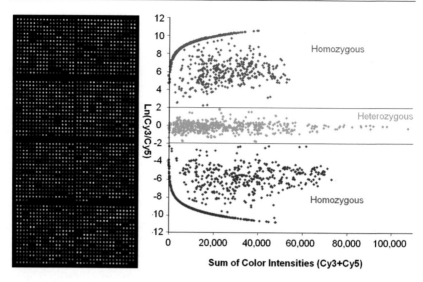

Fig. 3. Typical result from genotyping a genomic DNA from a human individual. (Left panel) A microarray image with a panel of 1172 SNPs. Each probe was printed twice and shown as neighboring spots. Red and green, homozygous; yellow, heterozygous; white, pink, and light green, spots with strong signal that have exceeded the linear range; and dark, low signal but does not necessarily mean no signal or too low for genotype calls. (Right panel) Scatter plot based on the color intensities from the microarray image on the left. Two horizontal lines are the cutoffs (natural logarithm ratios [Cy3/Cy5] of 2 and −2) dividing the spots into three genotype groups. (Adapted from ref. *36*.)

Because DNA sequences are double stranded, ssDNA can be generated in two directions with corresponding primers and can be used for independent genotyping with corresponding probes. Results generated with such a dual-probe method can be compared. Inconsistent genotypes can then be discarded to ensure a very high level of genotyping accuracy. A typical microarray image is shown in the left panel of Fig. 3. A scatter plot of the signal intensities in this image is shown in the right panel of Fig. 3.

Theoretically, when the template ssDNA is from a homozygous individual, a probe should predominantly incorporate one color (signal color that is specific) over the other (background color), whereas a probe hybridizing to ssDNA from a heterozygous individual should incorporate both colors equally. Experimentally, the color intensity is affected by various factors such as nonspecific hybridization, the bandwidth of the light filters, and the ratio between photomultiplier gains selected for each wavelength during scanning. Because of the impact of these experimental factors, three major issues need to be addressed when determining genotypes from the digitized data produced from a microarray image: normalization of the two color intensities, background subtraction of each color, and genotype determination.

We have taken advantage of our ability to analyze a large number of SNPs in a single assay and use homozygous SNPs as internal controls. Our computer program first sorts the SNPs based on the ratio of the two color intensities. For each human subject, the maximal fraction of heterozygous SNPs is expected to be 50%, and the other 50% would be homozygous with 25% for each of the two alleles. To be safe, we treat 20% of SNPs with the highest ratio and 20% with lowest ratio as homozygous.

A given homozygous SNP has two color intensities, the background color intensity and the signal color intensity. The background color intensity can be used for background subtraction. For a heterozygous SNP, the intensities of the two signal colors should be at a 1:1 ratio, but often deviate from this ratio because of experimental variables. Such a difference can be calibrated based on the signal color intensities of the two groups of homozygous SNPs.

After normalization and background subtraction, the genotypes are determined based on the natural logarithms of ratios (Ln[R]s) between the two normalized color intensities by using empirical linear values as cutoffs. These divide SNPs into three groups, two homozygous and one heterozygous for a diploid sample. The cutoff values were validated by comparing the microarray results obtained by using the dual-probe method and from with those obtained by using independent genotyping methods. For sperm samples, usually no SNPs should be in a heterozygous state, and therefore, the Ln(R)s for SNPs labeled predominantly with different colors are usually well separated on the scatter plots (Fig. 4).

4. APPLICATIONS OF HIGH-THROUGHPUT GENETIC ANALYSIS OF INDIVIDUAL SPERM

Because of the high level of sensitivity of our genotyping system, robust results can be obtained from 5 ng of human genomic DNA. With genomic DNA, the detection rate is usually higher than 97% with an accuracy of higher than 99.6%. When single sperm samples are used, the detection rate is usually approx 90% and the accuracy is comparable with that of genomic DNA. Very recently, we have shown that more than 2000 SNPs can be analyzed in a single assay with a detection rate and accuracy similar to the results for multiplexing approx 1000 SNPs (Luo and Li, unpublished data, 2004). The upper limit of the capacity for our genotyping system still needs to be tested. Using our high-throughput

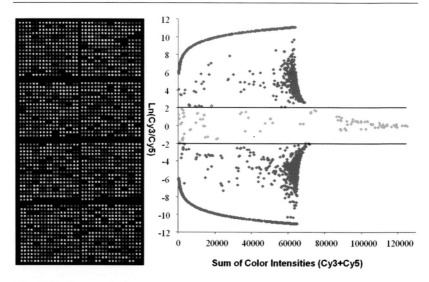

Fig. 4. Typical result from genotyping a single sperm. (Left panel) A microarray image with the panel of 1172 SNPs shown in Fig. 3. Each probe was printed twice and shown as neighboring spots. Red and green, homozygous; yellow, heterozygous; white, pink, and light green, spots with strong signal that have exceeded the linear range; and dark, low signal but does not necessarily mean no signal or too low for genotype calls. (Right panel) Scatter plot based on the color intensities from the microarray image on the left. Two horizontal lines are the cutoffs (natural logarithm ratios [Cy3/Cy5] of 2 and −2) dividing the spots into three genotype groups. Yellow spots are either from SNPs that were not real because of the presences of a small portion of SNPs consisting of paralogous sequence variants in the databases *(87,88)* or from a low level (3.91%) of contamination as demonstrated in the previous studies *(87,88)*, which has been shown to be from oligonucleotides synthesized by the current semi-open oligonucleotide synthesis system. Note: heterozygous SNPs are treated as noninformative in genetic analysis with single sperm.

genotyping system with single sperm as subjects, several studies have been completed in our laboratory (refs. *7, 9,* and *36*; Luo et al., unpublished data, 2005; Cui et al., unpublished data, 2005; Pramanik et al, unpublished data, 2005. Here, we review two studies that have been recently reported.

4.1. Determination of the Physical Structure of Chromosomal Regions With Highly Repetitive Sequences on Single Chromosomes

Microdeletion on the Y chromosome is the most common cause of human male infertility *(42–44)*. Precise and exhaustive identification of microdeletions requires screening with a high-marker density. With the conventional one-marker-per-assay approaches, such a screening is very expensive and unaffordable. With our high-throughput genotyping methods, a large number of markers can be included in the screening, making the exhaustive screen possible and practical.

Although no analysis on male infertility has been performed in our laboratory, the microarray approach that we use for analyzing the human *IGHV* region may be easily adapted for such purpose. Human *IGHV* region is a very complex chromosomal region. The region contains 123–129 gene segments *(45–51)*. Of the 123 *IGHV* gene segments described by Matsuda et al. *(50)*, 79 were pseudogenes and 44 gene segments had open reading frames. Of the 44 genes, 39 were expressed as heavy chain proteins and one as messenger RNA, while the remaining 4 were not found among cDNAs. However, the functional *IGHV* gene segments may vary from 38 to 46 depending on the haplotypes *(46)*. *IGHV* segments are also found at two other chromosomal locations, 15q11 and 16p11 *(45,52–54)*. In total, each human haploid genome contains approx 150 distinct immunoglobulin *IGHV* sequences *(45,47,49,52–54)* that are subdivided into seven families *(50,55–64)*. *IGHV* sequences in each family share more than 80% identity. Human *IGHV* segments of different families are highly interspersed *(47,49, 50,56,65–67)*.

Determination of the *IGHV* segment organization has been a slow process. The difficulty stems from the large number of *IGHV* sequences in each family sharing a high degree of identity; extensive polymorphisms with respect to the *IGHV* segment sequences, number, and composition; different chromosomal locations; and diploidy of the human genome. Completion of a physical map with complete sequence determined for the *IGHV* region is only the beginning for thorough understanding of the physical structure of the *IGHV* region because (1) if the map was constructed by using diploid materials, the organization of the *IGHV* gene segment in such a map may not represent the organization in any actual haplotype; (2) even if the map was constructed by using the materials from a single haplotype, because the *IGHV* region is highly diversified, a map for a single haplotype is far from sufficient for understanding the physical structure of the *IGHV* region; and (3) gene order is not the only aspect of understanding the physical structure of the *IGHV* region. Many other aspects, such as gene segment number and composition of the haplotypes, the content of sequence variation among the allelic sequences, and insertion/deletion and duplication polymorphisms among the haplotypes also need to be examined.

However, with single sperm as subjects, the experimental problems caused by the complexity of the *IGHV* region can be significantly simplified. This is because sperm cells only have one copy of the genome. Therefore, variations in the *IGHV* region among the haplotypes can be studied on an individual haplotype basis. The parental origins of the two haplotypes among the sperm from a single donor can also be easily determined by analysis of a few SNPs in a chromosome region. For study of highly repetitive regions, one of the major difficulties is discriminating between the allelic and interlocus differences, which become confusing in the effort to determine the physical structure of such a region. With sperm, interlocus differences can be found by analyzing multiple sperm of the same parental origins. Allelic differences can only be found between sperm groups of different parental origins. Before development of the microarray-based high-throughput genotyping methods, significant progress was made in using the early version of the multiplex amplification and genotyping methods to analyze the *IGHV* region *(5,8,23,24,68)*.

The microarray-based approach later allowed us to analyze the *IGHV* region in great detail by using a high-marker density along the length of the region *(9)*. For each *IGHV* gene, a segment of sequence was selected as a marker for detection. Marker sequences were amplified by a two-round PCR procedure as described earlier. Instead of arraying probes on to glass slides, multiplex PCR products from a group of single sperm samples from five individuals were spotted onto each microarray, allowing a large number of sperm to be analyzed simultaneously on each array. Two probes labeled with different fluorescent dyes, Cy3 and Cy5, were hybridized to a microarray. *IGHV* genes were detected based on the microarray signal. The parental origin of the haplotype in each sperm was determined by analysis of multiple SNPs in the region.

By analyzing 374 single sperm samples from five Caucasian males, three deletion/insertion polymorphisms (Del I–Del III) with deletion allele frequencies ranging from 0.1 to 0.3 were identified. Del I was reported in our previous publications as 35–40 Kb in size and affecting three *IGHV* genes (*IGHV1-8*, *IGHV3-9*, and *IGHV2-10*; ref. 8). Del II affects a region 2–18 Kb containing two pseudogenes *IGHV(II)-28.1* and *IGHV3-29*, and Del III spans approx 21–53 Kb involving genes *IGHV4-39*, *IGHV7-40*, *IGHV(II)-40-1*, and *IGHV3-41*. Deletion alleles of both Dels II and III were found in a heterozygous state, and therefore, could not be easily detected if haploid samples had not been used in the study. Results of the present study indicate that deletions/insertions together with other possible chromosomal rearrangements may play an important role in forming the genetic structure of the *IGHV* region, and may significantly contribute to antibody diversity. Because these three polymorphisms are located within or next to the 3'-half of the *IGHV* region, they may have an important role in the expressed *IGHV* gene repertoire during immune response.

4.2. Understanding the Contribution of Meiotic Recombination to Haplotype Structure Formation

It is known that in the human population, certain alleles of genetic markers within a short distance are in tight association (linkage disequilibrium [LD]) and LD becomes weak or disappears when the markers are located farther apart *(69)*. Chromosomal segments containing markers in LD are called haplotype blocks *(70)*. Haplotype blocks in the human genome were first described on a large scale for a 500-Kb region of chromosome 5q31 *(71)* and the entire chromosome 21 *(72)*, and subsequently in other regions of the genome *(73–76)*. Information on the haplotype structure of the human genome is of great interest because it can be used to significantly reduce the number of markers necessary for localizing genes responsible for complex diseases *(77–79)*. The progress of the International HapMap Project has resulted in the mapping of haplotype blocks across the entire human genome *(80)*. However, very little is known about the mechanisms underlying the formation of haplotype blocks. There is a strong belief that meiotic recombination plays a primary role in shaping LD observed in the human genome and therefore has a direct effect on the haplotype structure found in the human *(18,71,73,76,81–85)*. However, proving such a correlation requires direct evidence of the contribution of recombination on haplotype block formation. By using pooled sperm, a 216-Kb segment in the class II region of the major histocompatibility complex was studied *(82)*. Six recombination hotspots were precisely located within regions where LD breaks down.

To address the issues whether the human genome contains recombination hotspots in a similar pattern and/or density; and whether the hotspots fall between haplotype blocks, another region on chromosome 1q42.3 was analyzed *(81)*. The authors' approach allows them to focus on small subregions to learn a great deal about the mechanisms underlying meiotic recombination and its impact on the genetic structure of the human genome during evolution. However, by analysis of small regions, it is difficult to learn the distribution of recombination crossovers at levels higher than individual hotspots. In-depth study of a large chromosomal region is also necessary for this purpose. However, this is especially challenging because haplotype blocks are usually very

7. Greenawalt DM, Cui X, Wu Y, et al. Strong correlation between meiotic crossovers and haplotype structure in a 2.5-Mb region on the long arm of chromosome 21. Genome Res 2006;16:208–214.

8. Pramanik S, Li H. Direct detection of insertion/deletion polymorphisms in an autosomal region by analyzing high-density markers in individual spermatozoa. Am J Hum Genet 2002;71:1342–1352.

9. Chimge NO, Pramanik S, Hu G, et al. Determination of gene organization in the human IGHV region on single chromosomes. Genes Immun 2005;6:186–193.

10. Cui XF, Li HH, Goradia TM, et al. Single-sperm typing: determination of genetic distance between the G gamma-globin and parathyroid hormone loci by using the polymerase chain reaction and allele-specific oligomers. Proc Natl Acad Sci USA 1989;86:9389–9393.

11. Conner BJ, Reyes AA, Morin C, Itakura K, Teplitz RL, Wallace RB. Detection of sickle cell beta S-globin allele by hybridization with synthetic oligonucleotides. Proc Natl Acad Sci USA 1983;80:278–282.

12. Saiki RK, Bugawan TL, Horn GT, Mullis KB, Erlich HA. Analysis of enzymatically amplified beta-globin and HLA-DQ alpha DNA with allele-specific oligonucleotide probes. Nature 1986;324:163–166.

13. Li H, Cui X, Arnheim N. Direct electrophoretic detection of the allelic state of single DNA molecules in human sperm by using the polymerase chain reaction. Proc Natl Acad Sci USA 1990;87:4580–4584.

14. Goradia TM, Stanton VP, Jr, Cui XF, et al. Ordering three DNA polymorphisms on human chromosome 3 by sperm typing. Genomics 1991;10:748–755.

15. Hubert R, Stanton VP, Jr, Aburatani H, et al. Sperm typing allows accurate measurement of the recombination fraction between D3S2 and D3S3 on the short arm of human chromosome 3. Genomics 1992;12:683–687.

16. Cui X, Gerwin J, Navidi W, Li H, Kuehn M, Arnheim N. Gene-centromere linkage mapping by PCR analysis of individual oocytes. Genomics 1992;13:713–717.

17. Zhang L, Cui X, Schmitt K, Hubert R, Navidi W, Arnheim N. Whole genome amplification from a single cell: implications for genetic analysis. Proc Natl Acad Sci USA 1992;89:5847–5851.

18. Cullen M, Perfetto SP, Klitz W, Nelson G, Carrington M. High-resolution patterns of meiotic recombination across the human major histocompatibility complex. Am J Hum Genet 2002;71:759–776.

19. Fischer SG, Lerman LS. Separation of random fragments of DNA according to properties of their sequences. Proc Natl Acad Sci USA 1980;77:4420–4424.

20. Myers RM, Fischer SG, Maniatis T, Lerman LS. Modification of the melting properties of duplex DNA by attachment of a GC-rich DNA sequence as determined by denaturing gradient gel electrophoresis. Nucleic Acids Res 1985;13:3111–3129.

21. Fischer SG, Lerman LS. DNA fragments differing by single base-pair substitutions are separated in denaturing gradient gels: correspondence with melting theory. Proc Natl Acad Sci USA 1983;80:1579–1583.

22. Myers RM, Fischer SG, Lerman LS, Maniatis T. Nearly all single base substitutions in DNA fragments joined to a GC-clamp can be detected by denaturing gradient gel electrophoresis. Nucleic Acids Res 1985;13:3131–3145.

23. Li H, Cui X, Pramanik S, Chimge NO. Genetic diversity of the human immunoglobulin heavy chain VH region. Immunol Rev 2002;190:53–68.

24. Cui X, Li H. Determination of gene organization in individual haplotypes by analyzing single DNA fragments from single spermatozoa. Proc Natl Acad Sci USA 1998;95:10,791–10,796.

25. Lin Z, Cui X, Li H. Multiplex genotype determination at a large number of gene loci. Proc Natl Acad Sci USA 1996;93:2582–2587.
26. Edwards MC, Gibbs RA. Multiplex PCR: advantages, development, and applications. PCR Methods Appl 1994;3:S65–S75.
27. Shuber AP, Grondin VJ, Klinger KW. A simplified procedure for developing multiplex PCRs. Genome Res 1995;5:488–493.
28. Yeakley JM, Fan JB, Doucet D, et al. Profiling alternative splicing on fiber-optic arrays. Nat Biotechnol 2002;20:353–358.
29. Hardenbol P, Baner J, Jain M, et al. Multiplexed genotyping with sequence-tagged molecular inversion probes. Nat Biotechnol 2003;21:673–678.
30. Kennedy GC, Matsuzaki H, Dong S, et al. Large-scale genotyping of complex DNA. Nat Biotechnol 2003;21:1233–1237.
31. Matsuzaki H, Loi H, Dong S, et al. Parallel genotyping of over 10,000 SNPs using a one-primer assay on a high-density oligonucleotide array. Genome Res 2004;14: 414–425.
32. Fan J-B, Oliphant A, Shen R, et al. Highly parallel SNP genotyping. In: Cold Spring Harbor Symposia on Quantitative Biology. Cold Spring Harbor Laboratory Press, City: 2004;69–78.
33. Butcher LM, Meaburn E, Liu L, et al. Genotyping pooled DNA on microarrays: a systematic genome screen of thousands of SNPs in large samples to detect QTLs for complex traits. Behav Genet 2004;34:549–555.
34. Zhou X, Mok SC, Chen Z, Li Y, Wong DT. Concurrent analysis of loss of heterozygosity (LOH) and copy number abnormality (CNA) for oral premalignancy progression using the Affymetrix 10K SNP mapping array. Hum Genet 2004;115:327–330.
35. Zhou X, Li C, Mok SC, Chen Z, Wong DT. Whole genome loss of heterozygosity profiling on oral squamous cell carcinoma by high-density single nucleotide polymorphic allele (SNP) array. Cancer Genet Cytogenet 2004;151:82–84.
36. Wang HY, Luo M, Tereshchenko IV, et al. A genotyping system capable of simultaneously analyzing >1000 single nucleotide polymorphisms in a haploid genome. Genome Res 2005;15:276–283.
37. Shumaker JM, Metspalu A, Caskey CT. Mutation detection by solid phase primer extension. Hum Mutat 1996;7:346–354.
38. Lindblad-Toh K, Tanenbaum DM, Daly MJ, et al. Loss-of-heterozygosity analysis of small-cell lung carcinomas using single-nucleotide polymorphism arrays. Nat Biotechnol 2000;18:1001–1005.
39. Pastinen T, Kurg A, Metspalu A, Peltonen L, Syvanen AC. Minisequencing: a specific tool for DNA analysis and diagnostics on oligonucleotide arrays. Genome Res 1997;7:606–614.
40. Syvanen AC. From gels to chips: "minisequencing" primer extension for analysis of point mutations and single nucleotide polymorphisms. Hum Mutat 1999;13:1–10.
41. Pastinen T, Raitio M, Lindroos K, Tainola P, Peltonen L, Syvanen AC. A system for specific, high-throughput genotyping by allele-specific primer extension on microarrays. Genome Res 2000;10:1031–1042.
42. Aknin-Seifer IE, Lejeune H, Touraine RL, Levy R. Y chromosome microdeletion screening in infertile men in France: a survey of French practice based on 88 IVF centres. Hum Reprod 2004;19:788–793.
43. Vogt PH. AZF deletions and Y chromosomal haplogroups: history and update based on sequence. Hum Reprod Update 2005;11:319–336.
44. Ali S, Hasnain SE. Genomics of the human Y-chromosome. 1. Association with male infertility. Gene 2003;321:25–37.

45. Pallares N, Lefebvre S, Contet V, Matsuda F, Lefranc MP. The human immunoglobulin heavy variable genes. Exp Clin Immunogenet 1999;16:36–60.

46. Scaviner D, Barbie V, Ruiz M, Lefranc MP. Protein displays of the human immunoglobulin heavy, kappa and lambda variable and joining regions. Exp Clin Immunogenet 1999;16:234–240.

47. Cook GP, Tomlinson IM, Walter G, et al. A map of the human immunoglobulin VH locus completed by analysis of the telomeric region of chromosome 14q. Nat Genet 1994;7:162–168.

48. Cook GP, Tomlinson IM. The human immunoglobulin VH repertoire. Immunol Today 1995;16:237–242.

49. Matsuda F, Shin EK, Nagaoka H, et al. Structure and physical map of 64 variable segments in the 3′0.8-megabase region of the human immunoglobulin heavy-chain locus. Nat Genet 1993;3:88–94.

50. Matsuda F, Ishii K, Bourvagnet P, et al. The complete nucleotide sequence of the human immunoglobulin heavy chain variable region locus. J Exp Med 1998;188: 2151–2162.

51. Shin EK, Matsuda F, Nagaoka H, et al. Physical map of the 3′ region of the human immunoglobulin heavy chain locus: clustering of autoantibody-related variable segments in one haplotype. Embo J 1991;10:3641–3645.

52. Cherif D, Berger R. New localizations of VH sequences by in situ hybridization with biotinylated probes. Genes Chromosomes Cancer 1990;2:103–108.

53. Tomlinson IM, Cook GP, Carter NP, et al. Human immunoglobulin VH and D segments on chromosomes 15q11.2 and 16p11.2. Hum Mol Genet 1994;3:853–860.

54. Nagaoka H, Ozawa K, Matsuda F, et al. Recent translocation of variable and diversity segments of the human immunoglobulin heavy chain from chromosome 14 to chromosomes 15 and 16. Genomics 1994;22:189–197.

55. Lee KH, Matsuda F, Kinashi T, Kodaira M, Honjo T. A novel family of variable region genes of the human immunoglobulin heavy chain. J Mol Biol 1987;195: 761–768.

56. Berman JE, Mellis SJ, Pollock R, et al. Content and organization of the human Ig VH locus: definition of three new VH families and linkage to the Ig CH locus. EMBO J 1988;7:727–738.

57. Rabbitts TH, Matthyssens G, Hamlyn PH. Contribution of immunoglobulin heavy-chain variable-region genes to antibody diversity. Nature 1980;284:238–243.

58. Schroeder HW, Jr, Hillson JL, Perlmutter RM. Early restriction of the human antibody repertoire. Science 1987;238:791–793.

59. Humphries CG, Shen A, Kuziel WA, Capra JD, Blattner FR, Tucker PW. A new human immunoglobulin VH family preferentially rearranged in immature B-cell tumours. Nature 1988;331:446–449.

60. Buluwela L, Rabbitts TH. A VH gene is located within 95 Kb of the human immunoglobulin heavy chain constant region genes. Eur J Immunol 1988;18: 1843–1845.

61. van Dijk KW, Mortari F, Kirkham PM, Schroeder HW, Jr, Milner EC. The human immunoglobulin VH7 gene family consists of a small, polymorphic group of six to eight gene segments dispersed throughout the VH locus. Eur J Immunol 1993;23:832–839.

62. Tomlinson IM, Walter G, Marks JD, Llewelyn MB, Winter G. The repertoire of human germline VH sequences reveals about fifty groups of VH segments with different hypervariable loops. J Mol Biol 1992;227:776–798.

63. Kirkham PM, Mortari F, Newton JA, Schroeder HW, Jr. Immunoglobulin VH clan and family identity predicts variable domain structure and may influence antigen binding. Embo J 1992;11:603–609.

64. Mortari F, Newton JA, Wang JY, Schroeder HW, Jr. The human cord blood antibody repertoire. Frequent usage of the VH7 gene family. Eur J Immunol 1992;22: 241–245.

65. Kodaira M, Kinashi T, Umemura I, et al. Organization and evolution of variable region genes of the human immunoglobulin heavy chain. J Mol Biol 1986;190: 529–541.

66. Walter MA, Surti U, Hofker MH, Cox DW. The physical organization of the human immunoglobulin heavy chain gene complex. Embo J 1990;9:3303–3313.

67. Lefranc MP. Nomenclature of the human immunoglobulin heavy (IGH) genes. Exp Clin Immunogenet 2001;18:100–116.

68. Cui X, Li H. Human immunoglobulin VH4 sequences resolved by population-based analysis after enzymatic amplification and denaturing gradient gel electrophoresis. Eur J Immunogenet 2000;27:37–46.

69. Ardlie KG, Kruglyak L, Seielstad M. Patterns of linkage disequilibrium in the human genome. Nat Rev Genet 2002;3:299–309.

70. Wall JD, Pritchard JK. Haplotype blocks and linkage disequilibrium in the human genome. Nat Rev Genet 2003;4:587–597.

71. Daly MJ, Rioux JD, Schaffner SF, Hudson TJ, Lander ES. High-resolution haplotype structure in the human genome. Nat Genet 2001;29:229–232.

72. Patil N, Berno AJ, Hinds DA, et al. Blocks of limited haplotype diversity revealed by high-resolution scanning of human chromosome 21. Science 2001;294: 1719–1723.

73. Gabriel SB, Schaffner SF, Nguyen H, et al. The structure of haplotype blocks in the human genome. Science 2002;296:2225–2229.

74. Olivier M, Wang X, Cole R, et al. Haplotype analysis of the apolipoprotein gene cluster on human chromosome 11. Genomics 2004;83:912–923.

75. Stenzel A, Lu T, Koch WA, et al. Patterns of linkage disequilibrium in the MHC region on human chromosome 6p. Hum Genet 2004;114:377–385.

76. Twells RC, Mein CA, Phillips MS, et al. Haplotype structure, LD blocks, and uneven recombination within the LRP5 gene. Genome Res 2003;13:845–855.

77. Judson R, Salisbury B, Schneider J, Windemuth A, Stephens JC. How many SNPs does a genome-wide haplotype map require? Pharmacogenomics 2002; 3:379–391.

78. Phillips MS, Lawrence R, Sachidanandam R, et al. Chromosome-wide distribution of haplotype blocks and the role of recombination hot spots. Nat Genet 2003;33:382–387.

79. Wang N, Akey JM, Zhang K, Chakraborty R, Jin L. Distribution of recombination crossovers and the origin of haplotype blocks: the interplay of population history, recombination, and mutation. Am J Hum Genet 2002;71:1227–1234.

80. Consortium IH. The International HapMap Project. Nature 2003;426:789–796.

81. Jeffreys AJ, Neumann R, Panayi M, Myers S, Donnelly P. Human recombination hot spots hidden in regions of strong marker association. Nat Genet 2005;37: 601–606.

82. Jeffreys AJ, Kauppi L, Neumann R. Intensely punctate meiotic recombination in the class II region of the major histocompatibility complex. Nat Genet 2001;29: 217–222.

83. Crawford DC, Bhangale T, Li N, et al. Evidence for substantial fine-scale variation in recombination rates across the human genome. Nat Genet 2004;36:700–706.

84. McVean GA, Myers SR, Hunt S, Deloukas P, Bentley DR, Donnelly P. The fine-scale structure of recombination rate variation in the human genome. Science 2004;304:581–584.

85. Kauppi L, Sajantila A, Jeffreys AJ. Recombination hotspots rather than population history dominate linkage disequilibrium in the MHC class II region. Hum Mol Genet 2003;12:33–40.

86. Kong A, Gudbjartsson DF, Sainz J, et al. A high-resolution recombination map of the human genome. Nat Genet 2002;31:241–247.

87. Cheung J, Estivill X, Khaja R, et al. Genome-wide detection of segmental duplications and potential assembly errors in the human genome sequence. Genome Biol 2003;4:R25.

88. Fredman D, White SJ, Potter S, Eichler EE, Den Dunnen JT, Brookes AJ. Complex SNP-related sequence variation in segmental genome duplications. Nat Genet 2004;36:861–866.

5 Physiological and Proteomic Approaches to Understanding Human Sperm Function
Prefertilization Events

Sarah J. Conner, PhD,
Linda Lefièvre, PhD,
Jackson Kirkman-Brown, PhD,
Gisela S. M. Machado-Oliveira, BSc,
Frank Michelangeli, PhD,
Stephen J. Publicover, PhD,
and Christopher L. R. Barratt, PhD

Summary

Sperm dysfunction is the single most common defined cause of infertility. Approximately 1 in 15 men are subfertile and the condition is increasing in frequency. However, the diagnosis is poor and, excluding assisted conception, there is no treatment because of our limited understanding of the cellular, biochemical, and molecular functioning of the spermatozoon. The underlying premise of our research program is to establish a rudimentary understanding of the processes necessary for successful fertilization. We detail advances in our understanding of calcium signaling in the cell and outline genetic and proteomic technologies that are being used to improve the diagnosis of the condition.

Key Words: Proteomics; calcium signaling; zona pellucida; capacitation.

1. INTRODUCTION

This chapter discusses the premise that there is a clear need to significantly improve our understanding of the cellular basis of normal sperm function. This knowledge is fundamental for two key developments in

From: *The Genetics of Male Infertility*
Edited by: D.T. Carrell © Humana Press Inc., Totowa, NJ

male fertility: first, to provide the basis for effective diagnostic tools and, second, to facilitate the study of the physiology of abnormal/ dysfunctional cells that is central to developing rational, non-assisted reproduction technology (non-ART) therapy. We discuss the role of calcium in sperm function and question the exclusive use of in vitro experiments with no reference to the in vivo situation. Additionally, we highlight how our understanding of sperm zona binding has been questioned with the discovery of the "four zona proteins" model. Finally, we examine strategies to determine the dysfunction of spermatozoa, in particular the use of proteomics.

Epidemiological data shows that one in seven couples are classed as subfertile *(1,2)*. Sperm dysfunction is the single most common cause of infertility and affects approx 1 in 15 men *(3)*. Studies using semen assessment as the criteria for subfertility (sperm concentration $<20 \times 10^6$/mL) show that one in five 18 yr olds are classed as subfertile *(4)*. This is a high proportion of the population compared with other prevalent diseases, such as diabetes (2.8% of the population; ref. *5*). Thus, male subfertility is a very significant global problem and reports suggest that its prevalence is increasing *(6)*.

2. IMPROVING THE DIAGNOSIS OF MALE FERTILITY

There is a clear requirement to produce new and robust tests of sperm function to diagnose male infertility. The value of traditional semen parameters (concentration, motility, and morphology) in the diagnosis and prognosis of male infertility has been debated for almost 60 yr and, perhaps not surprisingly, the debate continues *(7)*. Suffice it to say traditional semen parameters provide some degree of prognostic and diagnostic information for the infertile couple *(8,9)*. However, it is only at the lower ranges of the spectrum that these parameters are most useful and even then they can only be used as guidance for couples and do not represent absolute values *(10)*.

Traditional semen analysis will therefore only be a limited first-line tool in the diagnosis of male infertility. Consequently, the emphasis has been on developing simple, robust, and effective tests of sperm function. Yet despite the plethora of potential assays available, results have been very disappointing *(11)*. Recent data suggest that only three potential tests of sperm function have sufficient data to support their routine use: penetration into cervical mucus (or substitutes; ref. *12*), measurement of reactive oxygen species production *(13)*, and estimate of sperm DNA damage *(14)*, however, promising initial data for the latter is now being questioned *(15,16)*.

After decades of research why are more effective and robust estimates of sperm function unavailable? The primary reason is our limited basic understanding of the functioning of the spermatozoon.

3. DEVELOPMENT OF EFFECTIVE DRUG-BASED NON-ART THERAPY

With such an important health issue as male infertility, we would expect a number of rational and effective treatments to be available. However, there are no drug treatments to enhance sperm function that have been shown to be effective in randomized controlled trials *(17,18)*. Thus, remarkably, the only treatment option for the subfertile man is in vitro fertilization (IVF) or intracytoplasmic sperm injection (collectively termed "assisted conception"). Assisted conception is very expensive, invasive, has limited success, a number of side effects, is not widely available, and poses significant concerns about the long-term health of children *(19,20)*. However, the number of patients treated with assisted conception is continually increasing. For example, in the United States there was a 78% increase in ART treatments from 1996 to 2002 *(21)* and currently, up to 4% of births are a result of ART *(4)*. Put simply, this means that, as a result of our ignorance of the causes of sperm dysfunction, we are currently subjecting an increasing number of women to inappropriate invasive therapy to treat their partners.

In summary, we need to understand in cellular, biochemical, genetic, and molecular terms how a sperm cell works to address the issues discussed previously *(22)*. Because the functioning of a spermatozoon is critically dependent on the tight regulation of calcium that, when disrupted, results in fertilization failure *(23)*, our research is focused on this area. We are attempting to study the regulation of calcium within the context of the journey a sperm makes in the female tract in the belief that this will lead us to a more comprehensive understanding.

4. UNDERSTANDING THE CALCIUM TOOLKIT AS A BASIC FUNCTION OF THE SPERMATOZOON

4.1. Functional Importance of Sperm Intracellular Calcium Concentration Signaling

Although there is little doubt that spermatozoa use a range of cell messengers, (e.g., cyclic adenosine monophosphate), data accumulated over the last few years have shown that intracellular calcium concentration ($[Ca^{2+}]_i$) plays a major role in all important sperm functions that occur after ejaculation *(24)*. However, in contrast to somatic cells

(25,26), an understanding of Ca^{2+}-signaling in the sperm cell (despite its great importance) is only now developing *(24,27)*. The simple pump-leak model is initially attractive for spermatozoa. Because of the small size of the cell, diffusion is unlikely to be a limiting factor and it is reasonable to assume that Ca^{2+}-influx from the extracellular compartment can effect a rapid rise in $[Ca^{2+}]_i$ in any part of the cytoplasm. However direct evidence for Ca^{2+} store mobilization in mammalian spermatozoa is now available (probably the acrosome) and activation of capacitative Ca^{2+} influx *(28–30)*. It has become apparent that a second, separately regulated store may exist, which functions primarily to regulate flagellar beat *(31,32)*. Thus sperm may possess a relatively complex Ca^{2+}-signaling apparatus including pump-leak and multiple stores (Fig. 1).

In the last few years there have been several developments in our understanding of calcium regulation by the spermatozoon *(33)*. In our laboratories, we have recently concentrated on role of Ca^{2+} clearance mechanisms in sperm. In most cells, Ca^{2+} clearance is undertaken to a great extent by adenosine 5'-triphosphate (ATP)-requiring Ca^{2+} pumps (Ca^{2+}-ATPases) or Na^+-Ca^{2+} exchangers, which extrude Ca^{2+} either out of the cell, or into intracellular Ca^{2+} stores *(34)*. Analysis of Ca^{2+} clearance in mouse sperm suggests that both Ca^{2+} pumps and Ca^{2+} exchangers are important contributors to Ca^{2+} clearance in mammalian sperm, although the relative importance of each is yet to be determined *(24)*.

4.2. Ca²⁺ Pumps

To date, three types of ATP-utilizing Ca^{2+} pumps have been identified: plasma membrane Ca^{2+} ATPase (PMCA), sarcoplasmic-endoplasmic Ca^{2+} ATPase (SERCA), and secretory pathway Ca^{2+} ATPase (SPCA; refs. *34* and *35*).

4.2.1. THE ROLE OF PMCA IN SPERM

PMCA protein is present in rat spermatids, mouse spermatozoa *(36,37)*, and sea urchin sperm *(38)*. PMCA4 is the main isoform present (>90% of the PMCA protein in sperm is PMCA4 *[39]*) and is primarily confined to the principal piece of the sperm flagellum *(37,39,40)*. Null mutants for PMCA isoforms have been created *(41)*. The major phenotype observed in PMCA4-null mice was male infertility, yet they showed normal spermatogenesis and mating behavior. The sperm, although appearing normal before capacitation, failed to respond to conditions that induce hyperactivated motility. After 90 min, most cells were non-motile, with a few showing very weak hyperactivated motility compared to wild-type *(39,41)*. Measurement of $[Ca^{2+}]_i$ showed that, after 60 min of incubation in capacitating medium, resting $[Ca^{2+}]_i$

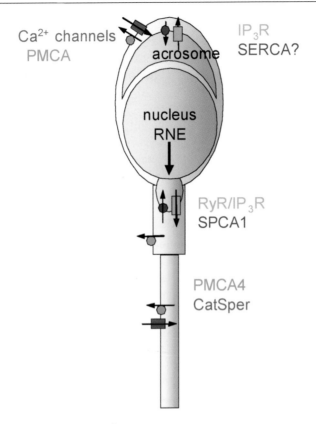

Fig. 1. Two-store model for Ca^{2+}-signaling in human spermatozoa. Plasma membrane Ca^{2+} adenosine 5′-triphosphatases (ATPases) and Na^+-Ca^{2+} exchangers are shown in green; Ca^{2+} channels in the plasma membrane are shown in red; sarcoplasmic-endoplasmic reticulum ATPases on intracellular stores are shown in blue, and channels for mobilization of stored Ca^{2+} are shown in orange. Identified or putative components of the Ca^{2+}-signaling toolkit are labeled (using the same color coding) adjacent to their localization *(24,103)*.

was increased from 157 to 370 nM in PMCA4-deficient sperm *(40)*. This effect could be mimicked using the PMCA inhibitor 5-(and -6)-carboxyeosin diacetate succinimidyl ester on wild-type mice. A similar failure of hyperactivated motility was observed.

4.2.2. THE ROLE OF SERCA IN SPERM

In contrast to the persuasive evidence for the importance of PMCA in sperm function, the activity of SERCA in mature sperm is controversial. In our laboratory, using an anti-SERCA antibody (which recognized all known mammalian SERCA isoforms), no cross-reactivity was detected in Western blots using human sperm *(42)*. Furthermore, thapsigargin only induced Ca^{2+}-mobilization and disruption of Ca^{2+}-signaling in sperm in the 1–10 µM range, which is far higher than concentrations used to specifically inhibit SERCA (43,44). Earlier studies on the effects of thapsigargin on the acrosome reaction and on $[Ca^{2+}]_i$ in sperm also showed that between 0.5 µM and more than 20 µM thapsigargin concentrations were required to induce this response. Thus, treatment of sperm with thapsigargin at concentrations sufficient to inhibit SERCAs is largely without effect, significant actions occurring only at high, "nonspecific" doses. Recently, Gunarante and Vaquier showed that sea urchin SERCA was present in the testis but not mature sperm, further questioning the role of SERCA in mature spermatozoa (38).

4.2.3. THE ROLE OF SPCA IN SPERM

In somatic cells, SPCA are found located on the Golgi apparatus or secretory vesicles (45,46) and are believed to control the levels of both Ca^{2+} and Mn^{2+} within the Golgi to regulate its function (34). We have shown that rat germ cells (spermatids) express the messenger RNA for SPCA1 (46). SPCA1 is also present in mature human sperm and is localized to the anterior midpiece, extending into the rear of the head (42), perhaps reflecting expression in the putative Ca^{2+} store of the redundant nuclear envelope (RNE; ref. 47).

In summary, there is strong evidence to indicate that sperm express both PMCA and SPCA and that these Ca^{2+} pumps play a major role in controlling sperm Ca^{2+} homeostasis. The role for SERCA in mature sperm is more tenuous, but there appears to be some evidence that it may play a role during spermatogenesis.

5. ACTIONS OF CA^{2+}-MOBILIZING AGONISTS: PROGESTERONE AS AN EXAMPLE

In human spermatozoa the $[Ca^{2+}]_i$ response to progesterone has been studied in great detail. In fact, human spermatozoa appear to be unusually sensitive to progesterone (48). When stimulated with 3 µM progesterone, believed to be representative of concentrations present in the vicinity of the oocyte-cumulus, human sperm generate a biphasic $[Ca^{2+}]_i$ response consisting of a transient (lasting 1–2 min) followed by a sustained elevation. Both parts of the response involve influx of extracellular Ca^{2+} and presumably reflect gating of membrane Ca^{2+}-permeable channels. However, the nature of the channels involved is largely unknown. We have suggested previously that the response to progesterone may be similar to that induced by zona pellucida (ZP), activating a voltage-operated calcium channel (VOCC; although probably not

T-type *[49,50]*) and possibly converging with the ZP-activated pathway on activation of store-operated influx *(22)*. Extracellular La^{3+} can completely inhibit the response to progesterone *(51)*, confirming the importance of membrane Ca^{2+} channels, and a late component of the initial $[Ca^{2+}]_i$ transient (that is particularly sensitive to occlusion by prior progesterone stimulation *[32]*) is sensitive to nifedipine *(48)*. However, the balance of evidence from studies that have specifically attempted to demonstrate a role for VOCCs in the response to progesterone does not support this model *(49,52–54)*. Stimulation of sperm from PLCδ4-knockout (KO) mice with 50–100 μM progesterone generates a response of reduced amplitude and greatly reduced duration compared with that of wild-type cells *(55)*, consistent with a requirement for emptying of an inositol 1,4,5 triphosphate (IP_3)-sensitive store, although the high doses required to evoke large responses in murine sperm may be acting by a different pathway than that normally studied in human spermatozoa, which saturates at approx 300 nM progesterone *(32,56)*. Attempts to demonstrate pharmacologically that the sustained elevation of $[Ca^{2+}]_i$ is a result of activation of store-operated channels have produced equivocal data *(32,42,49)*.

It has been shown that progesterone also activates repeated $[Ca^{2+}]_i$ oscillations in human spermatozoa that are the result of store mobilization *(32,57)*. If progesterone is applied as a gradient (to represent more closely the stimulus encountered as a spermatozoon approaches the oocyte) then the initial $[Ca^{2+}]_i$ transient, a characteristic of all previous studies, does not occur, but $[Ca^{2+}]_i$ oscillations occur in a large portion of cells *(32)*. Although IP_3 receptors (IP_3Rs) have been localized to this area of the sperm, the $[Ca^{2+}]_i$ oscillations are resistant to pharmacological treatments designed to inhibit phospholipase C (PLC) or IP_3Rs, suggesting that IP_3 generation is not required for their generation *(32)*. Instead, Ca^{2+} influx induced by progesterone apparently activates a ryanodine-like receptor located in the sperm neck/midpiece (probably on the RNE) leading to repetitive bursts of Ca^{2+}-induced Ca^{2+} release. Reuptake of Ca^{2+} during oscillations is thapsigargin-insensitive and apparently is dependent (at least in part) on activity of SPCA1 *(42)*.

6. SUMMARY: CA^{2+} SIGNALING TOOLKIT IN SPERM

On the basis of the data summarized previously, a complex model for sperm Ca^{2+}-homeostasis involving several types of Ca^{2+}-permeable channels in the plasma membrane and at least two stores is appropriate (Fig. 1). Furthermore, it is clear that these toolkit components are distributed to allow localization of $[Ca^{2+}]_i$ signals. In addition to a range of VOCCs, which are clearly localized to sperm regions, the CatSpers, which are essential for activation of hyperactivated mobility, are expressed specifically in the principal piece of the sperm tail, as is PMCA4. It appears that the acrosome functions as an IP_3-releasable store, activated by agonists linked to PLC. Recent studies suggest mobilization of acrosomal Ca^{2+} is intimately involved in activation of acrosome reaction (58,59). A separate store, probably the RNE, exists in the neck region of the sperm and plays a key role in regulation of flagellar beat mode.

7. THE INTERACTION BETWEEN HUMAN SPERMATOZOA AND THE FEMALE REPRODUCTIVE TRACT: WHAT CAN WE LEARN?

We already know that the journey of the sperm cell from the site of deposition to the site of fertilization is both dynamic (on the part of the sperm and the female tract) and highly complex (60–62), with the female tract clearly regulating the function of the sperm cell. However, the details of these interactions, especially in the human, are unknown.

There are a number of elegant in vivo investigations studying the transport of sperm in several species (e.g., pigs, hamsters, cows), which show that the female tract sequesters spermatozoa in a functional reservoir (primarily in the oviduct; ref. 61). However, the situation in the human may be somewhat different, because an oviductal reservoir in the human has yet to be discovered (63). Additionally, in vitro experiments using a series of oviductal tissues preparations (including explants) have shown that human sperm will bind to these tissues but with noticeably less tenacity than in animals. In fact, human spermatozoon will bind, release, then bind again, potentially repeating this cycle several times (64). In animals, binding to the oviduct acts to prolong the survival of the sperm cell, perhaps keeping it in a state of suspended animation.

In the human, it is not only the oviduct that may influence the physiological state of the sperm cell. Several experiments in the 1970s and 1980s have shown that cervical mucus acts to rapidly activate the sperm yet maintain it in a state ready for fertilization for several days (60). Such experiments reveal the strong influence of the female reproductive tract but at the same time make us aware of gaping holes in our understanding of the true biological basis of sperm activation (capacitation). For example, how is the process arrested/suspended? In fact, there is almost a complete divorce in thinking between researchers studying capacitation (in vitro) and what is likely to be happening in vivo. For our understanding to progress there needs to be a reconnection of the two schools. For example, it does not take 6–24 h to fully capacitate a human sperm cell. A sperm may, however, begin the process of capacitation very rapidly (e.g., when in cervical mucus), but then be prevented from further activation. The IVF system, specifically the culture medium, is designed to almost immediately maximize the fertilizing potential of the sperm, switching on a series of capacitation-related events very rapidly with no intention to put a break in the system *(65)*. Consequently, the differences in the systems (in vivo, in vitro in a research laboratory and IVF) need to be realized and used to complement our understanding. Almost all our knowledge about human sperm function has been gained from experiments in vitro with almost no regard to how the cell may behave in vivo. Perhaps this is why our understanding has remained at a low level. Probably we have been studying the spermatozoon in the wrong environment, in the wrong way, and at the wrong time.

8. HOW DO SPERM INTERACT WITH THE HUMAN ZP? THE "FOUR ZONA PROTEINS" MODEL

A number of studies have shown the importance of sperm zona binding as a prerequisite of normal sperm function *(66)*. However, the molecular details of this interaction remain a mystery. One reason for this is that we may have been using the wrong paradigm to study these interactions. Almost all our knowledge is based on the three zona protein model of the mouse (ZP1, ZP2, and ZP3). Using this model, ZP1 is thought to contribute to the structural integrity of the ZP matrix acting as a linker molecule between ZP filaments *(67)*. ZP2 has been found to be involved in the secondary binding for acrosome-reacted spermatozoa *(68–70)* and ZP3 is accepted to be the primary sperm receptor responsible for binding to intact capacitated spermatozoa and induction of the acrosome reaction *(71)*.

There are four ZP genes and four ZP proteins in the human *(72,73)*. This is very different from the mouse, in which only three proteins are present *(74)*. Accumulating evidence supports the four protein model as the prevalent structure for the ZP across vertebrates (Table 1). Mass spectrometry suggests that ZP4 levels in the human are equivalent to those of ZP3 and ZP2 with ZP1 being a more minor component *(72)*. Experiments have shown that mouse zonae humanized to express human ZP2 and ZP3 can bind mouse sperm but are unable to bind

Table 1
Expression of ZP Genes in Vertebrate Species Commonly Used in Research

	ZP1	ZP2	ZP3	ZP4
Human	•	•	•	•
Macaque	•	•	•	•
Pig		•	•	•
Cow		•	•	•
Rabbit		•	•	•
Mouse	•	•	•	Non-functional
Rat	•	•	•	•
Hamster			•	
Chicken	•	•	•	•

Blank boxes indicate that no gene has yet been identified but that the gene is not necessarily absent. Accession numbers: *human ZP1*, XM_172861; *human ZP2*, M90366; *human ZP3*, NM_007155; *human ZP4*, NM_021186; *macaque ZP1*, Y10381; *macaque ZP2*, Y10690; *macaque ZP3*, X82639; *macaque ZP4*, AY222647; *pig ZP2*, D45064; *pig ZP3*, NM_213893; *pig ZP4*, NM_214045; *cow ZP2*, NM_173973; *cow ZP3* NM_173974; *cow ZP4*, NM_173975; *rabbit ZP2*, L12167; *rabbit ZP3*, U05782; *rabbit ZP4*, M58160; *mouse ZP1*, NM_009580; *mouse ZP2*, NM_011775; *mouse ZP3*, NM_011776; *rat ZP1*, NM_053509; *rat ZP2*, NM_031150; *rat ZP3*, NM_053762; *rat ZP4*, NM_172330; *hamster ZP3*, M63629; *chicken ZP1*, NM_204683; *chicken ZP2*, AY268034; *chicken ZP3*, NM_204389; *chicken ZP4*, NM_204879 (73).

human sperm *(75)*. It is possible that this failure to bind is to the result of a requirement for species-specific glycosylation *(76)*. Alternatively, this result may reflect human sperm having evolved to bind to a ZP consisting of four ZP proteins rather than three. Further to this is the possibility that ZP4 is required for direct interaction as part of the sperm receptor on the ZP. Recombinant forms of human ZP3 and ZP4 have both been shown to induce human sperm to undergo the acrosome reaction, seemingly by independent pathways *(77,78)*. There is also data from a number of other species of mammal (macaque, cow, and rabbit) that supports the hypothesis that ZP4 has sperm binding activity *(79–81)*. In the pig, for example, the primary sperm receptor is a heterocomplex of ZP3 and ZP4 *(82)*.

Interestingly, four zona proteins are expressed in the rat ZP *(83)*. The rat may therefore represent a better animal model for human fertilization than the mouse. Whatever the model, it is clear that we need to understand how the four protein model relates to sperm interaction as a prerequisite to understanding sperm zona interaction in the human. Without acquiring this knowledge we are unlikely to make any real progress in studying sperm function/dysfunction.

9. METHODS TO DETERMINE THE PATHOLOGY OF SPERM DYSFUNCTION

9.1. Mouse Models for Male Infertility: The Role of KO Mice

With the increasing number of KO mice being generated with a male infertility phenotype (Fig. 2; refs. *84–86*) and the relative ease of screening men, we should expect that the causes of sperm dysfunction would be well known. However, although KO animals are very useful, there are specific difficulties translating findings in mice to men: (1) there is significant redundancy in the reproductive process, (2) the pathology, although similar, is not the same and very detailed studies are needed on both the mouse and man to determine the real differences, and (3) fertilization in humans has a number of very specific differences from that in mice *(22)*. Consequently, successful examples of identifying gene defects in subfertile men by screening for genes knocked out in mice are rare *(87)*. The usual case is that no mutations are found and much effort has been wasted (e.g., examination of men with globozoospermia for mutations in casein kinase IIα [encoded by *Csnk2a2* gene]; ref. *88*).

Thus alternative/complementary strategies to determine the defects in men with sperm dysfunction are required. Simplistically, differences between normal and dysfunctional cells can be examined using transcript or proteomic profiling. Whether sperm have functional messenger RNA is open to debate and thus a transcriptome approach may be limited *(89)*. However, spermatozoa, because they are transcriptionally inactive, are ideal cells for proteomics to examine normal cell function and changes associated with defined correlates of fertilization success *(90)*.

9.2. Proteomics for Understanding the Sperm Cell and Diagnosis of Sperm Dysfunction

Comprehensive and systematic identification and quantification of proteins expressed in cells and tissues are providing important and fascinating insights into the dynamics of cell function. For example, there has been a wealth of detailed proteomic studies to identify molecular signatures of disease states (e.g., phospho-protein networks in cancer cells; ref. *91*).

Although spermatozoa are ideal to study from a proteomic perspective, there have been relatively few studies examining the proteome of human spermatozoa *(90)*. Initial studies have used antisperm antibody sera in an attempt to detect potential sperm targets for male contraception. This is a logical approach because antisperm antibodies are associated with sterility, albeit in a very limited number of cases. Unfortunately, however, this rational approach has met with limited

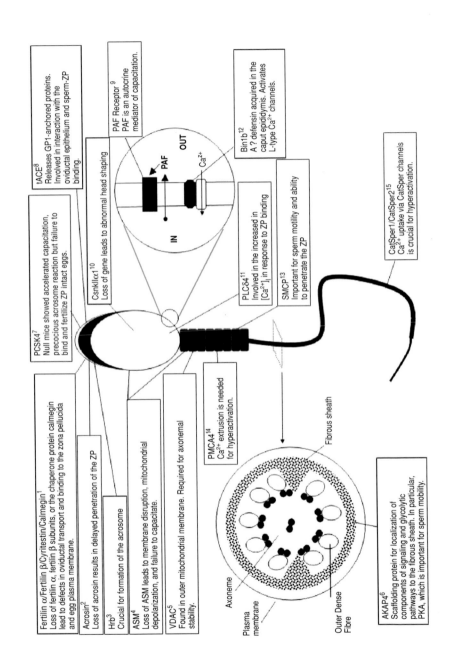

Fertilin α/Fertilin β/Cyritestin/Calmegin[1]
Loss of fertilin α, fertilin β subunits, or the chaperone protein calmegin lead to defects in oviductal transport and binding to the zona pellucida and egg plasma membrane.

Acrosin[2]
Loss of acrosin results in delayed penetration of the ZP

Hrb[3]
Crucial for formation of the acrosome

ASM[4]
Loss of ASM leads to membrane disruption, mitochondrial depolarization, and failure to capacitate.

VDAC[5]
Found in outer mitochondrial membrane. Required for axonemal stability.

AKAP4[6]
Scaffolding protein for localization of components of signaling and glycolytic pathways to the fibrous sheath. In particular, PKA, which is important for sperm mobility.

PCSK4[7]
Null mice showed accelerated capacitation, precocious acrosome reaction but failure to bind and fertilize ZP intact eggs.

tACE[8]
Releases GP1-anchored proteins. Involved in interaction with the oviductal epithelium and sperm-ZP binding.

PAF Receptor[9]
PAF is an autocrine mediator of capacitation.

Csnkll\alpha1[10]
Loss of gene leads to abnormal head shaping

Bin1b[12]
A ? defensin acquired in the caput epididymis. Activates L-type Ca^{2+} channels.

PLCδ4[11]
Involved in the increased in $[Ca^{2+}]_i$ in response to ZP binding

SMCP[13]
Important for sperm motility and ability to penetrate the ZP

PMCA4[14]
Ca^{2+} extrusion is needed for hyperactivation.

CatSper1/CatSper2[15]
Ca^{2+} uptake via CatSper channels is crucial for hyperactivation.

IN

OUT

PAF

Ca^{2+}

Fibrous sheath

Axoneme

Plasma membrane

Outer Dense Fibre

success *(92–94)* with very few robust candidate proteins being identified *(95)*.

Other than those previously mentioned, there have been very few studies that have employed proteomic approaches to examine male infertility. A small number of studies have attempted initial characterization of the sperm plasma membrane *(96)*. Further studies have examined specific processes, for example calcium-binding proteins and proteins that are tyrosine phosphorylated *(97,98)*. Interestingly, it has been more than 10 yr since the discovery of tyrosine phosphorylation as a putative marker of capacitation, yet the role of the proteins and their sequence of activation is very sketchy and, with the exception of the A kinase anchor proteins (AKAPs) (AKAP3 and AKAP4), only a small number of candidate proteins have been identified *(99)*. We are still a long way from obtaining even a minimal "picture" of events.

The slow progress/application of the proteomic revolution in human spermatozoa contrasts markedly with other fields. A relevant example is the large-scale proteomic studies on human cilia *(100)*. Estimates from *Chlamydomonas* suggest there are at least 250 flagellar proteins. In close agreement, Ostrowski and colleagues were able to identify 200 ciliary axonemal proteins, some of which were sperm/testis-specific (e.g., Sp17). However a combination of proteomic approaches is often required. For example, Ostrowski and colleagues *(100)* only identified 38 potential proteins using two-dimensional polyacrylamide gel electrophoresis. A number of proteins were not resolved (e.g., dynein heavy chains, which have a large molecular mass) and complementary approaches were needed to provide a detailed picture. One-dimensional gels identified another 110 proteins. A second approach involved isolated axonemes, followed by digestion and analysis directly by liquid chromatography/mass spectrometry (MS)/MS or multidimensional liquid chromatography/MS/MS. This led to the identification of a further 66 proteins.

In our laboratory, we have been using proteomic strategies to identify defects in sperm function responsible for fertilization *(101,102)*. Specifically we are interested in identifying differences in sperm protein expression between control (fertile) men and patients with spermatozoa that failed to fertilize oocytes in vitro. Our initial studies have focused

---

Fig. 2. *(Opposite page)* A diagrammatic representation of a spermatozoon illustrating the site of expression and effect of gene knockout experiments in the mouse. Particular emphasis is placed on the process of sperm capacitation, transport in the female tract and interaction with the zona pellucida. [1]*104–109*, [2]*110*, [3]*111*, [4]*112*, [5]*113*, [6]*114*, [7]*115*, [8]*116,117*, [9]*118*, [10]*119*, [11]*120*, [12]*121*, [13]*122*, [14]*39,40*, [15]*123–125*. (Adapted from refs. *126* and *127*.)

on a two-dimensional gel-based approach and developing a series of fertile controls (with several ejaculates) to determine if any differences observed in the patient samples are real. Initial results are interesting. To our surprise, there was relatively little intra- and interdonor variation (1.4 and 1.8% of the total number of spots identified, respectively; ref. *102*). However, differences between gels occur and when accounting for this, we have categorized one man *(102)* in which we have identified 20 differences from the control that we are confident represent true differences.

10. CONCLUSION

There is an urgent need to develop a more detailed understanding of the physiological, biochemical, and molecular functioning of the human sperm cell. We can use this knowledge as a platform to improve the diagnosis of male infertility and importantly to develop potential non-ART-based therapies. The tools at our disposal have never been more sophisticated and it is likely that rapid progress will be made in this area within the next 5 yr. Perhaps then we will see a decrease in the use of inappropriate ART treatment.

ACKNOWLEDGMENTS

This work was supported by funding from MRC, BBSRC, The Wellcome Trust, Lord Dowding Fund for Humane Research, Genosis (Ltd), and Fonds de recherche en santé du Québec.

The authors wish to thank all past members of the group who have contributed to our research. We would also like to acknowledge the staff in the Assisted Conception Unit for assistance with semen samples and providing human eggs. The authors would particularly like to thank all patients and donors who took part in our research and who continue to do so.

DISCLAIMER

Part of this chapter contains previous arguments and adaptations from manuscripts produced by our group in the last year *(24,62,73,103)*.

REFERENCES

1. Hull MG, Glazener CM, Kelly NJ, et al. Population study of causes, treatment, and outcome of infertility. Br Med J (Clin Res Ed) 1985;291:1693–1697.
2. Templeton A, Fraser C, Thompson B. The epidemiology of infertility in Aberdeen. BMJ 1990;301:148–152.
3. Human Fertilisation and Embryology Authority (HFEA) website. Available at: www.hfea.gov.uk. Accessed: 12/01/05.

4. Andersen AG, Jensen TK, Carlsen E, et al. High frequency of sub-optimal semen quality in an unselected population of young men. Hum Reprod 2000;15: 366–372.

5. Wild S, Roglic G, Green A, Sicree R, King H. Global prevalence of diabetes: estimates for the year 2000 and projections for 2030. Diabetes Care 2004;27: 1047–1053.

6. Sharpe RM, Irvine DS. How strong is the evidence of a link between environmental chemicals and adverse effects on human reproductive health? BMJ 2004;328: 447–451.

7. Bjorndahl L, Barratt CL. Semen analysis: setting standards for the measurement of sperm numbers. J Androl 2005;26:11.

8. Tomlinson MJ, Kessopoulou E, Barratt CL. The diagnostic and prognostic value of traditional semen parameters. J Androl 1999;20:588–593.

9. Larsen L, Scheike T, Jensen TK, et al. Computer-assisted semen analysis parameters as predictors for fertility of men from the general population. The Danish First Pregnancy Planner Study Team. Hum Reprod 2000;15:1562–1567.

10. Comhaire F. Clinical andrology: from evidence-base to ethics. The 'E' quintet in clinical andrology. Hum Reprod 2000;15:2067–2071.

11. Muller CH. Rationale, interpretation, validation, and uses of sperm function tests. J Androl 2000;21:10–30.

12. Ivic A, Onyeaka H, Girling A, et al. Critical evaluation of methylcellulose as an alternative medium in sperm migration tests. Hum Reprod 2002;17:143–149.

13. Aitken RJ, Baker MA, O'Bryan M. Shedding light on chemiluminescence: the application of chemiluminescence in diagnostic andrology. J Androl 2004;25: 455–465.

14. Seli E, Sakkas D. Spermatozoal nuclear determinants of reproductive outcome: implications for ART. Hum Reprod Update 2005;11:337–349.

15. Bungum M, Humaidan P, Spano M, Jepson K, Bungum L, Giwercman A. The predictive value of sperm chromatin structure assay (SCSA) parameters for the outcome of intrauterine insemination, IVF and ICSI. Hum Reprod 2004;19: 1401–1408.

16. Gandini L, Lombardo F, Paoli D, et al. Full-term pregnancies achieved with ICSI despite high levels of sperm chromatin damage. Hum Reprod 2004;19: 1409–1417.

17. Kamischke A, Nieschlag E. Diagnosis and Treatment of Male Infertility. Cambridge University Press, Cambridge; 2002.

18. Greco E, Romano S, Iacobelli M, et al. ICSI in cases of sperm DNA damage: beneficial effect of oral antioxidant treatment. Hum Reprod 2005;20:2590–2594.

19. Maher ER, Afnan M, Barratt CL. Epigenetic risks related to assisted reproductive technologies: epigenetics, imprinting, ART and icebergs? Hum Reprod 2003;18: 2508–2511.

20. Hansen M, Bower C, Milne E, de Klerk N, Kurinczuk JJ. Assisted reproductive technologies and the risk of birth defects—a systematic review. Hum Reprod 2005;20:328–338.

21. Centers for Disease Control and Prevention (CDC) website. Available at: www.cdc.gov. Accessed: 12/01/05.

22. Barratt CL, Publicover SJ. Interaction between sperm and zona pellucida in male fertility. Lancet 2001;358:1660–1662.

23. Krausz C, Bonaccorsi L, Maggio P, et al. Two functional assays of sperm responsiveness to progesterone and their predictive values in in-vitro fertilization. Hum Reprod 1996;11:1661–1667.

24. Jimenez-Gonzalez C, Michaelangeli F, Harper CV, Barratt CLR, Publicover S. Calcium signalling in human spermatozoa: a specialized "toolkit" of channels, transporters and stores. Hum Reprod Update 2006;12:253–267.

25. Berridge MJ. Unlocking the secrets of cell signaling. Annu Rev Physiol 2005;67:1–21.

26. Berridge MJ, Lipp P, Bootman MD. The versatility and universality of calcium signalling. Nat Rev Mol Cell Biol 2000;1:11–21.

27. Harper CV, Publicover SJ. Reassessing the role of progesterone in fertilization—compartmentalized calcium signalling in human spermatozoa? Hum Reprod 2005;20:2675–2680.

28. Blackmore PF. Thapsigargin elevates and potentiates the ability of progesterone to increase intracellular free calcium in human sperm: possible role of perinuclear calcium. Cell Calcium 1993;14:53–60.

29. O'Toole CM, Arnoult C, Darszon A, Steinhardt RA, Florman HM. Ca(2+) entry through store-operated channels in mouse sperm is initiated by egg ZP3 and drives the acrosome reaction. Mol Biol Cell 2000;11:1571–1584.

30. Evans JP, Florman HM. The state of the union: the cell biology of fertilization. Nat Cell Biol 2002;4:s57–s63.

31. Ho HC, Suarez SS. An inositol 1,4,5-trisphosphate receptor-gated intracellular Ca(2+) store is involved in regulating sperm hyperactivated motility. Biol Reprod 2001;65:1606–1615.

32. Harper CV, Barratt CL, Publicover SJ. Stimulation of human spermatozoa with progesterone gradients to simulate approach to the oocyte. Induction of [Ca(2+)](i) oscillations and cyclical transitions in flagellar beating. J Biol Chem 2004;279:46,315–43,325.

33. Darszon A, Nishigaki T, Wood C, Trevino CL, Felix R, Beltran C. Calcium channels and Ca2+ fluctuations in sperm physiology. Int Rev Cytol 2005;243:79–172.

34. Michelangeli F, Ogunbayo OA, Wootton LL. A plethora of interacting organellar Ca2+ stores. Curr Opin Cell Biol 2005;17:135–140.

35. Toyoshima C, Inesi G. Structural basis of ion pumping by Ca2+-ATPase of the sarcoplasmic reticulum. Annu Rev Biochem 2004;73:269–292.

36. Berrios J, Osses N, Opazo C, et al. Intracellular Ca2+ homeostasis in rat round spermatids. Biol Cell. 1998;90:391–398.

37. Wennemuth G, Babcock DF, Hille B. Calcium clearance mechanisms of mouse sperm. J Gen Physiol 2003;122:115–128.

38. Gunaratne HJ, Neill AT, Vacquier VD. Plasma membrane calcium ATPase is concentrated in the head of sea urchin spermatozoa. J Cell Physiol 2006;207:413–419.

39. Okunade GW, Miller ML, Pyne GJ, et al. Targeted ablation of plasma membrane Ca2+-ATPase (PMCA) 1 and 4 indicates a major housekeeping function for PMCA1 and a critical role in hyperactivated sperm motility and male fertility for PMCA4. J Biol Chem 2004;279:33,742–33,750.

40. Schuh K, Cartwright EJ, Jankevics E, et al. Plasma membrane Ca2+ ATPase 4 is required for sperm motility and male fertility. J Biol Chem 2004;279:28,220–28,226.

41. Prasad V, Okunade GW, Miller ML, Shull GE. Phenotypes of SERCA and PMCA knockout mice. Biochem Biophys Res Commun 2004;322:1192–1203.

42. Harper C, Wootton L, Michelangeli F, Lefievre L, Barratt C, Publicover S. Secretory pathway Ca(2+)-ATPase (SPCA1) Ca(2)+ pumps, not SERCAs, regulate complex [Ca(2+)](i) signals in human spermatozoa. J Cell Sci 2005;118:1673–1685.

43. Wictome M, Henderson I, Lee AG, East JM. Mechanism of inhibition of the calcium pump of sarcoplasmic reticulum by thapsigargin. Biochem J 1992;283: 525–529.
44. Brown GR, Benyon SL, Kirk CJ, et al. Characterisation of a novel Ca2+ pump inhibitor (bis-phenol) and its effects on intracellular Ca2+ mobilization. Biochim Biophys Acta 1994;1195:252–258.
45. Wuytack F, Raeymaekers L, Missiaen L. PMR1/SPCA Ca2+ pumps and the role of the Golgi apparatus as a Ca2+ store. Pflugers Arch 2003;446:148–153.
46. Wootton LL, Argent CC, Wheatley M, Michelangeli F. The expression, activity and localisation of the secretory pathway Ca2+ -ATPase (SPCA1) in different mammalian tissues. Biochim Biophys Acta 2004;1664:189–197.
47. Ho HC, Suarez SS. Characterization of the intracellular calcium store at the base of the sperm flagellum that regulates hyperactivated motility. Biol Reprod 2003;68:1590–1596.
48. Kirkman-Brown JC, Barratt CL, Publicover SJ. Nifedipine reveals the existence of two discrete components of the progesterone-induced [Ca2+]i transient in human spermatozoa. Dev Biol 2003;259:71–82.
49. Blackmore PF. Extragenomic actions of progesterone in human sperm and progesterone metabolites in human platelets. Steroids 1999;64:149–156.
50. Blackmore PF, Eisoldt S. The neoglycoprotein mannose-bovine serum albumin, but not progesterone, activates T-type calcium channels in human spermatozoa. Mol Hum Reprod 1999;5:498–506.
51. Blackmore PF, Beebe SJ, Danforth DR, Alexander N. Progesterone and 17 alpha-hydroxyprogesterone. Novel stimulators of calcium influx in human sperm. J Biol Chem 1990;265:1376–1380.
52. Garcia MA, Meizel S. Progesterone-mediated calcium influx and acrosome reaction of human spermatozoa: pharmacological investigation of T-type calcium channels. Biol Reprod 1999;60:102–109.
53. Bonaccorsi L, Forti G, Baldi E. Low-voltage-activated calcium channels are not involved in capacitation and biological response to progesterone in human sperm. Int J Androl 2001;24:341–351.
54. Fraire-Zamora JJ, Gonzalez-Martinez MT. Effect of intracellular pH on depolarization-evoked calcium influx in human sperm. Am J Physiol Cell Physiol 2004;287:C1688–C1696.
55. Fukami K, Yoshida M, Inoue T, et al. Phospholipase Cdelta4 is required for Ca2+ mobilization essential for acrosome reaction in sperm. J Cell Biol 2003;161:79–88.
56. Baldi E, Casano R, Falsetti C, Krausz C, Maggi M, Forti G. Intracellular calcium accumulation and responsiveness to progesterone in capacitating human spermatozoa. J Androl 1991;12:323–330.
57. Kirkman-Brown JC, Barratt CL, Publicover SJ. Slow calcium oscillations in human spermatozoa. Biochem J 2004;378:827–832.
58. De Blas G, Michaut M, Trevino CL, et al. The intraacrosomal calcium pool plays a direct role in acrosomal exocytosis. J Biol Chem 2002;277:49,326–49,331.
59. Herrick SB, Schweissinger DL, Kim SW, Bayan KR, Mann S, Cardullo RA. The acrosomal vesicle of mouse sperm is a calcium store. J Cell Physiol 2005;202: 663–671.
60. De Jonge C. Biological basis for human capacitation. Hum Reprod Update 2005;11:205–214.
61. Suarez SS, Pacey AA. Sperm transport in the female reproductive tract. Hum Reprod Update 2006;12:23–37.

62. Barratt CL, Kirkman-Brown J. Man-made versus female-made environment—will the real capacitation please stand up? Hum Reprod Update 2006;12:1–2.

63. Williams M, Hill CJ, Scudamore I, Dunphy B, Cooke ID, Barratt CL. Sperm numbers and distribution within the human fallopian tube around ovulation. Hum Reprod 1993;8:2019–2026.

64. Pacey AA, Davies N, Warren MA, Barratt CL, Cooke ID. Hyperactivation may assist human spermatozoa to detach from intimate association with the endosalpinx. Hum Reprod 1995;10:2603–2609.

65. Moseley FL, Jha KN, Bjorndahl L, et al. Protein tyrosine phosphorylation, hyperactivation and progesterone-induced acrosome reaction are enhanced in IVF media: an effect that is not associated with an increase in protein kinase A activation. Mol Hum Reprod 2005;11:523–529.

66. Liu de Y, Garrett C, Baker HW. Clinical application of sperm-oocyte interaction tests in in vitro fertilization—embryo transfer and intracytoplasmic sperm injection programs. Fertil Steril 2004;82:1251–1263.

67. Wassarman PM. Zona pellucida glycoproteins. Annu Rev Biochem 1988;57:415–442.

68. Bleil JD, Greve JM, Wassarman PM. Identification of a secondary sperm receptor in the mouse egg zona pellucida: role in maintenance of binding of acrosome-reacted sperm to eggs. Dev Biol 1988;128:376–385.

69. Mortillo S, Wassarman PM. Differential binding of gold-labeled zona pellucida glycoproteins mZP2 and mZP3 to mouse sperm membrane compartments. Development 1991;113:141–149.

70. Tsubamoto H, Hasegawa A, Nakata Y, Naito S, Yamasaki N, Koyama K. Expression of recombinant human zona pellucida protein 2 and its binding capacity to spermatozoa. Biol Reprod 1999;61:1649–1654.

71. Bleil JD, Wassarman PM. Sperm–egg interactions in the mouse: sequence of events and induction of the acrosome reaction by a zona pellucida glycoprotein. Dev Biol 1983;95:317–324.

72. Lefievre L, Conner SJ, Salpekar A, et al. Four zona pellucida glycoproteins are expressed in the human. Hum Reprod 2004;19:1580–1586.

73. Conner SJ, Lefievre L, Hughes DC, Barratt CL. Cracking the egg: increased complexity in the zona pellucida. Hum Reprod 2005;20:1148–1152.

74. Boja ES, Hoodbhoy T, Fales HM, Dean J. Structural characterization of native mouse zona pellucida proteins using mass spectrometry. J Biol Chem 2003;278:34,189–34,202.

75. Rankin TL, Coleman JS, Epifano O, et al. Fertility and taxon-specific sperm binding persist after replacement of mouse sperm receptors with human homologs. Dev Cell 2003;5:33–43.

76. Dell A, Chalabi S, Easton RL, et al. Murine and human zona pellucida 3 derived from mouse eggs express identical O-glycans. Proc Natl Acad Sci USA 2003;100:15,631–15,636.

77. Chakravarty S, Suraj K, Gupta SK. Baculovirus-expressed recombinant human zona pellucida glycoprotein-B induces acrosomal exocytosis in capacitated spermatozoa in addition to zona pellucida glycoprotein-C. Mol Hum Reprod 2005;11:365–372.

78. Caballero-Campo P, Chirinos M, Fan XJ, et al. Biological effects of recombinant human zona pellucida proteins on sperm function. Biol Reprod 2006;74:760–768.

79. Prasad SV, Wilkins B, Skinner SM, Dunbar BS. Evaluating zona pellucida structure and function using antibodies to rabbit 55 kDa ZP protein expressed in baculovirus expression system. Mol Reprod Dev 1996;43:519–529.

80. Topper EK, Kruijt L, Calvete J, Mann K, Topfer-Petersen E, Woelders H. Identification of bovine zona pellucida glycoproteins. Mol Reprod Dev 1997;46: 344–350.

81. Govind CK, Hasegawa A, Koyama K, Gupta SK. Delineation of a conserved B cell epitope on bonnet monkey (Macaca radiata) and human zona pellucida glycoprotein-B by monoclonal antibodies demonstrating inhibition of sperm–egg binding. Biol Reprod 2001;62:67–75.

82. Yurewicz EC, Sacco AG, Gupta SK, Xu N, Gage DA. Hetero-oligomerization-dependent binding of pig oocyte zona pellucida glycoproteins ZPB and ZPC to boar sperm membrane vesicles. J Biol Chem 1998;273:7488–7494.

83. Hoodbhoy T, Joshi S, Boja ES, Williams SA, Stanley P, Dean J. Human sperm do not bind to rat zonae pellucidae despite the presence of four homologous glyco-proteins. J Biol Chem 2005;280:12,721–12,731.

84. Matzuk MM, Lamb DJ. Genetic dissection of mammalian fertility pathways. Nat Cell Biol 2002;4:s41–s49.

85. GermOnline website. Available at: www.germonline.org. Accessed: 12/01/05.

86. Wiederkehr C, Basavaraj R, Sarrauste de Menthiere C, et al. Database model and specification of GermOnline Release 2.0, a cross-species community annotation knowledgebase on germ cell differentiation. Bioinformatics 2004;20: 808–811.

87. Miyamoto T, Hasuike S, Yogev L, et al. Azoospermia in patients heterozygous for a mutation in SYCP3. Lancet 2003;362:1714–1719.

88. Pirrello O, Machev N, Schimdt F, Terriou P, Menezo Y, Viville S. Search for mutations involved in human globozoospermia. Hum Reprod 2005;20: 1314–1318.

89. Ostermeier GC, Dix DJ, Miller D, Khatri P, Krawetz SA. Spermatozoal RNA profiles of normal fertile men. Lancet 2002;360:772–777.

90. Ainsworth C. Cell biology: the secret life of sperm. Nature 2005;436:770–771.

91. Irish JM, Hovland R, Krutzik PO, et al. Single cell profiling of potentiated phos-pho-protein networks in cancer cells. Cell 2004;118:217–228.

92. Naaby-Hansen S, Flickinger CJ, Herr JC. Two-dimensional gel electrophoretic analysis of vectorially labeled surface proteins of human spermatozoa. Biol Reprod 1997;56:771–787.

93. Shetty J, Naaby-Hansen S, Shibahara H, Bronson R, Flickinger CJ, Herr JC. Human sperm proteome: immunodominant sperm surface antigens identified with sera from infertile men and women. Biol Reprod 1999;61:61–69.

94. Shibahara H, Sato I, Shetty J, et al. Two-dimensional electrophoretic analysis of sperm antigens recognized by sperm immobilizing antibodies detected in infer-tile women. J Reprod Immunol 2002;53:1–12.

95. Bohring C, Krause W. Immune infertility: towards a better understanding of sperm (auto)-immunity. The value of proteomic analysis. Hum Reprod 2003;18:915–924.

96. Shetty J, Diekman AB, Jayes FC, et al. Differential extraction and enrichment of human sperm surface proteins in a proteome: identification of immunocontracep-tive candidates. Electrophoresis 2001;22:3053–3066.

97. Naaby-Hansen S, Mandal A, Wolkowicz MJ, et al. CABYR, a novel calcium-binding tyrosine phosphorylation-regulated fibrous sheath protein involved in capacitation. Dev Biol 2002;242:236–254.

98. Ficarro S, Chertihin O, Westbrook VA, et al. Phosphoproteome analysis of capac-itated human sperm. Evidence of tyrosine phosphorylation of a kinase-anchoring protein 3 and valosin-containing protein/p97 during capacitation. J Biol Chem 2003;278:11,579–11,589.

99. Naz RK, Rajesh PB. Role of tyrosine phosphorylation in sperm capacitation/ acrosome reaction. Reprod Biol Endocrinol 2004;2:75.
100. Ostrowski LE, Blackburn K, Radde KM, et al. A proteomic analysis of human cilia: identification of novel components. Mol Cell Proteomics 2002;1:451–465.
101. Lefievre L, Barratt CL, Harper CV, et al. Physiological and proteomic approaches to studying prefertilization events in the human. Reprod Biomed Online 2003;7:419–427.
102. Pixton KL, Deeks ED, Flesch FM, et al. Sperm proteome mapping of a patient who experienced failed fertilization at IVF reveals altered expression of at least 20 proteins compared with fertile donors: case report. Hum Reprod 2004;19: 1438–1447.
103. Publicover SJ, Barratt CL. Voltage-operated Ca2+ channels and the acrosome reaction: which channels are present and what do they do? Hum Reprod 1999;14: 873–879.
104. Ikawa M, Wada I, Kominami K, et al. The putative chaperone calmegin is required for sperm fertility. Nature 1997;387:607–611.
105. Cho C, Bunch DO, Faure JE, et al. Fertilization defects in sperm from mice lacking fertilin beta. Science 1998;281:1857–1859.
106. Cho C, Ge H, Branciforte D, Primakoff P, Myles DG. Analysis of mouse fertilin in wild-type and fertilin beta(–/–) sperm: evidence for C-terminal modification, alpha/beta dimerization, and lack of essential role of fertilin alpha in sperm–egg fusion. Dev Biol 2000;222:289–295.
107. Nishimura H, Cho C, Branciforte DR, Myles DG, Primakoff P. Analysis of loss of adhesive function in sperm lacking cyritestin or fertilin beta. Dev Biol 2001;233: 204–213.
108. Shamsadin R, Adham IM, Nayernia K, Heinlein UA, Oberwinkler H, Engel W. Male mice deficient for germ-cell cyritestin are infertile. Biol Reprod 1999;61: 1445–1451.
109. Kim E, Yamashita M, Nakanishi T, et al. Mouse sperm lacking ADAM1b/ADAM2 fertilin can fuse with the egg plasma membrane and effect fertilization. J Biol Chem 2006;281:5634–5639.
110. Baba T, Azuma S, Kashiwabara S, Toyoda Y. Sperm from mice carrying a targeted mutation of the acrosin gene can penetrate the oocyte zona pellucida and effect fertilization. J Biol Chem 1994;269:31,845–31,849.
111. Kang-Decker N, Mantchev GT, Juneja SC, McNiven MA, van Deursen JM. Lack of acrosome formation in Hrb-deficient mice. Science 2001;294:1531–1533.
112. Butler A, He X, Gordon RE, Wu HS, Gatt S, Schuchman EH. Reproductive pathology and sperm physiology in acid sphingomyelinase-deficient mice. Am J Pathol 2002;161:1061–1075.
113. Sampson MJ, Decker WK, Beaudet AL, et al. Immotile sperm and infertility in mice lacking mitochondrial voltage-dependent anion channel type 3. J Biol Chem 2001;276:39,206–39,212.
114. Miki K, Willis WD, Brown PR, Goulding EH, Fulcher KD, Eddy EM. Targeted disruption of the Akap4 gene causes defects in sperm flagellum and motility. Dev Biol 2002;248:331–342.
115. Gyamera-Acheampong C, Tantibhedhyangkul J, Weerachatyanukul W, et al. Sperm from mice genetically deficient for the PCSK4 proteinase exhibit accelerated capacitation, precocious acrosome reaction, reduced binding to egg zona pellucida, and impaired fertilizing ability. Biol Reprod 2005;4:666–673.
116. Hagaman JR, Moyer JS, Bachman ES, et al. Angiotensin-converting enzyme and male fertility. Proc Natl Acad Sci USA. 1998;95:2552–2557.

117. Kondoh G, Tojo H, Nakatani Y, et al. Angiotensin-converting enzyme is a GPI-anchored protein releasing factor crucial for fertilization. Nat Med 2005;11: 160–166.

118. Koizumi H, Yamaguchi N, Hattori M, et al. Targeted disruption of intracellular type I platelet activating factor-acetylhydrolase catalytic subunits causes severe impairment in spermatogenesis. J Biol Chem 2003;278:12,489–12,494.

119. Escalier D, Silvius D, Xu X. Spermatogenesis of mice lacking CK2alpha': failure of germ cell survival and characteristic modifications of the spermatid nucleus. Mol Reprod Dev 2003;66:190–201.

120. Fukami K, Nakao K, Inoue T, et al. Requirement of phospholipase Cdelta4 for the zona pellucida-induced acrosome reaction. Science 2001;292:920–923.

121. Zhou Q, Shima JE, Nie R, Friel PJ, Griswold MD. Androgen-regulated transcripts in the neonatal mouse testis as determined through microarray analysis. Biol Reprod 2005;72:1010–1019.

122. Nayernia K, Drabent B, Adham IM, et al. Male mice lacking three germ cell expressed genes are fertile. Biol Reprod 2003;69:1973–1978.

123. Carlson AE, Westenbroek RE, Quill T, et al. CatSper1 required for evoked Ca2+ entry and control of flagellar function in sperm. Proc Natl Acad Sci USA 2003;100:14,864–14,868.

124. Quill TA, Ren D, Clapham DE, Garbers DL. A voltage-gated ion channel expressed specifically in spermatozoa. Proc Natl Acad Sci USA 2001;98: 12,527–12,531.

125. Ren D, Navarro B, Perez G, et al. A sperm ion channel required for sperm motility and male fertility. Nature 2001;413:603–609.

126. Conner SJ, Barratt CLR. Genomic and proteomic approaches to defining sperm production and function-in The Sperm Cell-Production. Maturation, Fertilization, Regeneration. (Ed. De Jonge C and Barratt C) Cambridge University Press (Cambridge, UK) 2006 pp. 49–71.

127. Conner SJ, Lefièvre L, Kirkman-Brown J, et al. Understanding the physiology of pre-fertilization events in the human spermatozoa–a necessary prerequisite to developing rational therapy. Reproduction 2006, in press.

6 Genetics of Idiopathic Male Infertility

The Power of a Cross-Species Approach

Angshumoy Roy, MBBS, Yi-Nan Lin, MSC, and Martin M. Matzuk, MD, PhD

Summary

Nearly 7% of men suffer from male factor infertility. In one-fourth of infertile males, the etiology remains unexplained. Unlike other multifactorial disorders, gene–gene and gene–environment interactions in the regulation of male fertility have been poorly characterized. A candidate-gene approach that incorporates biological information from model organisms is likely to be critical in deciphering the genetic basis of idiopathic male fertility. Genes that fulfill essential roles in spermatogenesis often have orthologs in several species wherein they serve similar functions. By using a comparative cross-species approach, major susceptibility genes underlying male infertility can be identified in association studies. With a better understanding of the molecular regulation of spermatogenesis, proper diagnosis and treatment of male infertility should be realized in the foreseeable future.

Key Words: Infertility; idiopathic; candidate gene; spermatogenesis; *in silico*.

1. INTRODUCTION

Infertility is a major global health problem with wide-ranging socio-economic ramifications for the affected couple and the society at large. Clinically defined as an inability to conceive after 1 yr of unprotected intercourse, the worldwide estimates for the prevalence of infertility range from 10 to 15% *(1,2)*; significantly, in a 1982–1985 multicenter study conducted by the World Health Organization, the male partner was observed to have an abnormal semen analysis in approx 50% of the infertile couples investigated *(1)*. Whereas endocrine defects (e.g., gonadotropin deficiency or hyperprolactinemia), systemic disorders,

From: *The Genetics of Male Infertility*
Edited by: D.T. Carrell © Humana Press Inc., Totowa, NJ

erectile dysfunction, and ejaculatory inadequacy were present in a minor fraction of infertile males, approx 22% were classified as idiopathic, with idiopathic oligozoospermia ($<20 \times 10^6$ sperm/mL of semen) being the single most common diagnosis (11.2%) for a semen abnormality *(1)*.

A routine semen analysis *(3)* constitutes the mandatory first step in the evaluation of an infertile male. An initial semen evaluation, a detailed personal and family history, and a physical examination are usually followed by a work-up for specialized tests for sperm physiology, semen quality, and endocrine abnormalities, where appropriate *(4)*. If indicated, karyotyping for aneuploidies and screening for Y-chromosome microdeletions is also considered in selected patients *(4)*. Although novel tests of semen quality *(4,5)* have been introduced over the past decade to better characterize the heterogeneous nature of infertility, the prevalence of idiopathic infertility has remained more or less static.

As our understanding of the genetic regulation of gametogenesis and fertilization develops in the postgenomics era, it becomes intuitively apparent that a significant proportion of idiopathic cases are of genetic etiology. It has long been recognized that fertility or fecundity is a function of an individual's genetic makeup and his/her interaction with the environment. Subfertility is a multifactorial trait in which environmental toxins (e.g., lead, radiation, ethylene oxide) directly disrupt genes involved in gametogenesis or interact with multiple alleles that increase susceptibility to environmental modulation *(6)*. Association studies to detect familial segregation of male subfertility *(7,8)* have shown that male siblings of infertile males more often fail to sire offspring than control populations; segregation analysis has suggested an autosomal-recessive mode of inheritance for a majority of cases *(7)*. In addition, male infertility has also been identified as part of monogenic syndromes *(9)*, wherein it is a direct consequence of absence of gene function during spermatogenesis; however, idiopathic infertility is by definition nonsyndromic and is probably unrelated to these rare disorders.

More relevant have been the identification of microdeletions on the long arm of the Y chromosome (Yq dels) in azoospermic and severely oligozoospermic males. Since Tiepolo and Zuffardi *(10)* presented evidence in 1976 suggesting an association between Yq microdeletions and spermatogenic failure, an impressive body of evidence has accumulated *(11)* indicating that these lesions are present in approx 18% of males with idiopathic azoospermia *(12)*. Further evidence for a genetic basis of infertility comes from molecular genetic analysis of the cystic fibrosis transmembrane conductance regulator (*CFTR*) gene; approx 25% of patients with obstructive azoospermia have congenital bilateral absence of the vas deferens *(13)* and occasionally the unilateral form, anatomical defects that are associated with mutations in the *CFTR* gene in approx 80% of cases *(14)*.

The most conclusive evidence for the genetic basis of male idio-pathic infertility or subfertility comes from the vast number of mouse knockouts (KOs) with defects in fertility *(2,15)*. Several mouse models have been generated with isolated azoospermia (absence of sperm), oligozoospermia, asthenozoospermia (<50% motile sperm), or a combination of these defects. In this chapter, we discuss the relevance and importance of a cross-species approach to understanding the molecular genetics of idiopathic male infertility in humans, with particular reference to the laboratory mouse, *Mus mus-culus*. We exclude from our discussion forms of male infertility that are present as part of nonendocrine syndromes (e.g., Kartagener and Kallmann syndromes), endocrine disorders (pituitary failure, hyper-prolactinemia, sex steroid deficiencies), and chromosomal defects (e.g., Yq deletions). Also excluded are congenital bilateral absence of the vas deferens and congenital unilateral absence of the vas def-erens, which cause obstructive azoospermia primarily because of mutations in the *CFTR* gene, as described previously. We instead highlight a few studies in the mouse that have provided a basis for investigating humans with idiopathic male infertility and conclude with a general discussion on the vast array of novel technical and informatics tools that allow us to manipulate model organisms with greater ease and higher specificity.

2. GENETICS OF MALE IDIOPATHIC INFERTILITY: A CANDIDATE-GENE APPROACH

Classical genetic approaches have focused on linkage and associa-tion between markers and traits in large multigenerational pedigrees to map gene loci involved in the etiology of disease. This positional cloning approach, although tedious, has served researchers well in identifying causative genes for several monogenic disorders. For com-plex disorders such as infertility, in which several common variants are believed to modestly influence disease risk, traditional linkage analyses are less powerful *(16)* and have rarely been successfully used. In addi-tion, large families that segregate the infertility trait are seldom obtained, making linkage an ineffective tool *(17)* in studying infertility. The recent completion of phase I of the International HapMap Project *(18)* and the development of low-cost high-throughput genotyping technologies may eventually lead to genome-wide association studies in the future *(16)*; however, an additional deterrent to this approach in the study of male infertility lies with the genetic heterogeneity in sam-ple populations with infertility, which requires collection of large sam-ple sizes for achieving sufficient statistical power *(17)*.

Resequencing of candidate genes to detect allele frequency differences between cases and controls therefore remains the most practical approach to identifying infertility-associated disease genes in humans *(17)*. This candidate-gene approach has been fairly successful in other complex disorders but has several limitations for infertility research: the requirement for prior knowledge of the function and expression of the candidate gene so that biological plausibility of the role of the gene in causing the phenotype can be inferred and the effect of population stratification or ethnic admixture in cases and controls. Whereas the latter can be tackled through additional marker typing *(19)*, resolution of the former is exclusively dependent on our understanding of spermatogenesis in model organisms, particularly mice.

Thus, studies that have generated approx 100 mouse models of nonsyndromic male infertility with isolated defects in either sperm production, motility, or maturation *(2)* provide us with sufficient biological information to undertake a candidate approach in humans. Although single gene mutations in mice on homogeneous genetic backgrounds are not the best representative models for human infertility, which is supposedly complex in nature with multiple gene–environment interactions on essentially heterogeneous genetic backgrounds, these studies nevertheless uncover excellent candidate genes that serve essential and nonredundant roles at different steps of spermatogenesis.

3. MUTATIONS IN INFERTILE MALE PATIENTS: LESSONS FROM SELECTED MOUSE MODELS

Several comparative studies have illustrated the utility of choosing candidate genes for association studies in humans based on a defined function of the ortholog in mice. Homozygous deficiency for the synaptonemal complex protein 3 (SYCP3) leads to meiotic arrest and sterility in male mice. Failure of synaptonemal complex formation produces massive apoptotic cell death during the meiotic prophase in spermatocytes *(20)*. Interestingly, in a study of 19 infertile male patients with nonobstructive azoospermia, Miyamoto et al. *(21)* identified 2 unrelated patients of different ethnicity (2/19) with a 1-bp heterozygous deletion (643delA) in the human *SYCP3* gene that resulted in a frameshift mutation and a premature termination codon; the mutation was absent in 75 fertile control males. The authors also demonstrated defective binding of the mutant protein to the wild-type protein in an in vitro interaction assay. Although heterozygosity for a null mutation in *Sycp3* does not cause meiotic arrest in mice, the authors concluded that the mutant protein in the patients was producing a dominant negative effect on the wild-type protein. An alternative explanation could be the presence of multiple loci that interact with this allele to produce the phenotype in these patients. Regardless, the study demonstrates the feasibility of a candidate-gene approach to analyzing male infertility in humans.

The deleted in azoospermia-like (*Dazl*) gene is essential for differentiation of male germ cells; male mice that lack functional DAZL protein undergo germ cell loss and are sterile *(22)*. In an extensive study of 102 infertile men with oligozoospermia and/or asthenozoospermia, Tung et al. *(23)* sought to study the relationship between variants in the human *DAZL* gene and idiopathic oligoasthenozoospermia. The authors identified seven variants, six single-nucleotide polymorphisms (SNPs) in the 3′ untranslated region (UTR) and one nonsynonymous-coding SNP that were associated with the defects in the infertile men across different ethnic backgrounds. Surprisingly, the nonreference alleles of these SNPs showed positive association with increased sperm counts in these patients compared with controls, leading the authors to conclude that these UTR SNPs affect the function of the *DAZL* gene in a complex manner. Notably, however, the 200 controls chosen in this study represented a sample of the general population without characterization of their semen parameters, which might have led to the confounding effect.

Similar examples of correlation between mouse KOs and male patients relate to the basic nuclear proteins that compact DNA during spermiogenesis. After meiosis, histones are first replaced with transition nuclear protein (TNP)1 and TNP2 and then protamine (PRM)1 and PRM2 in two major chromatin remodeling steps designed to condense the sperm nucleus. Haploinsufficiency for either *Prm1* and *Prm2* in mice leads to male infertility in high-percentage chimeras *(24)*; heterozygous deficiency of either protamine leads to defective nuclear condensation and male sterility. Interestingly, PRM2 deficiency had been previously described in infertile men *(25)*; more recent studies have uncovered association of SNPs in human *PRM2* and male sterility. In one study *(26)*, a single missense mutation that introduced a premature termination codon in the *PRM2* gene was identified in 1 of 226 (0.4%) sterile male patients and not in 270 proven-fertile male controls. The resultant nonsense transcript was inferred to lead to haploinsufficiency for *PRM2*. The low frequency of the mutant allele in cases is probably due to the result of the flawed design of the association study: it included male sterile patients as a single group of cases without classifying them into different subgroups based on their semen analysis. Using more detailed semen analysis, including specialized tests to detect sperm DNA fragmentation and sperm morphology analysis, another group *(27)* studied only infertile males with normal sperm counts and increased DNA fragmentation and defective sperm morphology. Significantly, they found the association of a *PRM1* SNP in 3 of 30 (10%) cases, highlighting the critical value of proper phenotypic definition of patients and controls. However, this study used an extremely small control set ($n = 10$) of ethnically unmatched fertile males and lacked statistical verification of significance.

A similar study was designed to investigate the association between the human *TNP1* and *TNP2* loci and male infertility. In mice, loss of either *Tnp1* or *Tnp2* genes was found to cause male subfertility *(28,29)*. In a group of 282 infertile patients as cases, several SNPs were identified that were similar in frequency in cases and controls. However, a single patient with azoospermia was found to have a deletion in the promoter region that constitutes the binding site for the transcription factor cyclic adenosine monophosphate responsive element modulator *(30)*; this deletion in the cyclic adenosine monophosphate responsive element-binding promoter was absent from 266 controls.

Although these studies indicate the feasibility of association studies with a candidate-gene approach, most of these studies are underpowered to detect all the relevant causative alleles because of modest sample sizes or poor characterization of cases and controls. Future studies should focus on proper phenotypic classification of patients based on detailed semen analyses and a high-throughput strategy to study multilocus association, similar to one recent study that used selected markers to study association between components of estrogen signaling pathway and male idiopathic infertility *(31)*.

4. IDENTIFICATION OF NEW CANDIDATES CONSERVED ACROSS DIFFERENT VERTEBRATE LINEAGES USING TESTIS-SPECIFIC EXPRESSED SEQUENCE TAG LIBRARY SEARCHES

Although the studies of male reproductive genes conserved between humans and mice helped us to characterize their roles in male infertility, expanding the scope of cross-species analysis to include various mammalian lineages and beyond can provide further insights into the roles of conserved components in germ cell physiology. Because the continuation of life in higher organisms depends on the success of sexual reproduction, crucial gene functions and gene interactions during gametogenesis have been conserved under selective pressures that lead to the generation of functional gametes *(32,33)*. In other words, evolution has tested the dispensability of core reproductive genes, and the results are waiting to be deciphered by cross-species comparative genomics.

The cross-species comparative genomics approach was made possible by the methodological progress in high-throughput sequencing and the constantly improving bioinformatics tools tailored for the analysis of the vast amount of data. Expressed sequence tag (EST) libraries have been extensively used as the first step of large-scale gene discovery processes by cataloging the transcriptomes with short end-sequencing data of the cloned cDNA fragments *(34–36)*. After partitioning ESTs into nonredundant sets of gene-oriented clusters, such as UniGene entries, *in silico* subtraction can be used to extract genes preferentially expressed in target tissues from tissue-specific EST libraries *(37–40)*. Among them, testis-specific EST libraries catalog the genes actively expressed during spermatogenesis, and those from nonmammalian species are especially useful for identifying highly conserved reproductive genes (Table 1). Recently, abundant fathead minnow (*Pimephales promelas*) transcripts were deposited into the EST database as an effort to allow government and industry to develop tools to improve environmental toxicity monitoring in aquatic ecosystems. In fact, the large collections in the testis-specific EST library from fathead minnow (Table 1) also provided an excellent reference to identify conserved male reproductive genes showing preferential expression in testis. Compared to the approx 92 million yr of divergence within the mammalian lineage, the divergence time between mammal-bird, mammal-frog, and mammal-fish groups are 3.5–5 times longer (~310, ~360, and ~450 million yr, respectively; ref. *41*). If the preferential expression of orthologous genes in testis is conserved beyond the mammalian lineage, it would strongly suggest that these genes are indispensable during gametogenesis and their malfunction may cause male infertility.

Combining our accessibility to databases and other Internet-based tools, we can now easily identify new candidate genes and revisit known players involved in male reproduction. Using KO mice as models to mimic the disruption of male reproductive genes and to functionally dissect the genetic components of male infertility, our current approach begins with the identification of conserved testis-specific genes *(42)*. Here, we report the identification and computational analysis of *Klhl10 (43)*, a germ cell-specific gene identified in mice through *in silico* subtraction and validated through traditional expression analysis, as a step-by-step example to explain our cross-species gene characterization approach.

Table 1
Testis-Specific EST Libraries

Chicken (*Gallus gallus;* 21,447 total UniGene entries; refs. *48,49*)
    Lib.15562 WLtestis library (4891 sequences/2473 UniGene entries)
    Lib.15563 RJtestis library (5516 sequences/2294 UniGene entries)
    Lib.16173 Korean native chicken testis cDNA library (5069
    sequences/2159 UniGene entries)
Xenopus laevis (24,738 total UniGene entries)
    Lib.12882 NICHD_XGC_Te1 (2407 sequences/1095 UniGene
    entries)
    Lib.15412 NICHD_XGC_Te2N, normalized (11,700 sequences/3897
    UniGene entries)
    Lib.15418 NICHD_XGC_Te2 (12,231 sequences/2877 UniGene
    entries)
Xenopus tropicalis (15,440 total UniGene entries)
    Lib.16859 NIH_XGC_tropTe3 (21,384 sequences/3961 UniGene
    entries)
    Lib.16860 NIH_XGC_tropTe4 (22,173 sequences/4547 UniGene
    entries)
    Lib.16861 NIH_XGC_tropTe5 (21,812 sequences/4949 UniGene
    entries)
Rainbow trout (*Oncorhynchus mykiss*; 14,340 total UniGene entries)
    Lib.12452 AGENAE Rainbow trout normalized testis library (1039
    sequences/708 UniGene entries)
    Lib.15060 AGENAE Rainbow trout normalized testis library (11,503
    sequences/5906 UniGene entries)
Zebrafish (*Danio rerio*; 24,009 total UniGene entries; ref. *50*)
    Lib.9768 Gong zebrafish testis (8964 sequences/2531 UniGene
    entries)
    Lib.15929 Adult testis full-length (TLL) (2173 sequences/1127
    UniGene entries)
    Lib.15931 Adult testis normalized (TLL) (1680 sequences/938
    UniGene entries)
    Lib.15936 Adult testis ORESTES (TLL) (2646 sequences/708
    UniGene entries)
Fathead Minnow (*Pimephales promelas*; 249,938 total sequences; not
incorporated in UniGene database yet)
    7–8 mo adult testis (60,617 sequences/~11,500 initial clusters)
Ciona intestinalis (14,370 total UniGene entries; ref. *51*)
    Lib.10379 K. Inaba unpublished testis cDNA (9380 sequences/2112
    UniGene entries)

Testis-specific EST libraries (with >1000 sequences) available from species outside mammalian lineage as of January 2006. UniGene entry numbers, the nonredundant set of gene-oriented clusters, may be used for assessment of the coverage of the testis transcriptomes. Detailed information (except fathead minnow) can be found using library browser on the species-specific webpages of UniGene database (http://www. ncbi.nlm.nih.gov/entrez/query.fcgi?db=unigene).

1. Obtain the full-length cDNA sequence. After validation of the germ cell-specific expression of mouse *Klhl10*, we examined the 3′-end of *Klhl10* transcript for poly-A signal as an indication of completeness and used 5′-rapid amplification of 5′ complementary DNA ends (RACE) to obtain the 5′-UTR and the full coding region. We deposited the identified full-length sequence into GenBank database as nucleotide entries AY495337. The full-length cDNA sequences are crucial in the correct interpretation of gene structure for further analysis.

2. Identify the human ortholog. The translated *Klhl10* amino acid sequence was first used for the translated BLAST search against nucleotide database (tBLASTn) while limiting the search to *Mus musculus* to check for closely related genes in mouse transcriptome. The results showed that the closest homolog, *Klhl20*, shared only 37% protein identity in the matched region and it should not confuse further BLAST searches. After repeating tBLASTn search with *Klhl10* amino acid sequence limited to *Homo sapiens*, the matches with human cDNAs and ESTs suggested the presence of human ortholog of *Klhl10*. After aligning mouse *Klhl10* with all available cDNAs, ESTs, and genomic sequences, human *KLHL10* sequence was confirmed and deposited as AY495339. Similarly, searching with human *KLHL10* sequence returned matches with mouse *Klhl10*. Besides fulfilling the mutually best similarity criteria, the orthologous relationship was further confirmed by the shared gene order synteny around *Klhl10* (*Nt5c3l-Klhl10-Klhl11*), which can be visualized in Genome Browser (http://genome.ucsc.edu; ref. *44*).

3. Determine domain structures. The domain structures were examined by searching Pfam database (http://www.sanger.ac.uk/Software/Pfam/; ref. *45*) or Simple Modular Architecture Research Tool database (http://smart.embl-heidelberg.de/; ref. *46*). The searches with both mouse and human KLHL10 protein sequences identified BTB, BACK, and six Kelch repeats.

4. Extend searches in other species. To find *Klhl10* in other species, we began with translated mouse *Klhl10* amino acid sequence for tBLASTn to search the EST subset excluding mouse and human entries ([est_others] selected from the "CHOOSE DATABASE" option). After ruling out low-score matches by careful examination of the listed matches, the high-score matched ESTs can be grouped by species and assembled into longer contigs. The BLAST search process can then be repeated with assembled *Klhl10* contigs from other species until all EST matches were retrieved and assembled. These assembled *Klhl10* contigs can then be used computationally in gene prediction and experimentally in RACE-PCR cloning to obtain full-length sequences in those species. Interestingly, in species that have testis-specific EST

libraries, *Klhl10* mostly matched to testis-derived ESTs, suggesting conserved preferential expression in testis.

After retrieving all the available orthologs across distant lineages, the final prize lies in the information unlocked by cross-species comparison. Not only the alignment of amino acid sequences of conserved orthologs from distantly divergent species can show us the functionally constrained domains even in the absence of known protein domains, but the conserved orthologs can also provide common grounds to integrate the information from studies of male reproduction in a wide variety of species. Starting from these conserved reproductive genes, two-hybrid screening may build up the protein–protein interaction network and microarray gene profiling of KO animals may reveal the underlying genetic network.

5. CONCLUSIONS

Advances in assisted reproductive techniques (e.g., in vitro fertilization and intracytoplasmic sperm injection) have dramatically increased the chances of a successful pregnancy in a hitherto infertile couple *(47)*. However, several studies have raised questions regarding the safety of these procedures, particularly related to the transmissibility of undetected molecular defects to the offspring born from these techniques. The combination of a lack of informative tools and a slowly emerging understanding of the molecular basis of spermatogenesis has meant that the genetic basis of male factor infertility remains obscure. Although the drive to further improve assisted reproductive techniques carries on, emphasis also needs to be placed on developing newer methodologies to understand the molecular etiopathogenesis of infertility. The gap between the laboratory bench (and the mouse) and the patient can be effectively bridged by induction of diagnostic methods (semen analysis, imaging techniques, sperm RNA profiling, and so on) that harness the power of cutting-edge molecular genetic research with the simplicity of application that can be widely implemented in the clinic. Equipped with better knowledge, proper diagnosis and treatment of male infertility should be realized in the very near future.

6. REVIEW

Infertility is a genetically heterogeneous disorder with a multifactorial etiology. Using classical genetic strategies of linkage analysis to identify genes causing infertility is limited by the small family sizes in inherited forms of the disease. A candidate-gene approach to identify genes associated with disease relies heavily on biological information regarding the expression and function of the gene in model organisms. This strategy has been successfully used to identify several human genes (*SYCP3*, *DAZL*, *PRM1*, *PRM2*, and *TNP1*) that show association with several forms of idiopathic male infertility, as illustrated in this chapter. More than 100 genes can cause isolated infertility and subfertility in mice when mutated, suggesting that several more candidate genes should be tested in humans for association with male infertility. Furthermore, comparative analysis of genes in several model organisms can identify highly conserved genes that share similar spatiotemporal expression profiles and serve analogous roles, thereby making them the best candidate genes for analysis in humans. We review this cross-species approach in this chapter with examples highlighting the strengths and shortcomings of this strategy and conclude with a discussion of novel *in silico* tools that aid the researcher in identifying conserved genes across multiple mammalian and nonmammalian species.

7. ACKNOWLEDGMENTS

These studies were supported in part by National Institutes of Health Cooperative Centers Program in Reproductive Research (U54 HD07495) and Infertility (P01HD36289).

REFERENCES

1. World Health Organization. Towards more objectivity in diagnosis and management of male infertility. Int J Androl 1987;7:1–53.
2. Matzuk MM, Lamb DJ. Genetic dissection of mammalian fertility pathways. Nat Med 2002;8:S33–S40.
3. Special Programme of Research Development and Research Training in Human Reproduction (World Health Organization [WHO]). WHO laboratory manual for the examination of human semen and sperm–cervical mucus interaction, 3rd ed. Published on behalf of the World Health Organization by Cambridge University Press, Cambridge and New York; 1992.
4. Turek PJ. Practical approaches to the diagnosis and management of male infertility. Nat Clin Pract Urol 2005;2:226–238.
5. Weber RF, Dohle GR, Romijn JC. Clinical laboratory evaluation of male subfertility. Adv Clin Chem 2005;40:317–364.
6. Shah K, Sivapalan G, Gibbons N, Tempest H, Griffin DK. The genetic basis of infertility. Reproduction 2003;126:13–25.
7. Lilford R, Jones AM, Bishop DT, Thornton J, Mueller R. Case–control study of whether subfertility in men is familial. BMJ 1994;309:570–573.
8. van Golde RJ, van der Avoort IA, Tuerlings JH, et al. Phenotypic characteristics of male subfertility and its familial occurrence. J Androl 2004;25:819–823.
9. Meschede D, Horst J. The molecular genetics of male infertility. Mol Hum Reprod 1997;3:419–430.

10. Tiepolo L, Zuffardi O. Localization of factors controlling spermatogenesis in the nonfluorescent portion of the human Y chromosome long arm. Hum Genet 1976;34:119–124.
11. Huynh T, Mollard R, Trounson A. Selected genetic factors associated with male infertility. Hum Reprod Update 2002;8:183–198.
12. Foresta C, Moro E, Ferlin A. Y chromosome microdeletions and alterations of spermatogenesis. Endocr Rev 2001;22:226–239.
13. Patrizio P, Leonard DG. Mutations of the cystic fibrosis gene and congenital absence of the vas deferens. Results Probl Cell Differ 2000;28:175–186.
14. Stuhrmann M, Dork T. CFTR gene mutations and male infertility. Andrologia 2000;32:71–83.
15. Cooke HJ, Saunders PT. Mouse models of male infertility. Nat Rev Genet 2002;3:790–801.
16. Hirschhorn JN, Daly MJ. Genome-wide association studies for common diseases and complex traits. Nat Rev Genet 2005;6:95–108.
17. Gianotten J, Lombardi MP, Zwinderman AH, Lilford RJ, van der Veen F. Idiopathic impaired spermatogenesis: genetic epidemiology is unlikely to provide a short-cut to better understanding. Hum Reprod Update 2004;10:533–539.
18. Altshuler D, Brooks LD, Chakravarti A, Collins FS, Daly MJ, Donnelly P. A haplotype map of the human genome. Nature 2005;437:1299–1320.
19. Cardon LR, Bell JI. Association study designs for complex diseases. Nat Rev Genet 2001;2:91–99.
20. Yuan L, Liu JG, Zhao J, Brundell E, Daneholt B, Hoog C. The murine SCP3 gene is required for synaptonemal complex assembly, chromosome synapsis, and male fertility. Mol Cell 2000;5:73–83.
21. Miyamoto T, Hasuike S, Yogev L, et al. Azoospermia in patients heterozygous for a mutation in SYCP3. Lancet 2003;362:1714–1719.
22. Ruggiu M, Speed R, Taggart M, et al. The mouse Dazla gene encodes a cytoplasmic protein essential for gametogenesis. Nature 1997;389:73–77.
23. Tung JY, Rosen MP, Nelson LM, et al. Variants in deleted in AZoospermia-like (DAZL) are correlated with reproductive parameters in men and women. Hum Genet 2006;118:730–740.
24. Cho C, Willis WD, Goulding EH, et al. Haploinsufficiency of protamine-1 or -2 causes infertility in mice. Nat Genet 2001;28:82–86.
25. de Yebra L, Ballesca JL, Vanrell JA, Bassas L, Oliva R. Complete selective absence of protamine P2 in humans. J Biol Chem 1993;268:10,553–10,557.
26. Tanaka H, Miyagawa Y, Tsujimura A, Matsumiya K, Okuyama A, Nishimune Y. Single nucleotide polymorphisms in the protamine-1 and -2 genes of fertile and infertile human male populations. Mol Hum Reprod 2003;9:69–73.
27. Iguchi N, Yang S, Lamb DJ, Hecht NB. A protamine SNP: one genetic cause of male infertility. J Med Genet 2006;43:382–384.
28. Yu YE, Zhang Y, Unni E, et al. Abnormal spermatogenesis and reduced fertility in transition nuclear protein 1-deficient mice. Proc Natl Acad Sci USA 2000;97:4683–4688.
29. Zhao M, Shirley CR, Hayashi S, et al. Transition nuclear proteins are required for normal chromatin condensation and functional sperm development. Genesis 2004;38:200–213.
30. Miyagawa Y, Nishimura H, Tsujimura A, et al. Single-nucleotide polymorphisms and mutation analyses of the TNP1 and TNP2 genes of fertile and infertile human male populations. J Androl 2005;26:779–786.

31. Galan JJ, Buch B, Cruz N, et al. Multilocus analyses of estrogen-related genes reveal involvement of the ESR1 gene in male infertility and the polygenic nature of the pathology. Fertil Steril 2005;84:910–918.

32. Eddy EM, O'Brien DA. Gene expression during mammalian meiosis. Curr Top Dev Biol 1998;37:141–200.

33. Kleene KC. Sexual selection, genetic conflict, selfish genes, and the atypical patterns of gene expression in spermatogenic cells. Dev Biol 2005;277:16–26.

34. Adams MD, Kelley JM, Gocayne JD, et al. Complementary DNA sequencing: expressed sequence tags and human genome project. Science 1991;252: 1651–1656.

35. Okubo K, Hori N, Matoba R, et al. Large scale cDNA sequencing for analysis of quantitative and qualitative aspects of gene expression. Nat Genet 1992;2: 173–179.

36. Wilcox AS, Khan AS, Hopkins JA, Sikela JM. Use of 3′ untranslated sequences of human cDNAs for rapid chromosome assignment and conversion to STSs: implications for an expression map of the genome. Nucleic Acids Res 1991;19: 1837–1843.

37. Boguski MS, Schuler GD. ESTablishing a human transcript map. Nat Genet 1995;10:369–371.

38. Strausberg RL, Dahl CA, Klausner RD. New opportunities for uncovering the molecular basis of cancer. Nat Genet 1997;15:415–416.

39. Huminiecki L, Bicknell R. In silico cloning of novel endothelial-specific genes. Genome Res 2000;10:1796–1806.

40. Rajkovic A, Yan MSC, Klysik M, Matzuk M. Discovery of germ cell-specific transcripts by expressed sequence tag database analysis. Fertil Steril 2001;76:550–554.

41. Hedges SB. The origin and evolution of model organisms. Nat Rev Genet 2002;3:838–849.

42. Lin YN, Matzuk MM. High-throughput discovery of germ-cell-specific genes. Semin Reprod Med 2005;23:201–212.

43. Yan W, Ma L, Burns KH, Matzuk MM. Haploinsufficiency of kelch-like protein homolog 10 causes infertility in male mice. Proc Natl Acad Sci USA 2004;101:7793–7798.

44. Hinrichs AS, Karolchik D, Baertsch R, et al. The UCSC Genome Browser Database: update 2006. Nucleic Acids Res 2006;34:D590–D598.

45. Finn RD, Mistry J, Schuster-Bockler B, et al. Pfam: clans, web tools and services. Nucleic Acids Res 2006;34:D247–D251.

46. Letunic I, Copley RR, Schmidt S, et al. SMART 4.0: towards genomic data integration. Nucleic Acids Res 2004;32:D142–D144.

47. Devroey P, Van Steirteghem A. A review of ten years experience of ICSI. Hum Reprod Update 2004;10:19–28.

48. Savolainen P, Fitzsimmons C, Arvestad L, Andersson L, Lundeberg J. ESTs from brain and testis of White Leghorn and red junglefowl: annotation, bioinformatic classification of unknown transcripts and analysis of expression levels. Cytogenet Genome Res 2005;111:79–87.

49. Shin JH, Kim H, Song KD, et al. A set of testis-specific novel genes collected from a collection of Korean Native Chicken ESTs. Anim Genet 2005;36:346–348.

50. Zeng S, Gong Z. Expressed sequence tag analysis of expression profiles of zebrafish testis and ovary. Gene 2002;294:45–53.

51. Inaba K, Padma P, Satouh Y, et al. EST analysis of gene expression in testis of the ascidian Ciona intestinalis. Mol Reprod Dev 2002;62:431–445.

II MEIOSIS AND ERRORS OF MEIOSIS

7 The Immunocytogenetics of Human Male Meiosis
A Progress Report

Daniel Topping, MD,
Petrice Brown, MS,
and Terry Hassold, PhD

Summary

Recently, several components of the mammalian meiotic recombination pathway have been identified and new immunofluorescence approaches to the analysis of human meiosis have been developed. This has made it possible to directly examine the dynamics of chromosome behavior in meiosis I spermatocytes and address previously intractable questions, such as: How do chromosomes pair and synapse with one another? How does recombination occur? What is the relationship—if any—between abnormalities in meiosis and cases of unexplained male infertility? In this chapter, we discuss results from immunocytogenetic studies of human males, summarizing how they have contributed to our understanding of both normal and abnormal spermatogenesis.

Key Words: Meiosis; pachytene; synaptonemal complex; recombination; aneuploidy.

1. INTRODUCTION

The contribution of meiotic chromosome abnormalities to human male infertility has long been recognized. As early as 1959, human cytogeneticists documented the association between numerical sex chromosome abnormalities (i.e., 47,XXY) and failure to produce sperm *(1)*. Subsequently, cytogenetic analyses of males attending infertility clinics demonstrated that structural chromosome abnormalities (e.g., translocations) were also an important contributor to infertility *(2)*. The reason for these effects was revealed by conventional light and electron microscopic analyses of testicular biopsies in aneuploid or translocation-carrying individuals in studies conducted during the 1970s and 1980s. Specifically, germ cells with additional or rearranged chromosomes

From: *The Genetics of Male Infertility*
Edited by: D.T. Carrell © Humana Press Inc., Totowa, NJ

were found to have severe defects in orientation and movement of chromosomes during the earliest stages of meiosis, frequently resulting in meiotic arrest and germ cell death. Further, infertile individuals with apparently normal chromosome constitutions but with defects in homologous chromosome pairing and/or synapsis were also identified, suggesting that gene mutations as well as chromosome abnormalities might contribute to arrest at meiosis I (MI).

During the intervening two decades, we have witnessed remarkable advances in our understanding of the molecular basis for male infertility (e.g., the identification of *DAZ* mutations; refs. *3* and *4*), but there has been surprisingly little new information on the possible contribution of meiotic abnormalities to infertility. In large part, this reflects technical limitations: although we have been able to conduct routine karyotypic analyses and, occasionally, analyses of meiotic chromosome synapsis and pairing in infertile men, it has not been possible to simultaneously analyze meiotic chromosomes and chromosome-associated proteins.

Fortunately, this situation is now changing. The identification of mammalian homologs of meiosis-acting proteins of lower organisms and the introduction of novel immunofluorescence technology to meiotic analysis has made it possible to directly analyze protein localization patterns in meiocytes, leading to renewed interest in human meiosis research. Thus, beginning approx 10 yr ago, several groups initiated studies to characterize protein–DNA interactions in human male meiosis, using testicular biopsy material obtained from infertility clinics. In this chapter, we summarize some of the most important of these studies, first discussing the impact they have had on our understanding of normal male meiosis, and second their relevance to the etiology of idiopathic male infertility.

2. WHAT IMMUNOCYTOGENETICS HAS TAUGHT US ABOUT MALE MEIOSIS

Meiosis is the specialized cell process whereby an organism undergoes two nuclear divisions in preparation for gamete formation. In humans, this results in a reduction of chromosomes from the diploid (46) to the haploid (23) number, with each gamete containing one copy of each chromosome. In this fashion, genetic diversity is created because each daughter cell contains a different combination of alleles.

Several processes are unique to meiocytes. However, none are more profound than those that occur during prophase of MI, when homologous chromosomes are required to first find their partners, then become intimately associated with one another and finally exchange genetic

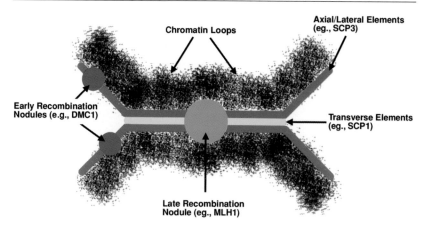

Fig. 1. The synaptonemal complex (SC) and associated recombination machinery proteins. The SC is a tripartite structure, consisting of two axial/lateral elements and the transverse filament in the central region. In leptotene, DNA from the two sister chromatids of each homolog becomes bound to the forming axial elements; by zygotene, the axial elements are completely formed. In zygotene, the transverse filament of the central region begins to bring the axial elements of each homolog into close register. By pachytene, the synaptic process is complete, with the chromosomal DNA bound to the fully-formed, mature SC; the axial elements are now referred to as lateral elements. Recombination occurs in the context of the SC, with "early" recombination nodules presumably representing sites of double strand breaks and "late" nodules a subset of those breaks that are processed as exchanges. Following pachytene, the SC dissolves, with the chiasmata (crossovers) acting to hold the homologs together until the metaphase/anaphase I transition.

Several of the components of the SC and the recombination machinery are now known, including SCP1 (a component of the transverse filament), SCP2, and SCP3 (components of the axial/lateral elements); DMC1 and RAD51 (components of early recombination nodules); and MLH1 (a component of late nodules). These can be detected cytologically using the appropriate antibodies; subsequently, specific chromosomes/chromosome regions can be identified with fluorescence *in situ* hybridization probes.

material, all in preparation for chromosome segregation at the first meiotic division. This series of events requires coordinated activity of a number of different protein families, two of which have been extensively studied in humans using immunocytogenetic methodology: synaptonemal complex proteins, responsible for linking pairs of homologous chromosomes, and recombination proteins, responsible for promoting exchanges (crossovers) between homologous chromosomes (Fig. 1).

2.1. Synaptonemal Complex Proteins

The synaptonemal complex (SC) is the prophase-specific supramolecular proteinaceous structure that forms between, and holds together,

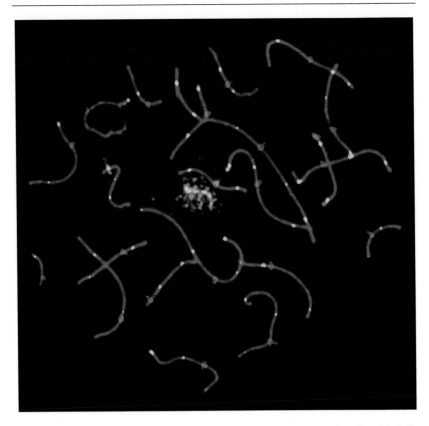

Fig. 2. Representative human pachytene stage spermatocyte, showing 23 fully formed synaptonemal complexes (SCs). SCs are detected by SCP3 (in red), centromeres by CREST (in blue), and sites of crossovers by MLH1 (in yellow). Two fluorescence *in situ* hybridization probes have been used to identify individual chromosomes: a paint probe for chromosome 22 (dispersed green signal) and a probe to the centromeric region of chromosome 18 (punctate green signal).

homologs (Fig. 1). Three component proteins of the SC have been identified: SCP1, SCP2, and SCP3. Of these, SCP3 has been the most useful in immunostaining studies because it localizes to the first-formed components of the SC (i.e., the axial elements; *see* Fig. 1) and thus can be used to monitor assembly and disassembly of the SC during prophase *(5–8)*. These and other studies have shown that, in the human male, short linear SCP3 fragments are first detectable in leptotene, coalescing to form full-length axial elements in zygotene, and by pachytene, the 46 axial elements have been "zipped up" by the transverse filament (i.e., by SCP1) to form 23 fully mature SCs (Fig. 2).

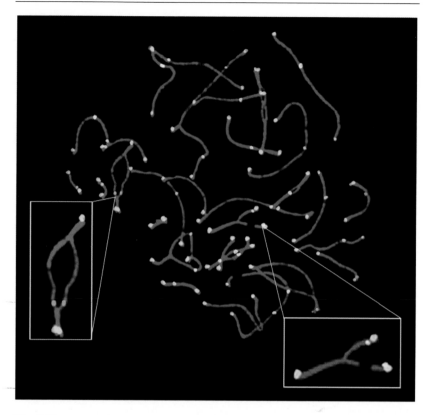

Fig. 3. Representative zygotene stage spermatocyte showing (left inset) a partially synapsed non-acrocentric chromosome with distally located regions of synapsis and an asynapsed interstitial region and (right inset) a partially synapsed acrocentric chromosome, with a region of synapsis extending from the distal region of the long arm toward the centromere, but with the proximal long arm and all of the short arm asynapsed.

Although these and other analyses have provided a broad outline of SC formation, few specifics have been available on the mechanics of human SC assembly. However, immunostaining studies of human males have finally begun to shed light on this process. Specifically, Brown et al. *(5)* analyzed formation of the SC in leptotene and zygotene spermatocytes from a series of control males (i.e., individuals with obstructive azoospermia [OA] in whom meiosis appeared unimpaired) and reported several general "rules" that apply to synapsis in males. Most importantly, the number of synaptic initiation sites appears to be tightly regulated in humans. On non-acrocentric chromosomes, there are invariably two sites per chromosome, one located near the short-arm telomere and one near the long-arm telomere; thus, there is one initiation site per chromosome arm (Fig. 3). In contrast, acrocentric chromosomes have only one site, located distally on the long arm (Fig. 3). For both types of chromosomes, synapsis then proceeds toward the centromere.

Brown et al. *(5)* found little evidence that specific p- or q-arm sequences affect progression of synapsis. However, surprisingly, the centromere appears to have an inhibitory effect. For example, when one arm of a non-acrocentric chromosome is "zippered up" before the other, the centromere appears to act as a "stop sign," preventing further movement from that arm. This inhibitory role is in contrast to observations from some model organisms, in which the centromere promotes homologous pairing *(9)*. Further, these results provide evidence for a basic difference between synapsis and meiotic recombination in the human (i.e., there is now considerable evidence that chiasma interference is unaffected by the centromere, although it impedes the spread of synapsis). Thus it appears that, at least in the pericentromeric region, synaptic progression and transmission of recombination pathway signals are controlled differently.

In other studies, Brown et al. *(5)* demonstrated that synapsis is initiated in subtelomeric regions, not at the telomere proper. Specifically, they used pantelomeric probes to localize the telomeric repeat sequences (TTAGGG) in leptotene cells. In the vast majority of cases, they found that synaptic initiation sites were located proximal to the telomeric signals. However, it is not yet clear whether there are specific sequences that seed synapsis, nor is it known whether the synaptic initiation sites are located in regions housing subtelomeric repeats or in unique sequences.

Finally, Brown et al. *(5)* conducted studies comparing the number and location of synaptic initiation with the number and location of crossovers. The two processes share several features: for both, there appears to be a single "obligatory" event on p- and q-arms of non-acrocentric chromosomes and on q-arms of acrocentric chromsomes; both are excluded from the p-arms of acrocentric chromosomes and both are preferentially distally located on chromosome arms *(5,7,10)*. Thus, an obvious question is whether any, most, or all synaptic initiation sites are subsequently translated into crossovers. Although the answer to this question is not yet certain, the initial evidence suggests that the answer is no. That is, the number of crossovers (~45–50 per cell) exceeds that of synaptic initiation sites (~40 per cell), crossovers appear to be more proximally positioned than are initiation sites and, as discussed earlier, the centromere affects the two processes differently. Nevertheless, it may still be that some subset of initiation sites are associated with the formation of crossovers. Detailed mapping of synaptic initiation sites and crossovers on individual chromosomes should allow us to directly test this possibility.

2.2. Recombination Proteins

Cytological identification of crossovers provides two important advantages over traditional, genetic linkage-based analysis of meiotic recombination: first, the ability to simultaneously visualize exchanges on each chromosome in a meiocyte and second, the ability to detect all exchanges in the cell (i.e., because only two of the four products are meiosis are recovered in gametes, linkage analysis can only detect one-half of all exchanges). However, until recently, the only available cytological methodology involved analysis of diakinesis/metaphase I preparations, an approach limited by the paucity of cells at the appropriate stage and by technical difficulties associated with generating good-quality images. Thus, relatively little information was generated with this approach.

With the advent of immunostaining technology, there was considerable optimism that crossover-associated proteins might be identified in pachytene cells, providing an alternative approach to diakinesis/metaphase I preparations. This optimism was realized about 10 yr ago, when analyses of mouse meiocytes suggested that the DNA mismatch repair protein MLH1 might colocalize with sites of crossover in pachytene cells *(11)*. Subsequent studies demonstrated that this was indeed the case both for mice and humans (*see*, e.g., Fig. 3; refs. *6, 8, 11,* and *12*). For example, human analyses of a series of control males *(7)* demonstrated that: the number of MLH1 foci per pachytene spermatocyte fit expectations from genetic linkage analyses, the foci were distally positioned, consistent with available data from linkage studies, and consistent with basic meiotic principles, the foci displayed positive interference (i.e., the presence of one focus reduced the likelihood that a second focus would be positioned nearby). These observations have now been confirmed by several groups *(6,8,13–19)* making it clear that MLH1 can serve as a marker for crossovers in studies of pachytene spermatocytes.

This observation has provided an important new tool to address questions that were previously intractable. For example, it has allowed us to directly examine possible interindividual variation, and to ask whether factors such as age might affect recombination levels. The answers to each of these two questions have been somewhat surprising. First, given the well-known association between disturbances in meiotic recombination and nondisjunction at MI *(20)*, it might have been expected that recombination levels would be homogeneous among males. In fact, several studies have now demonstrated that apparently normal males may average as few as 45 exchanges per cell, whereas others may average as many as 55 per cell (i.e., an approx 20% difference). Whether or not this results in differences in the levels of aneuploid sperm between low and high "recombinators" is not yet known. Similarly, because the level of meiotic nondisjunction increases modestly with paternal age *(21)*, an age-related reduction in recombination might have been expected. In fact, the available data from MLH1 studies provides little evidence for such an effect *(6,12,22)*.

This approach has also allowed us to characterize the distribution of exchanges on individual chromosomes. These analyses indicate that, except for the short arms of acrocentric chromosomes, each chromosome arm contains at least one MLH1 focus (crossover). The human male complement contains 17 non-acrocentric autosomes, 5 acrocentric autosomes, and the sex chromosome pair, implying a minimum of 40 exchanges per cell. The fact that, normally, between 45 and 50 exchanges are identified in pachytene spermatocytes indicates that cells typically contain 40 "mandatory" and between 5 and 10 "optional" exchanges.

This approach also provides an important tool to identify the underlying factors that control the number and location of exchanges in meiocytes. Initial immunocytogenetic studies have led to the identification of both chromosome-specific and genome-wide influences. For example, Sun et al. *(23)* recently demonstrated a *cis* effect, as they found that small synaptic defects (e.g., "splits" or "gaps") on individual SCs reduced the overall level of recombination on those chromosomes. Lynn et al. *(7)* identified an important genome-wide effect, finding that the overall level of recombination in a cell was proportional to the length of the SCs; that is, the SC appears to "measure" genetic length, with cells containing longer SCs having more MLH1 foci than cells with shorter SCs. This suggests that the SC may be responsible for setting the number of exchanges per cell, although it is also possible that it is simply reacting to upstream effectors. By analyzing the number and location of earlier-acting recombination proteins (e.g., SPO11, DMC1, RAD51, MSH4, MSH5), it should be possible to distinguish between these alternatives. Indeed, in an initial study of the temporal progression of meiosis in human males, Martin et al. *(24)* have used just such an approach in examining several different recombination-associated proteins.

Finally, this approach has allowed us to examine the temporal relationship between synapsis and recombination. For many years it was assumed that the SC is indispensable for recombination (i.e., that recombination occurs only in the context of the mature, tripartite SC).

However, studies of model organisms have provided conflicting results: in some (e.g., yeast and mouse) the recombination pathway is initiated before the establishment of the mature SC, whereas in others (e.g., *Drosophila*) synapsis follows recombination (for review, *see* ref. *12*). Initial observations from the human male indicate that humans follow the yeast paradigm, because recombination proteins such as RAD51 are present in leptotene, long before the mature SC is evident *(5)*.

3. IMMUNOCYTOGENETICS AND THE ETIOLOGY OF MALE INFERTILITY

In the preceding discussion, the observations were based on analyses of meiosis in "control" males (i.e., individuals attending infertility clinics because of OA). However, several groups have now applied immunocytogenetic methodology to study individuals with nonobstructive azoospermia (NOA). In general, these investigations have addressed two major questions: What portion, if any, of cases of NOA are attributable to meiotic arrest in germ cell development? In cases of NOA in which cells proceed through meiosis, is there an increase in errors of synapsis and/or recombination?

Preliminary data relating to these questions are provided in Table 1, which summarizes four recent immunocytogenetic studies of MI in NOA individuals *(6,14,25)*. Most importantly, the studies suggest that abnormalities leading to meiotic arrest are an important contributor to NOA of unexplained origin. Combining the data from the four studies, it appears that approx 10% of all NOA is associated with meiotic arrest phenotypes. Further, if cases without any obvious germ cells (i.e., case with only Sertoli cells evident) are excluded, the portion of cases resulting from meiotic arrest increases to nearly 20% of NOA. Thus, in instances in which testicular biopsies are obtained for diagnostic purposes, immunostaining may actually be as informative as other standard diagnostic assays (e.g., karyotyping).

Virtually no information is yet available on the underlying causes of these meiotic arrest phenoypes, but preliminary data from our laboratory suggest that there are likely to be multiple reasons. Specifically, in an initial analysis of three cases (Table 2; ref. *19*), we found subtle differences among individuals in the "end-stage" germ cells that were present in the seminiferous tubules. Specifically, although spermatocytes in all three cases appeared to progress normally to zygotene, one had fully formed axial elements but there was no evidence for synapsis, one had partially synapsed SCs but no evidence for MLH1 localization, and one had partially synapsed SCs in the presence of MLH1 foci (a representative

Table 1
Summary of Results of Immunocytogenetic Studies of Individuals with Nonobstructive Azoospermia

Reference	Total no. of patients	No. of patients with Sertoli cells only	No. of patients with meiotic arrest	No. of patients with post-pachytene cells	In patients with post-pachytene cells	
					Decreased no. of MLH1 foci?	Increase in synaptic defects?
25[a]	18[a]	8 (44%)	1 (6%)	9 (50%)	Yes	Yes
6	40	21 (53%)	4 (10%)	15 (37%)	Yes	Yes
14[b]	12	0 (0%)	0 (0%)	12 (100%)	No	No
19	26	9 (35%)	3 (12%)	14 (54%)	No	No

[a]Eight of these 18 individuals are also represented in the data set of ref. 6.
[b]Study population included one normospermic individual and seven individuals with either asthenoteratospermia or asthenospermia in addition to four individuals with nonobstructive azoospermia.

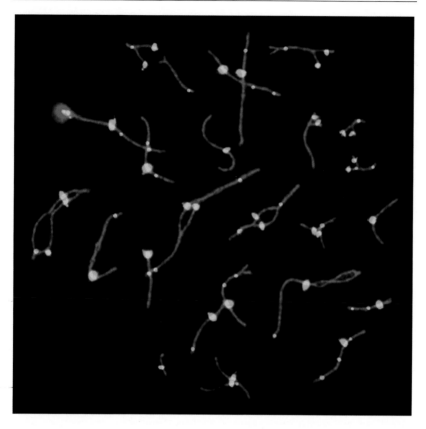

Fig. 4. Representative "end-stage" germ cell from an individual with a meiotic arrest phenotype. Note the presence of MLH1 foci (in yellow), despite the presence of multiple partially synapsed synaptonemal complexes. Synaptonemal complexes are detected by SCP3 (in red) and centromeric regions by CREST (in blue).

"end-stage" cell from this case is provided in Fig. 4). Clearly, in future analyses cases of meiotic arrest, it will be important to carefully examine the phenotypes of these "end-stage" cells, because this will be a crucial first step in the identification of the responsible molecular lesions.

The second question—whether there are disturbances in synapsis and/or recombination in individuals with NOA—also has important clinical ramifications. That is, abnormalities in either process will likely increase the rate of aneuploid sperm; thus, it is important to know whether there is an increase in such abnormalities in some, many, or all individuals with NOA in whom testicular sperm are evident. Unfortunately, the present data set is equivocal (Table 1). Two of the four studies reported increases in synaptic defects and decreases in recombination, whereas the other two failed to find an effect. Clearly, additional analyses of a more extensive series of cases will be needed to address this question.

Table 2
Variation in Meiotic Arrest Phenotypes in Three Individuals
With Nonobstructive Azoospermia

Phenotype	Patient 1	Patient 2	Patient 3
Presence of early markers of recombination	√	√	√
Presence of full-length axial elements	√	√	√
Presence of partially synapsed SCs	—	√	√
Presence of MLH1 foci	—	—	√
Presence of fully synapsed SCs	—	—	—

4. CONCLUSION

From the preceding discussion, it is obvious that immunocytoge-netic analysis of human spermatogenesis is in its infancy. Nevertheless, the initial results have already have been instructive. In studies of normal males, they have provided us with a general set of "rules" for synapsis of homologs; they have allowed us examine the distribution of crossovers in individual spermatocytes and the extent of variation in recombination among individuals; and they have pro-vided an approach to examine factors that may influence either synapsis or recombination. Further, in cases of abnormal spermato-genesis, immunocytogenetic methodology has provided a new approach to the study of unexplained infertility. The initial results on this front are also encouraging, suggesting that immunocytogenetics may uncover the reason for infertility in as many as 10% of all cases of NOA. Clearly, there are limitations to immunocytogenetic analy-sis of spermatogenesis: most importantly, the approach requires acquisition of testicular tissue, material that is not easily obtained. Nevertheless, the initial results suggest that even small data sets will produce large advances in our understanding of both normal and abnormal human spermatogenesis.

ACKNOWLEDGMENTS

Research conducted in the Hassold laboratory and discussed in this chapter was supported by National Institutes of Health grant HD42720.

REFERENCES

1. Jacobs PA, Strong JA. A case of human intersexuality having a possible XXY sex-determining mechanism. Nature 1959;183:302–303.
2. Chandley AC. The chromosomal basis of human infertility. Br Med Bull, 35, 181–186.
3. Cooke HJ. Y chromosome and male infertility. Rev Reprod 1999;4:5–10.
4. Fox MS, Reijo Pera RA. Male infertility, genetic analysis of the DAZ genes on the human Y chromosome and genetic analysis of DNA repair. Mol Cell Endocrinol 2001;184:41–49.
5. Brown PW, Judis L, Chan ER, et al. Meiotic synapsis proceeds from a limited number of subtelomeric sites in the human male. Am J Hum Genet 2005;77:556–566.
6. Gonsalves J, Sun F, Schlegel PN, et al. Defective recombination in infertile men. Hum Mol Genet 2004;13:2875–2883.
7. Lynn A, Koehle KE, Judis L, et al. Covariation of synaptonemal complex length and mammalian meiotic exchange rates. Science 2002;296:2222–2225.
8. Sun F, Trpkov K, Rademaker A, Ko E, Martin RH. Variation in meiotic recombination frequencies among human males. Hum Genet 2005;116:172–178.
9. Dernburg AF, Sedat JW, Hawley RS. Direct evidence of a role for heterochromatin in meiotic chromosome segregation. Cell 1996;86:135–146.
10. Broman KW, Weber, JL. Characterization of human crossover interference. Am J Hum Genet 2000;66:1911–1926.
11. Baker SM, Plug AW, Prolla TA, et al. Involvement of mouse Mlh1 in DNA mismatch repair and meiotic crossing over. Nat Genet 1996;13:336–342.
12. Lynn A, Ashley T, Hassold T. Variation in human meiotic recombination. Annu Rev Genomics Hum Genet 2004;5:317–349.
13. Barlow AL, Hulten, MA. Crossing over analysis at pachytene in man. Eur J Hum Genet 1998;6:350–358.
14. Codina-Pascual M, Oliver-Bonet M, Navarro J, et al. Synapsis and meiotic recombination analyses: MLH1 focus in the XY pair as an indicator. Hum Reprod 2005;20:2133–2139.
15. Oliver-Bonet M, Benet J, Sun F, et al. Meiotic studies in two human reciprocal translocations and their association with spermatogenic failure. Hum Reprod 2005;20:683–688.
16. Sun F, Kozak G, Scott S, et al. Meiotic defects in a man with non-obstructive azoospermia: case report. Hum Reprod 2004;19:1770–1773.
17. Sun F, Trpkov K, Rademaker A, et al. The effect of cold storage on recombination frequencies in human male testicular cells. Cytogenet Genome Res 2004;106: 39–42.
18. Tease C, Hulten MA. Inter-sex variation in synaptonemal complex lengths largely determine the different recombination rates in male and female germ cells. Cytogenet Genome Res 2004;107:208–215.
19. Topping D, Brown P, Judis L, et al. Synaptic defects at meiosis I and non-obstructive azoospermia. Hum Reprod, in press.
20. Hassold T, Sherman S, Hunt P. Counting cross-overs: characterizing meiotic recombination in mammals. Hum Mol Genet 2000;9:2409–2419.
21. Shi Q, Martin RH. Aneuploidy in human sperm: a review of the frequency and distribution of aneuploidy, effects of donor age and lifestyle factors. Cytogenet Cell Genet 2000;90:219–226.
22. Hassold T, Judis L, Chan ER, Schwartz S, Sefte A, Lynn A. Cytological studies of meiotic recombination in human males. Cytogenet Genome Res 2004;107: 249–255.

23. Sun F, Oliver-Bonet M, Liehr T, et al. Discontinuities and unsynapsed regions in meiotic chromosomes have a cis effect on meiotic recombination patterns in normal human males. Hum Mol Genet 2005;14:3013–3018.
24. Oliver-Bonet M, Turek PJ, Sun F, Ko E, Martin RH. Temporal progression of recombination in human males. Mol Hum Reprod 2005;11:517–522.
25. Sun F, Greene C, Turek PJ, Ko E, Rademaker A, Martin RH. Immunofluorescent synaptonemal complex analysis in azoospermic men. Cytogenet Genome Res 2005;111:366–370.

8   The Clinical Relevance of Sperm Aneuploidy

Renee H. Martin, PhD, FCCMG

Summary

The relevance and predictive capabilities of sperm aneuploidy frequencies have been assessed in normal men, men with a constitutional chromosomal abnormality, and infertile men with a normal karyotype. Sperm aneuploidy assessment by fluorescence *in situ* hybridization analysis (FISH) appears to be valuable and reliable. A number of studies have demonstrated that increased frequencies of aneuploidy in human sperm are mirrored by similar frequencies in embryos, fetuses, and newborns. It has been suggested that sperm aneuploidy should be employed as a routine screen before intracytoplasmic sperm injection treatment. This may be most valuable for the groups at highest risk, namely patients with Klinefelter syndrome; structural chromosomal abnormalities; macrocephalic, multinucleated, and multiflagellate sperm; and men with nonobstructive azoospermia. FISH analysis of sperm in these men should aid in counseling and decision making by the couples.

Key Words: Aneuploidy; meiosis; recombination; FISH; translocation.

1. INTRODUCTION

The analysis of sperm aneuploidy has been possible for decades, but many people wonder about the relevance of sperm aneuploidy frequencies and how predictive they are of aneuploidy in a conceptus or child. This chapter discusses the relevance of sperm aneuploidy in normal men, men with constitutional chromosomal abnormalities, and infertile men, and how it relates to risks of chromosomally abnormal children.

2. NORMAL MEN

The study of chromosome abnormalities in human sperm first became possible in 1978 with the advent of the human sperm–hamster oocyte fusion system *(1)*. Laboratories in Canada *(1,2)*, the United States *(3)*, Japan *(4)*, and Spain *(5)* provided strikingly consistent estimates of 1–2%

From: *The Genetics of Male Infertility*
Edited by: D.T. Carrell © Humana Press Inc., Totowa, NJ

aneuploid sperm in normal control donors. We were interested in using this technique to study the distribution of chromosome abnormalities to provide clues about the etiology of nondisjunction. All chromosomes were clearly susceptible to nondisjunction, but we determined that the G group chromosomes (chromosomes 21 and 22) and the sex chromosomes had a significantly elevated frequency of aneuploidy compared with other chromosomes (6). The increased susceptibility of these chromosomes is probably related to the fact that they generally only have one crossover and a lack of recombination is clearly linked to nondisjunction in humans (7,8). Human sperm karyotyping, using the hamster system, provides detailed information about each individual chromosome, permitting analysis of both numerical and structural abnormalities. However, there are significant disadvantages to this approach: sperm must be capable of fertilizing hamster oocytes; the technique is very difficult, time-consuming, and expensive; and the data yield is small. In fact, only 12 laboratories worldwide have had success with this technique despite many efforts.

Fluorescence *in situ* hybridization (FISH) analysis with chromosome-specific DNA probes was developed in the 1990s, providing a faster, cheaper, easier alternative for detecting aneuploidy in human sperm (9–11). Also, sperm hampered by abnormalities in motility or other aspects of fertilization can be assessed using FISH analysis (12–14). This is a simple technique that has been embraced by many laboratories, but it must be remembered that it is indirect: fluorescent signals, rather than chromosomes, are counted (*see* Fig. 1). We see considerable variability in aneuploidy frequencies for individual chromosomes among different studies. For example, for chromosome 21, the lowest disomy (two copies of chromosome 21) frequency has been reported as 0.05% (15) and the highest as 0.95% (16). It is unlikely that these differences arise only from interindividual variation in disomy. Rather, different approaches in the experimental design, different probes, and scoring criteria used are regarded as being responsible (for a review, *see* ref. 17). This makes it essential for each study to have controls analyzed in the same laboratory.

In a composite analysis of the distribution of disomy frequencies in studies on normal men, the mean disomy frequency for autosomes was 0.15 and 0.26% for sex chromosomes (18). Our laboratory has determined that most autosomes have a similar frequency of nondisjunction, but chromosome 21 and the sex chromosomes have a significantly increased frequency (19,20). These results corroborate our earlier studies in human sperm karyotypes (6). This has also been confirmed by other groups (21,22).

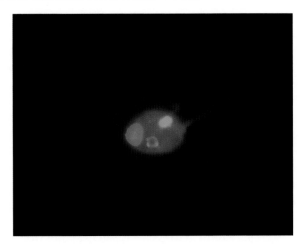

Fig. 1. Abnormal 24,XY sperm, with one red Yq12 signal and one centromere-specific green X signal. The presence of the single blue satellite III chromosome 1 signal, an internal control, indicates that this sperm is disomic rather than diploid.

3. MEN WITH CONSTITUTIONAL CHROMOSOME ABNORMALITIES

Constitutional chromosome abnormalities are relatively common in humans. These can be numerical chromosome abnormalities, such as men with an extra chromosome or structural abnormalities, such as translocations. Many of these abnormalities are associated with infertility and an increased risk of pregnancy loss. The frequency of constitutional chromosomal abnormalities in infertile men varies between 2 and 14%, depending on the severity of the infertility and the nature of the pathology *(23)*. Constitutional abnormalities have been studied using the hamster oocytes system, which provides precision in the human sperm karyotypes *(24,25)*. In the past decade, FISH analysis has been utilized with centromeric and telomeric probes to determine chromosome segregations and take advantage of the larger sample sizes *(26,27)*.

4. SEX CHROMOSOMAL ABNORMALITIES

Men with a 47,XYY karyotype generally produce normal children but there has been no systematic study of children born to those men. Theoretically, 50% of the sperm cells should be abnormal. In a study of 75 sperm karyotypes from a 47,XYY male, we found no sperm disomic for a sex chromosome *(28)*. Our results supported the hypothesis that the extra sex chromosome is eliminated during spermatogenesis.

FISH analysis on the same male with 10,000 sperm studied demonstrated a small but significant increase for XY disomy to 0.6% *(29)*. Similar FISH studies by other laboratories have demonstrated increased frequencies of sperm aneuploidy for the sex chromosomes ranging from 0.3 to 15% (refs. *30* and *31*; *see* ref. *32* for a review). However, when only the stringent three-color FISH studies are assessed, the frequency of 24,YY or 24,XY sperm was 1% or lower *(32)*. Thus, analysis of sperm chromosomal aneuploidy has largely been reassuring for these men.

Men with Klinefelter syndrome (47,XXY) or mosaic variants (e.g., 47,XXY/46,XY) generally have severe oligozoospermia or azoospermia and sperm can sometimes be obtained by a testicular biopsy. FISH analysis has demonstrated that the frequency of aneuploidy for the sex chromosomes varies from 1.5 to 7% *(33, 34)* in sperm from Klinefelter mosaics and 2 to 25% *(35, 36)* in the sperm of men who appear to have a nonmosaic 47,XXY karyotype (for a review, *see* ref. *23*). Chromosomally normal offspring as well as conceptions with a 47,XXY karyotype have been reported in Klinefelter syndrome males who have fathered a pregnancy through intracytoplasmic sperm injection (ICSI; ref. *23*). From both mouse *(37)* and human studies *(38)*, it appears likely that the extra sex chromosome is generally eliminated during meiosis (as in 47,XYY) but the abnormal testicular environment still leads to an increased frequency of aneuploidy sperm and embryos. Staessen et al. *(39)* have reported on ICSI and preimplantation genetic diagnosis (PGD) performed in 32 cycles of 20 couples with spermatozoa from nonmosaic Klinefelter patients. They found a significantly higher frequency of both sex chromosomal (13.2%) and autosomal (15.6%) abnormalities compared with a control group adjusted for age (3.1 and 5.2%). The three- to fourfold increase in chromosomal abnormalities in embryos is consistent with some of the sperm chromosome studies in these men, but there seems to be considerable variability in the frequency of sperm chromosome abnormalities in men with Klinefelter syndrome.

5. TRANSLOCATIONS

Robertsonian translocation carriers have a fusion of the long arms of two acrocentric chromosomes resulting in a balanced state with 45 chromosomes. Pairing of the chromosomes at meiosis can lead to chromosomally balanced and unbalanced gametes. Sperm karyotyping studies have demonstrated that 3 to 27% of the spermatozoa are unbalanced *(40)*. FISH studies in 23 Robertsonian translocation heterozygotes have shown similar frequencies of imbalance varying from 7 to 36% *(41,42)*.

Reciprocal translocations occur when there are exchanges of chromosome material between any chromosomes. During meiosis, four chromosomes must pair in reciprocal translocation heterozygotes and the resulting segregations have a higher frequency of unbalanced chromosomes than Robertsonian translocations. Sperm karyotyping studies of more than 30 reciprocal translocation heterozygotes have shown that 19–77% of spermatozoa are unbalanced *(24)*. FISH analyses of chromosome segregations in more than 30 carriers have reported frequencies of unbalanced chromosomes ranging from 37% *(43)* to 79% *(27)*. In one study, four male family members of a kindred segregating a chromosome 15;17 translocation were studied by FISH analysis *(44)*. The segregation patterns were very similar in all four men, with approx 50% of sperm chromosomally unbalanced. Also, Morel et al. *(43)* found similar frequencies of imbalance of 37 and 43% in two brothers heterozygous for a chromosome 7;8 translocation. These studies demonstrate that the risk of meiotic imbalance is primarily determined by the characteristics of the chromosomes involved and the breakpoint positions. They also demonstrate the reproducibility of the method. Because the frequency of chromosome abnormality is very high, some men carrying reciprocal translocations have undergone PGD to implant only chromosomally normal or balanced embryos. Studies comparing the frequency of chromosome abnormalities in sperm and embryos from reciprocal translocation carriers show a very close agreement in the abnormality frequencies *(45)*.

6. INVERSIONS

Inversion occurs when there are two chromosome breaks in the same chromosome and the segment heals in an inverted manner. During meiosis, the inverted chromosome may pair with a normal chromosome by an inversion loop. If an uneven number of crossovers occur in this loop, half of the gametes will be chromosomally unbalanced. There have been seven inversion heterozygotes studied by the sperm karyotyping technique with frequencies of chromosome imbalance varying from 0 to 31% *(46,47)*. There have been six studies of inversion heterozygotes by FISH analysis with 1 to 54% unbalanced sperm *(48,49)*. Thus, there is a considerable variation in the frequency of abnormal sperm produced by inversions and sperm aneuploidy testing is valuable to determine which inversion carriers have a significant risk.

7. INFERTILE MEN WITH A 46,XY KARYOTYPE

It is clear from the studies discussed earlier that men with a constitutional chromosomal abnormality have an increased risk for sperm chromosomal anomalies. However, it has also been determined that infertile men with a normal somatic karyotype produce sperm with an increased frequency of chromosome abnormalities. There have been more than 30 FISH studies of sperm chromosome abnormalities in 46,XY infertile men and the great majority have demonstrated a significantly increased frequency of aneuploidy for the autosomes and particularly for the sex chromosomes (for a review, *see* ref. *23*). Most studies have reported the increase of sperm chromosome abnormalities in infertile men to be about three times higher than control donors *(50–52)*. Reports based on prenatal diagnosis *(53)* of ICSI pregnancies and newborns *(54)* have indicated the risk of *de-novo* chromosome abnormalities to be approx 2 to 3%, which is threefold higher than normal pregnancies. Thus, the increased frequency of chromosome abnormalities in ICSI pregnancies and newborns mirrors the increased frequency observed in sperm of the infertile ICSI patients. Furthermore, studies have indicated that these chromosome abnormalities are of paternal origin *(55)*, underscoring the fact that chromosomally abnormal sperm in ICSI patients become chromosomally abnormal fetuses and children. We have found that this increased frequency of sperm chromosome abnormalities in 46,XY infertile men is observed for all types of abnormal semen profiles: oligozoospermia *(56)*, teratozoospermia *(57)*, aesthenozoospermia *(13)*, and azoospermia *(58)*. Many of these men have approximately three times the risk observed in control donors, although a number of studies suggest that the risk is higher for azoospermia with sperm retrieved from a testicular biopsy *(59,60)*. One important exception to this rule is men with a high percentage of macrocephalic, multinucleated, and multiflagellate sperm. A number of studies have reported very high frequencies of aneuploidy and polyploidy sperm in these men (50–100%; refs. *61–64*).

8. SPERM SELECTION BASED ON CHROMOSOMAL CONTENT

To many people, it seems intuitive that sperm selection must exist. After all, with millions of sperm to choose from, surely the best (i.e., most chromosomally normal) should have an advantage in developing into a mature sperm and fertilizing an oocyte. However, there is very little evidence that this is the case. In fact, the evidence against sperm selection is quite compelling. Most striking is the evidence from constitutional chromosomal abnormalities, such as translocations. Reciprocal translocations lead to a very high frequency of chromosome imbalance, with an average of 50% unbalanced sperm *(24,65)*. These can often be very abnormal after adjacent 2 or 3:1 segregation with the equivalent of an extra chromosome. The fact that we find such a high frequency of chromosome abnormalities in sperm argues against selection during spermatogenesis. Also, the theoretical expectations of the various segregations are generally observed *(43,66)*; for example, an equal frequency of balanced and normal chromosomes are seen in sperm after alternate segregation and similarly an equal frequency of the two outcomes expected from adjacent 1 segregation are observed, although some clearly have more chromosomal imbalance. Oliver-Bonet et al. studied human translocations at different spermatogenic stages (metaphase I, II, and mature sperm) and found no evidence of selection based on chromosomal content *(67)*. Furthermore, PGD studies have demonstrated the same frequency of aneuploidy in early embryos as in sperm, demonstrating that fertilization is not a barrier to chromosomally unbalanced sperm *(45)*. The selection occurs after this stage because the chromosome imbalance interferes with the normal embryological development so that by the time of the prenatal diagnosis at approx 16 wk gestation, only 11% of fetuses from male translocation carriers are chromosomally unbalanced *(68)*. Most studies in mice *(69,70)* and hamsters *(71)* have also shown no evidence for sperm selection.

9. RETROSPECTIVE STUDIES RELATING ANEUPLOIDY IN SPERM AND OFFSPRING

A number of studies have analyzed populations of paternally derived aneuploid children and then studied the fathers to determine if sperm aneuploidy was significantly elevated. Blanco et al. studied a population with a high prevalence of Down syndrome *(21)*. They determined that the two cases of paternally derived trisomy 21 had fathers with significantly increased disomy 21 sperm. Further studies showed that these men had generalized tendencies to meiotic nondisjunction, because other chromosomes had elevated aneuploidy frequencies *(72)*. In a similar study, however, Hixon et al. did not find a significantly elevated frequency of disomy 21 sperm in cases of Down syndrome of paternal origin *(73)*. Martinez-Pasarell et al. *(74,75)* found a significantly increased frequency of sex chromosomal aneuploidy in sperm from fathers of paternally derived Turner syndrome patients and Tang et al. *(76)* found an exceedingly high frequency of sex chromosomal nullisomy (19.6%) and XY disomy (18.6%) in the infertile father of a 45,X abortus, shown to be caused by a lack of paternal X chromosome. Eskenazi et al. *(77)* studied children with Klinefelter syndrome and found that paternally derived cases had higher frequencies of XY sperm than maternally derived cases. Thus, the majority of studies show an elevated frequency of chromosomally abnormal sperm in fathers of paternally derived aneuploid offspring.

10. PROSPECTIVE STUDIES RELATING ANEUPLOIDY IN SPERM AND OFFSPRING

In the first publication of an increased frequency of sperm chromosome abnormalities in infertile men with a normal karyotype, we reported on one male who had a frequency of 24,XY sperm that was ninefold higher than controls *(46)*. This man subsequently had ICSI and fathered a pregnancy that resulted in a 47,XXY fetus *(78)*. Nagvenkar et al. *(79)* studied men with severe oligozoospermia and normal fertility and related the sperm aneuploidy frequency to the outcome after ICSI. They found a significantly higher frequency of sex chromosomal disomy in the severe oligozoospermia group and this correlated with a lower pregnancy and live birth rate. Petit et al. *(80)* studied sperm aneuploidy in three groups of men with different ICSI outcomes: group A had at least four ICSI treatments without a pregnancy, group B had a pregnancy after one to three ICSI attempts, and group C consisted of a fertile control group. FISH analysis for chromosomes 8, 9, 13, 18, 21, X and Y demonstrated a higher aneuploidy frequency in group A compared with group B, and group B compared with group C. They suggested that sperm aneuploidy could be used as a predictive test before ICSI to improve genetic counseling for patients.

Gianaroli et al. *(81)* studied sperm aneuploidy and correlated it to results in blastomeres after PGD in couples in which the female partner was younger than 36 yr old. They found a higher incidence of monosomies and trisomies in embryos from microepididymal sperm aspiration and testicular sperm extraction sperm and aneuploidy for the sex chromosomes increased proportionally to the severity of the male-factor condition. These authors suggested that it is important to include sperm FISH analysis in preliminary tests given to infertile couples, especially in the case of repeated in vitro fertilization failures. These preliminary studies suggest a correlation between sperm aneuploidy frequencies and ICSI outcome.

10.1. Should Sperm Aneuploidy Testing Be Recommended for Infertile Men With a 46,XY Karyotype?

After a decade of analysis, it is clear that infertile men with a normal somatic karyotype have an increased risk of sperm aneuploidy. The magnitude of this risk has varied from 2- to 10-fold that of control donors. However, most studies have shown an increase of approximately threefold *(46–48)*, which mirrors the risk observed in newborns after ICSI. Is this enough of a risk to consider advocating sperm aneuploidy testing for all male-factor infertility patients? It is certainly important that all patients be informed of the risk but it is unlikely that patients would be dissuaded from treatment as a result. Sperm aneuploidy testing might be worthwhile if it uncovered some men with a very high frequency of sperm aneuploidy. However, these men appear to be relatively rare. In my laboratory, there were 6 of 66 infertile patients (with a normal karyotype) who had an XY disomy frequency that was at least fivefold greater than controls and 2 of 66 men with frequencies more than 10-fold higher (unpublished results). Thus, the majority of men have moderately increased risk. Although a number of studies have advocated routine sperm aneuploidy testing in infertile men with a normal karyotype, it is unlikely that this would uncover many men with a substantially increased risk of aneuploid children.

11. IS TESTING RECOMMENDED FOR MEN WITH NONOBSTRUCTIVE AZOOSPERMIA?

We have demonstrated that men with nonobstructive azoospermia have severe meiotic abnormalities including chromosome pairing and synapsis defects and a significant decrease in the frequency of recombination *(82–84)*. Because chromosome pairing and recombination is intimately linked with the normal segregation of chromosomes *(7,8)*, these defects may be responsible for the increased frequency of aneuploidy observed in testicular sperm from these men *(55–57)*. It is difficult to study sperm aneuploidy in men with nonobstructive azoospermia because, generally, such a small number of sperm are retrieved. However, when it is possible, it is certainly worthwhile. The new immunocytogenetic techniques, which allow analysis of chromosome synapsis and recombination, are also very valuable (*see* Fig. 2); presently, they are only available on a research basis in a few laboratories worldwide.

12. CONCLUSION

FISH analysis of sperm aneuploidy is clearly a valuable and reliable technique. A number of studies have shown that increased frequencies of aneuploidy in human sperm are mirrored by similar increases in

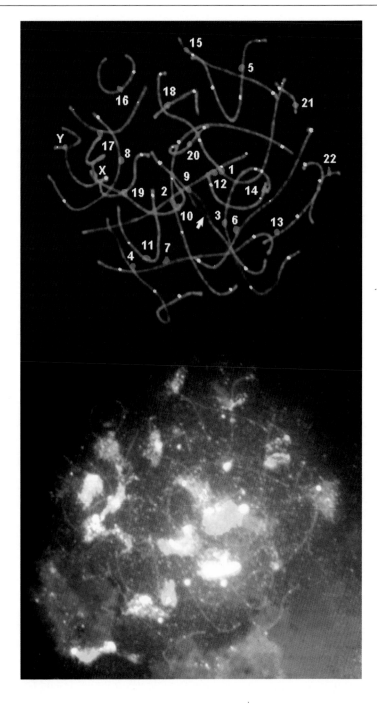

early embryos, fetuses, newborns, and children. As a result, there have been suggestions that sperm aneuploidy should be employed routinely for all infertile men before ICSI treatment. Because most infertile patients are likely to have only a moderate increase in sperm aneuploidy, it may be effective to target those groups at highest risk:

1. Patients with Klinefelter syndrome.
2. Patients with structural chromosomal abnormalities, such as translocations and inversions.
3. Men with a high proportion of macrocephalic, multinucleated, and multiflagellate sperm.
4. Men with nonobstructive azoospermia, when enough sperm are retrieved from the testicular biopsy.

Patients in these four groups have quite variable frequencies of sperm aneuploidy and thus FISH analysis of sperm could aid in counseling and decision making. The couple might then be reassured by a low risk or, in the event of a high risk, decide against ICSI treatment or proceed with ICSI combined with PGD.

ACKNOWLEDGMENTS

Renée H. Martin holds the Canada Research Chair in Genetics and this research is supported by grant MA-7961 from the Canadian Institutes of Health Research.

The expertise and assistance of Evelyn Ko, Fei Sun, and Nadine Gammon are gratefully acknowledged.

REFERENCES

1. Martin R. Genetic screening for gamete donors. Fertil Steril 1987;48:347–348.
2. Martin R, Balkan W, Burns K, Rademaker A, Lin C, Rudd N. The chromosome constitution of 1000 human spermatozoa. Hum Genet 1983;63:305–309.
3. Brandriff B, Gordon L, Ashworth L, et al. Chromosomes of human sperm: variability among normal individuals. Hum Genet 1985;70:18–24.
4. Mikamo K, Kamiguchi Y, Tateno H. Spontaneous and in vitro radiation-induced chromosome aberrations in human spermatozoa: application of a new method. In: Mendelsohn ML, Albertini RJ, eds. Mutation and the Environment Part B: Metabolism, Testing Methods, and Chromosomes. John Wiley and Sons, Inc., Toronto; 1990:447–456.

Fig. 2. *(Opposite page)* (Upper) Pachytene spermatocyte from a nonobstructive azoospermic patient, with synaptonemal complexes (SCs) shown in red, centromeres in blue, and MLH1 (recombination) foci in yellow. Note that SC 9 has an unpaired chromosome region (arrow). (Lower) Subsequent centromeric multicolor fluorescence in situ hybridization analysis allows identification of individual chromosomes so that MLH1 foci can be analyzed for each SC.

5. Templado C, Marquez C, Munne S, et al. An analysis of human sperm chromosome aneuploidy. Cytogenet Cell Genet 1996;74:194–200.

6. Martin R, Rademaker A. The frequency of aneuploidy among individual chromosomes in 6,821 human sperm chromosome complements. Cytogenet Cell Genet 1990;53:103–107.

7. Savage A, Petersen M, Pettay D, et al. Elucidating the mechanisms of paternal nondisjunction of chromosome 21 in humans. Hum Mol Gen 1998;7:1221–1227.

8. Shi Q, Spriggs E, Field L, Ko E, Barclay L, Martin R. Single sperm typing demonstrates that reduced recombination is associated with the production of aneuploid 24,XY human sperm. Amer J Med Genet 2001;99:34–38.

9. Martin R, Ko E, Chan K. Detection of aneuploidy in human interphase spermatozoa by fluorescence in situ hybridization (FISH). Cytogenet Cell Genet 1993;64:23–26.

10. Martin R, Spriggs E, Rademaker A. Multicolor fluorescence in situ hybridization analysis of aneuploidy and diploidy frequencies in 225,846 sperm from 10 normal men. Biol Reprod 1996;54:394–398.

11. Wyrobek A, Robbins W, Mehraein Y, Pinkel D, Weier H. Detection of sex chromosomal aneuploidies X-X, Y-Y, and X-Y in human sperm using two-chromosome fluorescence in situ hybridization. Amer J Med Genet 1994;53:1–7.

12. Martin R, Ernst S, Rademaker A, Barclay L, Ko E, Summers N. Analysis of sperm chromosome complements before, during, and after chemotherapy. Cancer Genet Cytogenet 1999;108:133–136.

13. Hristova R, Ko E, Greene C, Rademaker A, Chernos J, Martin R. Chromosome abnormalities in sperm from infertile men with aesthenoteratozoospermia. Biol Reprod 2002;66:1781–1783.

14. Robbins WA, Meistrich ML, Moore D, et al. Chemotherapy induces transient sex chromosomal and autosomal aneuploidy in human sperm. Nature Genet 1997;16:74–78.

15. Van Hummelen P, Lowe X, Wyrobek A. Simultaneous detection of structural and numerical chromosome abnormalities in sperm of healthy men by multicolor fluorescence in situ hybridization. Hum Genet 1996;98:608–615.

16. Rousseaux S, Hazzouri M, Pelletier R, Monteil M, Usson Y, Sele B. Disomy rates for chromosomes 14 and 21 studied by fluorescent in-situ hybridization in spermatozoa from three men over 60 years of age. Mol Hum Reprod 1998;4:695–699.

17. Egozcue J, Blanco J, Vidal F. Chromosome studies in human sperm nuclei using fluorescence in-situ hybridization (FISH). Hum Reprod Update 1997;3:441–452.

18. Shi Q, Martin R. Aneuploidy in human sperm: a review of the frequency and distribution of aneuploidy, effects of donor age and lifestyle factors. Cytogenet Cell Genet 2000;90:219–226.

19. Spriggs E, Rademaker A, Martin R. Aneuploidy in human sperm: the use of multicolor FISH to test various theories of nondisjunction. Am J Hum Gen 1996;58:356–362.

20. Shi Q, Martin R. Spontaneous frequencies of aneuploid and diploid sperm in 10 normal Chinese men: assessed by multicolor fluorescence in situ hybridization. Cytogenet Cell Genet 2000;90:79–83.

21. Blanco J, Gabau E, Gomez D, et al. Chromosome 21 disomy in the spermatozoa of the fathers of children with trisomy 21, in a population with a high prevalence of Down syndrome: increased incidence in cases of paternal origin. Am J Hum Gen 1998;63:1067–1072.

22. Williams BJ, Ballenger CA, Malter HE, et al. Non-disjunction in human sperm: results of fluorescence in situ hybridization studies using two and three probes. Hum Mol Gen 1993;2:1929–1936.

23. Shi Q, Martin R. Aneuploidy in human spermatozoa: FISH analysis in men with constitutional chromosomal abnormalities, and in infertile men. Reproduction 2001;121:655–666.

24. Martin R, Spriggs E. Sperm chromosome complements in a man heterozygous for a reciprocal translocation 46,XY,t(9;13)(q21.1;q21.2) and a review of the literature. Clin Genet 1995;47:42–46.

25. Martin R. Sperm chromosome analysis in a man heterozygous for a paracentric inversion of chromosome 14 (q24.1q32.1). Am J Hum Gen 1999;64:1480–1484.

26. Giltay J, Kastrop P, Tiemessen C, van Inzen W, Scheres JM, Pearson P. Sperm analysis in a subfertile male with a Y;16 translocation, using four-color FISH. Cytogenet Cell Genet 1999;84:67–72.

27. Geneix A, Schubert B, Force A, Rodet K, Briancon G, Boucher D. Sperm analysis by FISH in a case of t(17;22)(q11;q12) balanced transloction. Hum Reprod 2002; 17:325–331.

28. Benet J, Martin R. Sperm chromosome complements in a 47,XYY man. Hum Genet 1988;78:313–315.

29. Martin R, McInnes B, Rademaker A. Analysis of aneuploidy for chromosomes 13, 21, X and Y by multicolour fluorescence in situ hybridisation (FISH) in a 47,XYY male. Zygote 1999;7:131–134.

30. Chevret E, Rousseaux S, Monteil M, et al. Meiotic behaviour of sex chromosomes investigated by three-colour FISH on 35,142 sperm nuclei from two 47,XYY males. Hum Genet 1997;99:407–412.

31. Mercier S, Morel F, Roux C, Clavequin M, Bresson J. Analysis of the sex chromosomal equipment in spermatozoa of a 47,XYY male using two-colour fluorescence in-situ hybridization. Molecular Human Reproduction 1996;2:485–488.

32. Shi Q, Martin R. Multicolor fluorescence in situ hybridization analysis of meiotic chromosome segregation in a 47,XYY male and a review of the literature. Amer J Med Genet 2000;93:40–46.

33. Lim A, Fong Y, Yu S. Estimates of sperm sex chromosome disomy and diploidy rates in a 47,XXY/46,XY mosaic Klinefelter patient. Hum Genet 1999;104: 405–409.

34. Kruse R, Guttenbach M, Shartmann B, et al. Genetic counselling in a patient with XXY/XXXY/XY mosaic Klinefelter's syndrome: estimate of sex chromosome aberrations in sperm before intracytoplasmic sperm injection. Fertil Steril 1998;69:432–485.

35. Rives N, Joly G, Machy A, Simeon N, Leclerc P, Mace B. Assessment of sex chromosome aneuploidy in sperm nuclei from 47,XXY and 46,XY/47,XXY males: comparison with fertile and infertile males with normal karyotype. Molecular Human Reproduction 2000;6:107–112.

36. Estop A, Munne S, Cieply K, Vandermark K, Lamb A, Fisch H. Meiotic products of a Klinefelter 47,XXY male as determined by sperm fluorescence in-situ hybridization analysis. Hum Reprod 1998;13:124–127.

37. Mroz K, Hassold TJ, Hunt PA. Meiotic aneuploidy in the XXY mouse: evidence that a compromised testicular environment increases the incidence of meiotic errors. Hum Reprod 1999;14:1151–1156.

38. Blanco J, Egozcue J, Vidal F. Meiotic behaviour of the sex chromosomes in three patients with sex chromosome anomalies (47,XXY, mosaic 46,XY/47,XXY and 47,XYY) assessed by fluorescence in-situ hybridization. Hum Reprod 2001; 16:887–892.

39. Staessen C, Tournaye H, Van Assche E, et al. PGD in 47,XXY Klinefelter's syndrome patients. Hum Reprod Update 2003;9:319–330.

40. Martin R. Sperm cell—genetic aspects. In: Grudzinskas JG, Yovich JL, Simpson JL, Chard T, eds. Gametes: The Spermatozoon (Cambridge Reviews in Human Reproduction). Cambridge University Press, Cambridge; 1995:104–121.
41. Fryndman N, Romana S, Le Lorc'h M, Vekemans M, Fryndman R, Tachdjian G. Assisting reproduction of infertile men carrying a Robertsonian translocation. Hum Reprod 2001;16:2274–2277.
42. Mennicke K, Diercks P, Schlieker H, et al. Molecular cytogenetic diagnostics in sperm. Int J Androl 1997;20:11–19.
43. Morel F, Douet-Guilbert N, Roux C, et al. Meiotic segregation of a t(7;8)(q11.21;cen) translocation in two carrier brothers. Fertil Steril 2004;81:682–685.
44. Cora T, Acar H, Kaynak M. Molecular cytogenetic detection of meiotic segregation patterns in sperm nuclei of carriers of 46,XY,t(15;17)(q21;q25). J Androl 2002;23:793–798.
45. Escudero T, Abdelhadi I, Sandalinas M, Munne S. Predictive value of sperm fluorescence in situ hybridization analysis on the outcome of preimplantation genetic diagnosis for translocations. Fertil Steril 2003;79:1528–1534.
46. Martin R. Sperm chromosome analysis in a man heterozygous for a paracentric inversion of chromosome 7 (q11q22). Hum Genet 1986;73:97–100.
47. Martin R. Cytogenetic analysis of sperm from a man heterozygous for a pericentric inversion, inv (3) (p25q21). Am J Hum Gen 1991;48:856–861.
48. Jaarola M, Martin R, Ashley T. Direct evidence for suppression of recombination within two pericentric inversions in humans: a new sperm-FISH technique. Am J Hum Gen 1998;63:218–224.
49. Anton E, Blanco J, Egozcue J, Vidal F. Risk assessment and segregation analysis in a pericentric inversion inv6p23q25 carrier using FISH on decondensed sperm nuclei. Cytogenet Genome Res 2002;97:149–154.
50. Acar H, Kilinc M, Cora T, Aktan M, Taskapu H. Incidence of chromosome 8,10,X and Y aneuploidies in sperm nucleus of infertile men detected by FISH. Urologia Internationalis 2000;64:202–208.
51. Lahdetie J, Larsen S, Harkonen K. Analysis of chromosome aneuploidy in sperm by fluorescence in situ hybridization—a new approach to the study of male fertility in environmental exposures. Asclepios. Scand J Work Environ Health 1999;25:26–27.
52. Moosani N, Pattinson H, Carter M, Cox D, Rademaker A, Martin R. Chromosomal analysis of sperm from men with idiopathic infertility using sperm karyotyping and fluorescence in situ hybridization. Fertil Steril 1995;64:811–817.
53. Van Steirteghem A, Bonduelle M, Devroey P, Liebaers I. Follow-up of children born after ICSI. Hum Reprod Update 2002;8:111–116.
54. Aboulghar H, Aboulghar M, Manour R, Serour G, Amin Y, Al-Inany H. A prospective controlled study of karyotyping for 430 consecutive babies conceived through intracytoplasmic sperm injection. Fertil Steril 2001;76:249–254.
55. Van Opstal D, Los F, Ramlakhan S, et al. Determination of the parent of origin in nine cases of prenatally detected chromosome aberrations found after intracytoplasmic sperm injection. Hum Reprod 1997;12:682–686.
56. Martin RH, Rademaker AW, Greene C, et al. A comparison of the frequency of sperm chromosome abnormalities in men with mild, moderate, and severe oligozoospermia. Biol Reprod 2003;69:535–539.
57. Templado C, Hoang T, Greene C, Rademaker A, Chernos J, Martin R. Aneuploid spermatozoa in infertile men: teratozoospermia. Mol Reprod Dev 2002;61:200–204.
58. Martin RH, Greene C, Rademaker A, Ko E, Chernos J. Analysis of aneuploidy in spermatozoa from testicular biopsies from men with nonobstructive azoospermia. J Androl 2003;24:100–103.

59. Bernardini L, Gianaroli L, Fortini D, et al. Frequency of hyper-, hypohaploidy and diploidy in ejaculate, epididymal and testicular germ cells of infertile patients. Hum Reprod 2000;15:2165–2172.

60. Palermo G, Colombero L, Hariprashad J, Schlegel P, Rosenwaks Z. Chromosome analysis of epididymal and testicular sperm in azoospermic patients undergoing ICSI. Hum Reprod 2002;17:570–575.

61. Benzacken B, Gavelle FM, Martin-Pont B, et al. Familial sperm polyploidy induced by genetic spermatogenesis failure: case report. Hum Reprod 2001;16:2646–2651.

62. Devillard F, Metzler-Guillemain C, Pelletier R, et al. Polyploidy in large-headed sperm: FISH study of three cases. Hum Reprod 2002;17:1292–1298.

63. In't Veld PA, Broekmans FJ, de France HF, Pearson PL, Pieters MH, van Kooij RJ. Intracytoplasmic sperm injection (ICSI) and chromosomally abnormal spermatozoa. Hum Reprod 1997;12:752–754.

64. Lewis-Jones I, Aziz N, Sheshadri S, Douglas H, Howard P. Sperm chromosomal abnormalities are linked to sperm morphological deformities. Fertil Steril 2003; 79:212–215.

65. Morel F, Douet-Guilbert N, Le Bris MJ, et al. Meiotic segregation of translocations during male gametogenesis. Int J Androl 2004;27:200–212.

66. Oliver-Bonet M, Navarro J, Carrera M, Egozcue J, Benet J. Aneuploid and unbalanced sperm in two translocation carriers: evaluation of the genetic risk. molecular and Human Reproduction 2002;8:958–963.

67. Oliver-Bonet M, Navarro J, Codina-Pascual M, et al. From spermatocytes to sperm: meiotic behaviour of human male reciprocal translocations. Hum Reprod 2004;19:2515–2522.

68. Boué H, Gallano P. A collaborative study of the segregation of inherited chromosome structural rearrangements in 1356 prenatal diagnoses. Prenatal Diagnosis 1984;4:45–67.

69. Epstein CJ, Travis B. Preimplantation lethality of monosomy for mouse chromosome 19. Nature 1979;280:144–145.

70. Marchetti F, Wyrobek AJ. Mechanisms and consequences of paternally-transmitted chromosomal abnormalities. Birth Defects Research (Part C) 2005;75:112–129.

71. Sonta S. Transmission of chromosomal abnormalities: participation of chromosomally unbalanced gametes in fertilization and early development of unbalanced embryos in the Chinese hamster. Mutat Res 2002;504:193–202.

72. Soares S, Templado C, Blanco J, Egozcue J, Vidal F. Numerical chromosome abnormalities in the spermatozoa of the fathers of children with trisomy 21 of paternal origin: generalized tendency to meiotic non-disjunction. Hum Genet 2001;108:134–139.

73. Hixon M, Millie E, Judis L, et al. FISH studies of the sperm of fathers of paternally derived cases of trisomy 21: no evidence for an increase in aneuploidy. Hum Genet 1998;103:654–657.

74. Martinez-Pasarell O, Nogues C, Bosch M, Egozcue J, Templado C. Analysis of sex chromosome aneuploidy in sperm from fathers of Turner syndrome patients. Hum Genet 1999;104:345–349.

75. Martinez-Pasarell O, Templado C, Vicens-Calvet E, Egozcue J, Nogues C. Paternal sex chromosome aneuploidy as a possible origin of Turner syndrome in monozygotic twins. Hum Reprod 1999;14:2735–2738.

76. Tang SS, Gao H, Robinson WP, Ho Yuen B, Ma S. An association between sex chromosomal aneuploidy in sperm and an abortus with 45,X of paternal origin: possible transmission of chromosomal abnormalities through ICSI. Hum Reprod 2004;19: 147–151.

77. Eskenazi B, Wyrobek AJ, Kidd SA, et al. Sperm aneuploidy in fathers of children with paternally and maternally inherited Klinefelter syndrome. Hum Reprod 2002;17:576–583.

78. Moosani N, Chernos J, Lowry R, Martin R, Rademaker A. A 47,XXY fetus resulting from ICSI in a man with an elevated frequency of 24,XY spermatozoa. Hum Reprod 1999;14:1137–1138.

79. Nagvenkar P, Zaveri K, Hinduja I. Comparison of the sperm aneuploidy rate in severe oligozoospermic and oligozoospermic men and its relation to intracytoplasmic sperm injection outcome. Fertil Steril 2005;84:925–931.

80. Petit FM, Frydman N, Benkhalifa M, et al. Could sperm aneuploidy rate determination be used as a predictive test before intracytoplasmic sperm injection? J Androl 2005;26:235–241.

81. Gianaroli L, Magli MC, Ferraretti AP. Sperm and blastomere aneuploidy detection in reproductive genetics and medicine. J Histochem Cytochem 2005;53:261–267.

82. Gonsalves J, Sun F, Schlegal P, et al. Defective recombination in infertile men. Hum Mol Gen 2004;13:2875–2883.

83. Sun F, Greene C, Turek PJ, Ko E, Rademaker A, Martin RH. Immunofluorescent synaptonemal complex analysis in azoospermic men. Cytogenet Genome Res 2005;111:366–370.

84. Sun F, Kozak G, Scott S, et al. Meiotic defects in a man with non-obstructive azoospermia: case report. Hum Reprod 2004;19:1770–1773.

9 DNA Repair Genes and Genomic Instability in Severe Male Factor Infertility

Francesca K. E. Gordon, BS
and Dolores J. Lamb, PhD

Summary

The maintenance of genomic integrity is of key importance for gametogenesis. Nevertheless, the processes of DNA replication, mitosis, and meiosis are surprisingly error-prone and subject to damage. Accordingly, a series of DNA repair mechanisms have evolved that recognize and repair DNA damage and DNA replication errors to maintain the fidelity of the DNA sequence. Gradually translating findings from targeted gene deletion and mutant mouse models to human male infertility, we have learned that the processes of mitosis and meiosis require proper functioning of the entire DNA repair mechanism in the cell for normal fertility to be present in the male. This chapter focuses on our current understanding of the processes required for the maintenance of DNA integrity during spermatogensis.

Key Words: DNA repair; meiosis; synaptonemal complex; SPO 11; spermatogenesis.

1. INTRODUCTION

Despite the relatively common incidence of male infertility, relatively little is known about the etiology. From a therapeutic perspective, spermatogenic defects are among the most severe of these impairments, presenting as severe oligozoospermia (<1 million sperm per milliliter of ejaculate) and nonobstructive azoospermia (ejaculate with no sperm in the absence of genital tract obstruction).

Nonobstructive azoospermia may result from genetic and environmental factors. Exposure to toxins, legal or illegal drugs, and trauma to the testes can reduce or ablate sperm count and/or viability, either temporarily or permanently *(1–3)*. Numerical and structural sex chromosomal

From: *The Genetics of Male Infertility*
Edited by: D.T. Carrell © Humana Press Inc., Totowa, NJ

anomalies are associated with male infertility. Men with Klinefelter's syndrome (47,XXY), the most common cause of nonobstructive azoospermia, are azoospermic as a result of hypogonadism and chromosomal disjunction during meiosis *(4)*. Individuals with more subtle defects, like Y-chromosome microdeletions, may not present with phenotypic abnormalities, aside from spermatogenic defects that vary in severity with the location of the microdeletion *(5,6)*. Gross autosomal rearrangements, such as reciprocal translocations or unbalanced translocations, are associated with azoospermia as a result of chromosomal disjunction during meiosis I *(7,8)*.

A diverse array of genetic disorders cause infertility in the male *(9)*. Targeted gene deletion in mouse models defined key pathways required for normal male fertility, although translation of these findings to the clinic is slow. Fertility genes affecting the somatic cells of the testis include agents such as growth factors and their receptors, genes involved in hormone biosynthesis, metabolism and action, cell adhesion and tight junctions, and signal transduction pathways. Spermatogonia also require proper growth factor and receptor function, as well as expression of genes involved in the regulation of stem cells, mitosis, and apoptosis. Spermatocytes have entered the meiotic pathway and, not surprisingly, expression of proteins required for chromosome pairing and synapsis, homologous recombination, genomic integrity, and DNA replication and repair are necessary. Other genes affect spermatid differentiation include those required for cell remodeling, chromatin packaging, nuclear condensation, and spermiation. This chapter focuses on the contribution of proteins required for mitosis and meiosis during spermatogenesis, in particular those involved in homologous recombination and DNA repair, and the consequence(s) of mutations in these genes for the successful completion of this process and fertility.

An understanding of spermatogenesis is necessary to appreciate the importance of DNA repair pathway proteins in male germ cell development. Spermatogenesis requires primordial germ cell proliferation and later, the presence of spermatogonial stem cells in the testis, as well as the highly proliferative type A spermatogonia, a few of which differentiate to become type B spermatogonial—the cells destined to enter the meiotic pathway. Meiosis occurs during the spermatocyte stage and involves two divisions that ultimately produce a haploid spermatid that in turn undergoes extensive differentiation and morphology changes to become a mature spermatozoon. Thus, genes controlling genetic fidelity are of importance in both mitosis and meiosis during spermatogenesis.

Meiosis I differs from meiosis II and mitosis because it involves a reduction in the number of chromosomes per cell and an exchange of genetic material between homologous chromosomes or homologous recombination. This provides the basis for the continual mixing of the gene pool and evolution of the species (Fig. 1).

This exchange of genetic material occurs during prophase I and requires proper functioning of the mismatch repair proteins as demonstrated by work in humans, mice, and *Saccharomyces cerevisiae* *(10–13)*. Prophase I is further subdivided into leptotene, zygotene, pachytene, diplotene, and diakinesis (Fig. 2A). Chromosomes thicken and homologs begin to synapse during leptotene. Recombination is also initiated at this stage by formation of double-stranded breaks (DSBs; refs. *14* and *15*). Pairing of homologous chromosomes to facilitate recombination is stabilized by synaptonemal complex (SC) formation, which is complete during zygotene *(16–18)*.

A host of factors expressed during this phase of prophase I coordinates processing of DSBs into single-end invasions (SEIs) and then into holliday junctions (HJs; Fig. 1; refs. *16–21*). Resolution of HJs occurs during the pachytene stage of spermatogenesis *(11,17,19,22–25)*, completing exchange of genetic material between homologs. The SC then dissolves during diplotene, causing the chromosomes to separate where crossover has not occurred *(15)*. Further condensation occurs during diakinesis, making the tetrads clearly visible. As in mitotic metaphase, chromosomes line up on the metaphase plate. However, sister chromatids attach to the same pole rather than different poles as they do in mitotic metaphase. One copy of each chromosome moves to opposite poles of the primary spermatocyte during anaphase I. Like the events during mitosis, the nuclear envelope reforms and gradually generates two separate cells during telophase I. The only difference is that during meiosis the two daughter cells are haploid instead of diploid.

Gene expression is required for each step of this process and the following discussion provides a brief overview of some of the key factors important for progression through meiotic prophase I.

2. DEFECTIVE MITOSIS BECAUSE OF DNA REPAIR DEFECTS AND GERM CELL LOSS LEADING TO MALE INFERTILITY

2.1. Defective Recombination and Male Infertility

Studies in a number of model organisms define a series of meiotic checkpoints that arrest spermatogenesis when defective recombination is present, leading to male infertility. Men with maturation arrest pathology on testis biopsy show histology suggestive of this type of

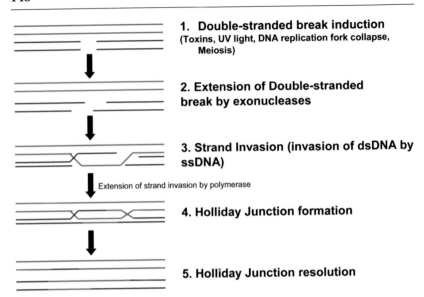

1. **Double-stranded break induction**
(Toxins, UV light, DNA replication fork collapse, Meiosis)

2. **Extension of Double-stranded break by exonucleases**

3. **Strand Invasion (invasion of dsDNA by ssDNA)**

Extension of strand invasion by polymerase

4. **Holliday Junction formation**

5. **Holliday Junction resolution**

Fig. 1. A generalized model of homologous recombination. A double-stranded break is induced by UV light, irradiation, free-radicals, toxins or factors expressed in the early stages of Meiosis I. This promotes exchange of genetic material between homologous chromosomes (1). Exonucleases together with other factors create regions of single-stranded extension of the break on one homolog. Proteins which bind to this piece of single-stranded DNA catalyze its invasion of the double-stranded homolog generating an intermediate single-end invasion structure (2). These single-stranded regions invade the intact double-stranded homologous chromosome (3). DNA Polymerase extends the site of this invasion. Mismatch repair proteins and associated factors bind to the single-end invasion structure and promotes both conversion of this structure into a Holliday Junction (4) and resolution of the Holliday Junction (5). Resolution of the Holliday junction into two separate double-stranded homologs completes the process of homologous recombination.

defect. This led Reijo-Pera, Martin, and colleagues to examine the frequency and location of recombination events in men with maturation arrest compared with those with histologically normal spermatogenesis (26,27). Nearly half of the infertile patients examined showed measurable defects in recombination during spermatogenesis, suggesting that men with arrest at the zygotene stage of prophase in meiosis I have a phenotype similar to that seen in mice with mutations in recombination genes, as described later. For these men, genetic checkpoints stop spermatogenesis when faulty meiotic recombination is present and eliminate the defective cells through apoptosis (27). Accordingly, it is important to translate the findings in the animal models to human infertility to define this etiology, because patients with nonobstructive azoospermia are candidates for treatment with an assisted reproductive technology.

2.1.1. INITIATION OF EVENTS REQUIRED FOR MEIOTIC RECOMBINATION: SPO11 AND RELATED PROTEINS

SPO11 is a topoisomerase variant required for the initiation of homologous recombination. Human and mouse SPO11 are about 80% homologous, but are quite different from other eukaryotic homologs. In both yeast and mammals, DSB initiation during leptotene requires SPO11, as demonstrated by recombination and synapsis defects in both organisms when expression of this gene is ablated *(15)*. In mice, disruption of *Spo11* results in defective meiosis and in both males and females *(28,29)*. DSB breaks do not form. Homologous recombination synapsis defects are present in the *Spo11–/–* mice resulting in apoptosis during early spermatocyte prophase. Interestingly, disruption of *Atm (30,31)*, *Dmc1 (32,33)*, *Mei1 (34,35)*, and *Morc (36)* result in an altered SPO11 localization and/or expression suggesting that SPO11 may have additional roles in synapsis. Not surprisingly, targeted deletion of these genes in other mouse models result in similar spermatogenic deficiencies. Likewise, the *Mei1* mutant mouse shows similarities to the *Spo11*-deficient mice, suggesting that it may work together with Spo11 in DSB formation.

SPO11 is then displaced from the DSB site by Mre11, which is abundantly expressed during early meiotic prophase *(37)*. Mutation of *Mre11* blocks meiotic recombination. This protein works in a multiprotein complex including RAD50, p200, p400, and NBS1, all of which are required for meiotic recombination. Other proteins (reviewed in ref. *15*) in complex with MRE11 generate 3′ overhangs from DSBs, providing substrates for factors like Rad51 involved in SEI formation *(13,15)*. Rad51 functions in recombination and DNA repair of DSBs that occur in meiosis, although the *Rad51* deletion is a preimplantation lethal mutation indicating a key role early in development.

2.1.2. SC PROTEINS

When the homologous chromosomes must pair and recombine, the chromosomes link through a supramolecular proteinacious structure (comprised of a complex aggregate of SYCP1, 2, and 3 proteins) known as the SC. SC formation facilitates recombination by stabilizing interaction between homologs and through interaction with proteins involved in recombination, such as Msh4-Msh5 and Rad 51 *(13,16,20)*.

Experimental models have used *S. cerevisiase* where SC formation is better understood than in mammals. These organisms are easier to genetically manipulate. In both yeast and mammals, this structure is comprised of lateral elements, central elements, and transverse elements that link the first two (Fig. 2; ref. *18*). The Zmm-family

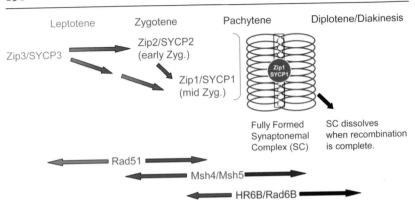

Fig. 2. Overview of synaptonemal complex formation in propase I. The synapton-menal complex forms during Leptotene and Zygotene and both stabilizes pairing of homologous chromosomes and interacts with proteins such as Rad51, Msh4-Msh5, and HR6B/Rad6 to facilitate recombination. Zip3/SYCP3 expression begins during Leptotene. It promotes association of Zip2/SYCP2 with chromosomes during early Zygotene which drives Zip1/SYCP1 polymerization along the length of each pair of homologs during mid-Zygotene. SYCP3 is first expressed and associates with condensing chromatids during Leptotene. It directs interaction of SYCP2 with the lateral element of the homologous pair during early Zygotene. Both SYCP2 and SYCP3 on the lateral element of each homologous pair then mediate association of SYCP1 with the central element. The synaptonemal complex persists through Pachytene and dissolves in Diplotene/Diakinesis when recombination is complete and spermatocyte development progresses to Metaphase I.

proteins, Zip1, Zip2, and Zip3, are the main SC structural proteins in yeast. Zip3 directs association of Zip2 with chromosomes, promoting Zip1 polymerization along the length of the homolog and presumably at the center where it makes up the central element *(16,20)*. Zmm-family proteins interact physically and genetically with Mre11, Msh4, and Msh5, which are important for recombination, suggesting an additional role for these structural proteins in progression through prophase I *(20)*.

Mammalian core SC proteins SCP1, 2, and 3 have minimal struc-tural homology but considerable secondary structure and functional homology with Zmm-family proteins. The lateral elements of the SC are formed by SCP2 and SCP3 and the central and transverse elements are composed of SCP1 polymers *(18)*. Spermatocytes in the *Sycp1*-null mice are arrested at pachytene, with a few cells reaching diplotene stage of meiosis. *Scp2* has not been deleted in mice, but it expressed during the meiotic prophase in the rat *(38)*. Targeted deletion of *Sycp3* results in male sterility because of apoptosis during meiotic prophase as a result synapsis failure *(39,40)*. The azoospermic phenotype of men with mutant SYCP3, the human homolog of SCP3, because of failed synapsis during prophase I indicates that mammalian SCP proteins facilitate chromosomal synapsis and recombination in a similar way to Zmm-family proteins in yeast *(41)*.

FKBP6 is another protein that localizes to the regions of chromosome synapsis and deletion of this gene results in the absence of normal pachytene spermatocytes and evidence of abnormal chromosome pairing and misalignments between homologous chromosomes *(42)*. Deletion of exon 8 of *Fkbp6* is the basis of the aspermia mutation observed in rats *(42)*.

2.1.3. RAD51

Rad51 expression is initiated during leptotene and peaks during mid- to late-zygotene (Fig. 3; ref. *17*). Given this window of expression, it is not surprising that Rad51 interacts with factors important in synapsis and SEI formation. A physical interaction between Zip3 and Rad51 has been observed despite little co-localization of these factors *(16)*. Because SC formation ends in late zygotene, it is possible that little co-localization between Rad51 and Zip3 is observed because of differences of peak expression times of these factors. Alternatively, Rad51 and Zip3 co-localization may only be observed at sites of recombination. SEI formation occurs during zygotene, which coincides with peak expression of Rad51. Other studies demonstrate that Rad51 forms a filament on single-stranded DNA and catalyzes strand exchange with homologous double-stranded DNA *(20,21)*. The Msh4-Msh5 (Fig. 5) heterodimer may stabilize this process, consistent with similarities in spatial and temporal expression patterns between these factors *(13,17)*.

2.1.4. MSH4-MSH5 HETERODIMER

The meiosis-specific expression of the homologs of the *Escherichia coli* MutHLS system is of particular interest. Mammalian *Msh4* and *Msh5* are expressed exclusively in germ cells and have a high homology to these same factors in yeast at core functional regions: the DNA-binding helix-loop-helix motif and the adenosine triphosphatase region *(10,43–45)*. MSH4 is meiosis-specific but is not involved in mismatch correction. The role of this protein is to ensure reciprocal recombination and segregation at meiosis I. MLH3 is also present in spermatocytes and co-immunoprecipitates with MSH4.

Msh4 or *Msh5* knockout mice exhibit chromosomal pairing and form DSBs but cannot complete synapsis resulting in a failure of primary spermatocytes at the zygotene/pachytene checkpoint *(10,13)*. These results

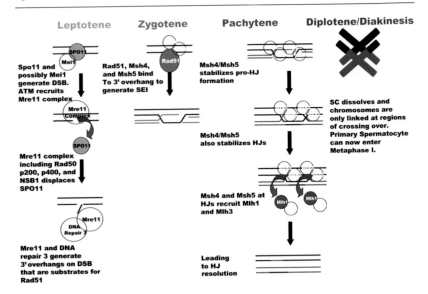

Fig. 3. Overview of homologous recombination during prophase I of meiosis I. Double-stranded breaks are induced by SPO11 and possibly Mei1. ATM is recruited to the double-stranded break where it recruits the Mre11 complex, displacing SPO11. The Mre11 complex generates the 3 single-stranded overhang that is the substrate for Rad51 which catalyzes formation of the single-end invasion intermediate along with Msh4 and Msh5. The Msh4-Msh5 heterodimer then mediates conversion of the single-end invasion intermediate to a proto-Holliday junction and then to a Holliday junction. It then recruits the Mlh1-Mlh3 heterodimer to the Holliday junction to mediate resolution of this structure. The Synatonemal complex then dissolves during Diplotene/Diakinesis leaving only the sites of crossover linked on homologous chromosomes. Once Holliday junctions are resolved and the synaptonemal complexes degrade, the germ cell is ready to transition to Metaphase I.

are consistent with other studies that define the function of Msh4-Msh5 in detail.

Msh4-Msh5 co-localize in vivo with Rad51 in mammals *(17)* and Rad51 and Zmm-family proteins in yeast *(10,16)*, indicating that Msh4-Msh5 is vital for the completion of synapsis that must take place before the transition into pachytene. Expression of Msh4 peaks during mid- to late-zygotene along with Rad51, suggesting that the Msh4-Msh5 heterocomplex acts in concert with Rad51 to promote SEI formation *(17)*. Msh4-Msh5 also seems to promote HJ formation through stabilization of an intermediate proto-HJ (pHJ) structure *(13,19)*. The Msh4-Msh5 heterocomplex binds with high affinity to a pHJ, triggering the exchange of adenosine 5′-diphosphate for adenosine 5′-triphosphate at the adenosine 5′-triphosphate-binding site, causing a sliding clamp to bind to the pHJ. This binding event stabilizes the pHJ and facilitates extension of the 3'-end by DNA polymerase, generating two adjacent HJs, which promotes the loading of more clamps onto the structure *(19)*. Msh4-Msh5 heterodimers recruit Mlh1-Mlh3 heterodimers to resolve the HJ and complete recombination *(17,19)*.

2.1.5. MLH3 AND MLH1

Mlh3 encodes a DNA repair protein that interacts with MLH1. Together they play a role in the maintenance of genomic integrity. Studies suggest a functional redundancy of this protein with Pms1 and Pms2. Targeted deletion of *Mlh3* in mice results in an arrest at metaphase with apoptosis *(46)*. Primary spermatocytes of *Mlh3* knockout mice fail at metaphase because of misaggregation of chromosomes. Mlh1–/– germ cells, in contrast, fail at the end of prophase I, suggesting that Mlh3 binds to recombination sites and subsequently recruits Mlh1 *(11)*. The presence of an Mlh1-binding site on Mlh3 *(46)* and later work showing a delay in co-localization of Mlh1 and Mlh3 at Msh4-postive foci during pachytene confirms these findings (Fig. 3; refs. *17* and *22*). Mlh1 and Mlh3 localize to recombination nodules during pachytene and diplotene, where they facilitate recombination and chaismata separation. During the progression from diplotene to metaphase 1, the number of Mlh1-Mlh3 foci decreased to zero, suggesting that these proteins are involved in resolution of chiasmata and prophase I to metaphase I transition *(22)*.

Recent data indicating that Mlh1-Mlh3 heterodimers resolve HJs during mid- to late-pachytene is bolstered by findings from earlier studies and from results in humans *(11,12,22,24)*. Genetic analysis in yeast and co-immunoprecipitation with mammalian proteins demonstrate both a physical and genetic interaction between Msh4 and Mlh3 that is further substantiated by co-localization experiments in mammalian germ cells *(17,24)*.

Loss of *MLH1* expression in human males results in a phenotype of azoospermia similar to that observed in mice *(11,47)*. Another study found that men with nonobstructive azoospermia had a smaller number of Mlh1-positive foci and less primary spermatids at the pachytene stage of meiosis. There were also more gaps (discontinuities) and splits (unpaired chromosomes) in men with nonobstructive azoospermia than in normal controls or men with obstructive azoospermia *(12)*, suggesting that reduced Mlh1 expression adversely affects recombination and may promote germ cell failure. Progression of germ cells through meiosis I was also absent in individuals with a truncation in SYCP3, the human homolog of SCP3. The C-terminal region of

SYCP3 was shortened in these individuals, preventing association with other SYCP3 proteins and presumably ablating SC formation. Mismatch repair mutations are observed in men with nonobstructive azoospermia that match results obtained from mouse studies, indicating that these mutations could account for some previously inexplicable cases of azoospermia.

3. OTHER DNA REPAIR-RELATED PROTEINS AND MALE INFERTILITY

3.1. Retinoblastoma

Mutational inactivation of Rb1 causes alteration or ablation of Rb protein expression leading to development of retinoblastoma (RB), a highly malignant pediatric ocular cancer. Loss of functional Rb leads to tumorogenesis via loss of cell cycle control (48,49) or impairment of the DNA damage repair pathway (50,51). O6-methylguanine-DNA methyltransferase (MGMT) is involved in the repair of DSBs induced by alkylating agents in vitro (52) and is important for the recognition of these lesions by mismatch repair proteins in vivo (53,54). The MGMT promoter is hyper-methylated in some patients with RB, leading to reduced or absent MGMT expression and consequent reduction in DNA damage repair (50).

Not surprisingly, patients with RB also display similar Mlh1 deficiencies, also resulting from Mlh1 promoter hyper-methylation (51). Inactivation of Mlh1 in RB patients can lead to microsatellite instability as well as reduction in DNA damage repair, both of which promote cancer progression as demonstrated by findings of Mlh1 and Msh2 and other DNA damage repair pathway proteins such as Mlh3 in hereditary nonpolyposis colon cancer lineages (51,55–57). Results from these studies demonstrate that the Rb protein interacts with mismatch repair pathway proteins during DNA damage repair in somatic cells.

3.2. The Ubiquitin–Proteasome Pathway

The ubiquitin–proteasome pathway is important for protein degradation (58) and other cellular processes including chromatin remodeling (59,60). Ubiquitination of a protein substrate requires the action of three enzymes: a ubiquitin-activating enzyme (E1) that converts ubiquitin into a form in which it can bind, a ubiquitin-conjugating enzyme (E2) that brings the ubiquitin molecule to its target, and finally a ubiquitin ligase (E3) that catalyzes binding of ubiquitin with the substrate (61). The testis is one of the regions of maximal ubiquitin–proteasome pathway activity in mammals (62) where it functions in chromatin condensation during meiotic prophase I and in postmeiotic chromatin condensation during spermiation *(63,64)*.

3.2.1. HRAD6B UBIQUITIN-CONJUGATING ENZYME (HR6B)

Immature male mice deficient in the Hr6b ubiquitin-conjugating enzyme experience germ cell failure in the first wave of spermatogenesis coincident with meiosis I. Pachytene spermatocytes show less condensed chromatin leading to an overall reduction in SC width and premature breakdown of these complexes at telomeres *(63)*. These results indicate that chromatin condensation during synapsis is important for proper SC formation and maintenance.

Homologous recombination was increased in *hr6b–/–* primary spermatocytes as indicated by an increased number of Mlh1-positive foci. This increase in recombination can be explained by increased accessibility of SPO11 to chromatin to initiate DSBs as a result of looser chromatin structure *(63)*.

HR6B, also known as Rad6B, is also involved in DNA damage repair in somatic cells (Fig. 4). Rad6B is recruited to chromatin upon DNA damage by exogenous (UV light, toxin exposure) or endogenous (free radical) agents by the RING finger protein Rad18 *(65,66)*. Rad6 associates with DNA where it mediates both error-free and error-prone postreplication repair, which is a different mechanism of DNA damage repair than mismatch repair *(65)*. Both Rad6 and Rad18 mutants in yeast can be suppressed by Srs2, which is involved in DNA damage repair through homologous recombination. It is possible that this suppressor mutation is effective because it allows DNA damage repair by homologous recombination to compensate for damaged post-replication repair *(67)*. Mammalian *Rad18–/–* ES cells also have increased sister chromatid exchange indicative of increased homologous recombination because of loss of Rad18 expression. Sister chromatid exchange increases still further in Rad18 knockout embryonic stem cells when they are exposed to UV light or toxins, suggesting that homologous recombination can compensate in part for an impaired postreplication repair pathway *(66)*.

3.2.2. THE FANCONI ANEMIA PROTEIN COMPLEX GENES AND DEFECTIVE GERM CELL PROLIFERATION

Fanconi anemia genes play an important role in male and female fertility. This is of importance because Fanconi anemia is a DNA damage repair disease. These proteins function in the response pathway that involves the BRCA1 and BRCA2 breast cancer susceptibility genes. Patients with Fanconi anemia are sensitive to DNA cross-linking agents. One of the most important steps in the pathway involves the

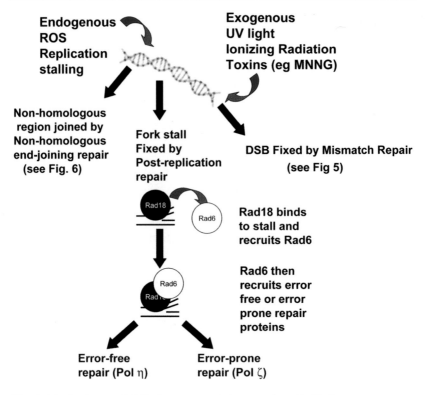

Fig. 4. Mechanisms of DNA damage repair in somatic cells. Endogenous stresses (free radicals) or exogenous agents (UV light, Ionizing radiation, toxins) cause DNA damage that the cell must either repair or undergo apoptosis to preserve integrity of its genome. Cells can repair this damage by double-stranded break repair (*see* Fig. 5), nonhomlogous end joining (*see* Fig. 6), or post-replication repair. Post-replication repair fixes lesions in DNA that result in stalled replication forks. Rad18 binds to the stalled replication fork and recruits Rad6. Rad6 then recruits either DNA polymerase η to promote error-free repair or DNA polymerase ζ that promotes error-prone repair.

mono-ubiquitination of FANCD2 that changes the subcellular localization of this protein to distinct foci in the nucleus. Targeted deletion of the Franca genes results in germ cell deficiencies resulting from defective proliferation of the germ cells *(68–74)*.

Nadler and Braun showed that loss of the Fanconi anemia complementation group C locus (Fancc) results in germ cell loss that occurs at the time of the mitotic proliferation of the primordial germ cells *(72)*. Similarly, *Pog* gene defects, which underlie the germ cell deficient *(gcd)* mutant mouse phenotype, are consistent with an association with Fanconi anemia *(70,75)*. *Pog* or *PHF9* encodes an E3 ubiquitin ligase associated with Fanconi anemia. It is thought

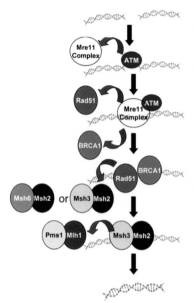

Double Standed Break induced by endogenous or exogenous agents

ATM binds to the DSB and recruits the Mre11 complex

Mre11 complex then recruits Rad51, BRCA1, and other proteins to the DSB site to initiate homologous recombination

Rad51 and BRCA1 recruit Msh2/Msh3 heterodimer or Msh2/Msh6 heterodimer to stabilize HJ formation

Msh2/Msh3 heterodimer recruits Mlh1/Pms1 heterodimer which resolves HJs

Break is repaired and cell can resume normal processes

Fig. 5. Endogenous or exogenous agents can cause double-stranded break repair in somatic cells. Induction of a double-stranded break leads to activation of ATM and its movement to the site of DNA damage where it recruits the Mre11 complex. The Mre11 complex then recruits Rad51, BRCA1, and other factors to the double-stranded break to initiate homologous recombination. Rad51 and BRCA1 in turn recruit either an Msh2-Msh6 or an Msh2-Msh3 heterodimer to the site of recombination where it helps stabilize Holliday junction formation and to recruit Mlh1-Pms1. Thus, Msh2-Msh3 (or Msh2-Msh6) catalyzes the resolution of this structure. These factors then resolve the Holliday junction and repair the break allowing the cell cycle to progress.

that this is a component of the Fanconi anemia protein core complex, possibly a catalytic subunit, required for FANCD2 monoubiquitination *(70)*.

3.3. Ataxia Telangiectasia/ATR

Men with ataxia telangiectasia (ATM) have gonadal atrophy and azoospermia because of failure of primary spermatocytes at the leptotene/zygotene transition *(76)*. This phenotype is identical to the mouse phenotype *(30)*. ATM is expressed in germ cells from B-type spermatagonia through pachytene *(77)*. ATM self-activates by autophosphorylation in the presence of DSBs, whether they are induced by SPO11 in meiosis or by exogenous factors in somatic cells *(78,79)* (Fig. 5). Because ATM is a kinase, it then phosphorylates Histone H2AX, which then becomes a substrate for the Mre11 complex during

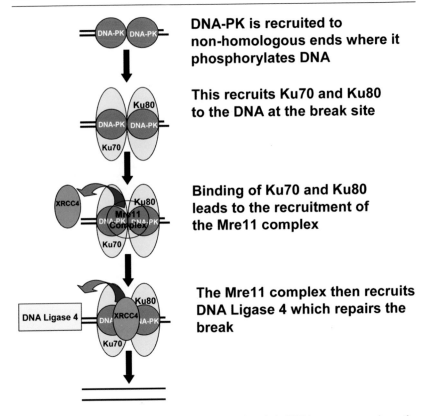

DNA-PK is recruited to non-homologous ends where it phosphorylates DNA

This recruits Ku70 and Ku80 to the DNA at the break site

Binding of Ku70 and Ku80 leads to the recruitment of the Mre11 complex

The Mre11 complex then recruits DNA Ligase 4 which repairs the break

Fig. 6. Nonhomologous end joining repair. A break in DNA can occur where the ends are not complimentary. In this case, DNA phosphokinase (DNA-PK) binds to and phosphorylates histones at the non-homologous break site. Binding of DNA-PK recruits Ku70 and Ku80 which leads to the recruitment of the Mre11 complex. Association of the Mre11 complex with Ku70 and Ku80 recruits XRCC4 which recruits DNA ligase 4 to the break site.

meiosis I or BRCA 1 and 2 during somatic DNA damage repair *(80,81)* (Fig. 6).

4. CONCLUSION

This chapter highlights the many genes involved in meiosis required for DNA repair, recombination, and replication. Research in this area is advancing rapidly, yet despite significant gaps in our knowledge, it is clear that defects in genes required for homologous recombination and DNA repair are integral to the maintenance of genomic integrity, as well as to the process of spermatogenesis. It is likely that a significant percentage of men with nonobstructive azoospermia harbor genetic defects in some of these functionally important genes. Mutations in genes required to maintain the fidelity of the genome might have implications for these patients in later life. In addition, the current practice of using the assisted reproductive technologies to achieve pregnancy for the severe male-factor couples with nonobstructive azoospermia may require additional evaluation of safety and efficacy for the offspring of this select patient population.

5. ACKNOWLEDGMENTS

This work was supported in part by PO1 HD 36289 to DJL from National Institutes of Health.

REFERENCES

1. Filho DW, Torres MA, Bordin AL, Crezcynski-Pasa TB, Boveris A. Spermatic cord torsion, reactive oxygen and nitrogen species and ischemia-reperfusion injury. Mol Aspects Med 2004;25:199–210.
2. Paul M, Himmelstein J. Reproductive hazards in the workplace: what the practitioner needs to know about chemical exposures. Obstet Gynecol 1988;71:921–938.
3. Bracken MB, Eskenazi B, Sachse K, McSharry JE, Hellenbrand K, Leo-Summers L. Association of cocaine use with sperm concentration, motility, and morphology. Fertil Steril 1990;53:315–322.
4. Lanfranco F, Kamischke A, Zitzmann M, Nieschlag E. Klinefelter's syndrome. Lancet 2004;364:273–283.
5. Brandell RA, Mielnik A, Liotta D, et al. AZFb deletions predict the absence of spermatozoa with testicular sperm extraction: preliminary report of a prognostic genetic test. Hum Reprod 1998;13:2812–2815.
6. Foresta C, Moro E, Ferlin A. Y chromosome microdeletions and alterations of spermatogenesis. Endocr Rev 2001;22:226–239.
7. Eaker S, Pyle A, Cobb J, Handel MA. Evidence for meiotic spindle checkpoint from analysis of spermatocytes from Robertsonian-chromosome heterozygous mice. J Cell Sci 2001;114:2953–2965.
8. Lyon MF, Ward HC, Simpson GM. A genetic method for measuring non-disjunction in mice with Robertsonian translocations. Genet Res 1975;26:283–295.
9. Matzuk MM, Lamb DJ. Genetic dissection of mammalian fertility pathways. Nat Cell Biol 2002;4:S41–S49.
10. de Vries SS, Baart EB, Dekker M, et al. Mouse MutS-like protein Msh5 is required for proper chromosome synapsis in male and female meiosis. Genes Dev 1999;13:523–531.
11. Lipkin SM, Moens PB, Wang V, et al. Meiotic arrest and aneuploidy in MLH3-deficient mice. Nat Genet 2002;31:385–390.
12. Sun F, Greene C, Turek PJ, Ko E, Rademaker A, Martin RH. Immunofluorescent synaptonemal complex analysis in azoospermic men. Cytogenet Genome Res 2005;111:366–370.
13. Svetlanov A, Cohen PE. Mismatch repair proteins, meiosis, and mice: understanding the complexities of mammalian meiosis. Exp Cell Res 2004;296:71–79.
14. Costa Y, Speed R, Ollinger R, et al. Two novel proteins recruited by synaptonemal complex protein 1 (SYCP1) are at the centre of meiosis. J Cell Sci 2005;118:2755–2762.

15. Richardson C, Horikoshi N, Pandita TK. The role of the DNA double-strand break response network in meiosis. DNA Repair (Amst) 2004;3:1149–1164.
16. Agarwal S, Roeder GS. Zip3 provides a link between recombination enzymes and synaptonemal complex proteins. Cell 2000;102:245–255.
17. Oliver-Bonet M, Turek PJ, Sun F, Ko E, Martin RH. Temporal progression of recombination in human males. Mol Hum Reprod 2005;11:517–522.
18. Ollinger R, Alsheimer M, Benavente R. Mammalian protein SCP1 forms synaptonemal complex-like structures in the absence of meiotic chromosomes. Mol Biol Cell 2005;16:212–217.
19. Snowden T, Acharya S, Butz C, Berardini M, Fishel R. hMSH4–hMSH5 recognizes Holliday Junctions and forms a meiosis-specific sliding clamp that embraces homologous chromosomes. Mol Cell 2004;15:437–451.
20. Borner GV, Kleckner N, Hunter N. Crossover/noncrossover differentiation, synaptonemal complex formation, and regulatory surveillance at the leptotene/zygotene transition of meiosis. Cell 2004;117:29–45.
21. Fukuda T, Ohya Y. Recruitment of RecA homologs Dmc1p and Rad51p to the double-strand break repair site initiated by meiosis-specific endonuclease VDE (PI-SceI). Mol Genet Genomics 2006;275:204–214.
22. Marcon E, Moens P. MLH1p and MLH3p localize to precociously induced chiasmata of okadaic-acid-treated mouse spermatocytes. Genetics 2003;165: 2283–2287.
23. Santucci-Darmanin S, Walpita D, Lespinasse F, Desnuelle C, Ashley T, Paquis-Flucklinger V. MSH4 acts in conjunction with MLH1 during mammalian meiosis. FASEB J 2000;14:1539–1547.
24. Santucci-Darmanin S, Neyton S, Lespinasse F, Saunieres A, Gaudray P, Paquis-Flucklinger V. The DNA mismatch-repair MLH3 protein interacts with MSH4 in meiotic cells, supporting a role for this MutL homolog in mammalian meiotic recombination. Hum Mol Genet 2002;11:1697–1706.
25. Wang TF, Kung WM. Supercomplex formation between Mlh1–Mlh3 and Sgs1–Top3 heterocomplexes in meiotic yeast cells. Biochem Biophys Res Commun 2002;296:949–953.
26. Gonsalves J, Turek PJ, Schlegel PN, Hopps CV, Weier JF, Pera RA. Recombination in men with Klinefelter syndrome. Reproduction 2005;130:223–229.
27. Gonsalves J, Sun F, Schlegel PN, et al. Defective recombination in infertile men. Hum Mol Genet 2004;13:2875–2883.
28. Baudat F, Manova K, Yuen JP, Jasin M, Keeney S. Chromosome synapsis defects and sexually dimorphic meiotic progression in mice lacking Spo11. Mol Cell 2000;6:989–998.
29. Romanienko PJ, Camerini-Otero RD. The mouse Spo11 gene is required for meiotic chromosome synapsis. Mol Cell 2000;6:975–987.
30. Barlow C, Hirotsune S, Paylor R, et al. Atm-deficient mice: a paradigm of ataxia telangiectasia. Cell 1996;86:159–171.
31. Elson A, Wang Y, Daugherty CJ, et al. Pleiotropic defects in ataxia-telangiectasia protein-deficient mice. Proc Natl Acad Sci USA 1996;93:13,084–13,089.
32. Yoshida K, Kondoh G, Matsuda Y, Habu T, Nishimune Y, Morita T. The mouse RecA-like gene Dmc1 is required for homologous chromosome synapsis during meiosis. Mol Cell 1998;1:707–718.
33. Pittman DL, Cobb J, Schimenti KJ, et al. Meiotic prophase arrest with failure of chromosome synapsis in mice deficient for Dmc1, a germline-specific RecA homolog. Mol Cell 1998;1:697–705.

34. Libby BJ, Reinholdt LG, Schimenti JC. Positional cloning and characterization of Mei1, a vertebrate-specific gene required for normal meiotic chromosome synapsis in mice. Proc Natl Acad Sci USA 2003;100:15,706–15,711.

35. Libby BJ, De La FR, O'Brien MJ, et al. The mouse meiotic mutation mei1 disrupts chromosome synapsis with sexually dimorphic consequences for meiotic progression. Dev Biol 2002;242:174–187.

36. Inoue N, Hess KD, Moreadith RW, et al. New gene family defined by MORC, a nuclear protein required for mouse spermatogenesis. Hum Mol Genet 1999;8: 1201–1207.

37. Goedecke W, Eijpe M, Offenberg HH, van AM, Heyting C. Mre11 and Ku70 interact in somatic cells, but are differentially expressed in early meiosis. Nat Genet 1999;23:194–198.

38. Offenberg HH, Schalk JA, Meuwissen RL, et al. SCP2: a major protein component of the axial elements of synaptonemal complexes of the rat. Nucleic Acids Res 1998;26:2572–2579.

39. Yuan L, Liu JG, Hoja MR, Wilbertz J, Nordqvist K, Hoog C. Female germ cell aneuploidy and embryo death in mice lacking the meiosis-specific protein SCP3. Science 2002;296:1115–1118.

40. Yuan L, Liu JG, Zhao J, Brundell E, Daneholt B, Hoog C. The murine SCP3 gene is required for synaptonemal complex assembly, chromosome synapsis, and male fertility. Mol Cell 2000;5:73–83.

41. Miyamoto T, Hasuike S, Yogev L, et al. Azoospermia in patients heterozygous for a mutation in SYCP3. Lancet 2003;362:1714–1719.

42. Crackower MA, Kolas NK, Noguchi J, et al. Essential role of Fkbp6 in male fertility and homologous chromosome pairing in meiosis. Science 2003;300:1291–1295.

43. Her C, Wu X, Bailey SM, Doggett NA. Mouse MutS homolog 4 is predominantly expressed in testis and interacts with MutS homolog 5. Mamm Genome 2001; 12:73–76.

44. Winand NJ, Panzer JA, Kolodner RD. Cloning and characterization of the human and Caenorhabditis elegans homologs of the Saccharomyces cerevisiae MSH5 gene. Genomics 1998;53:69–80.

45. Paquis-Flucklinger V, Santucci-Darmanin S, Paul R, Saunieres A, Turc-Carel C, Desnuelle C. Cloning and expression analysis of a meiosis-specific MutS homolog: the human MSH4 gene. Genomics 1997;44:188–194.

46. Lipkin SM, Wang V, Jacoby R, et al. MLH3: a DNA mismatch repair gene associated with mammalian microsatellite instability. Nat Genet 2000;24:27–35.

47. Maduro MR, Casella R, Kim E, et al. Microsatellite instability and defects in mismatch repair proteins: a new aetiology for Sertoli cell-only syndrome. Mol Hum Reprod 2003;9:61–68.

48. Weinberg RA. The retinoblastoma protein and cell cycle control. Cell 1995; 81:323–330.

49. Zhang HS, Postigo AA, Dean DC. Active transcriptional repression by the Rb-E2F complex mediates G1 arrest triggered by p16INK4a, TGFbeta, and contact inhibition. Cell 1999;97:53–61.

50. Choy KW, Pang CP, To KF, Yu CB, Ng JS, Lam DS. Impaired expression and promotor hypermethylation of O6-methylguanine-DNA methyltransferase in retinoblastoma tissues. Invest Ophthalmol Vis Sci 2002;43:1344–1349.

51. Choy KW, Pang CP, Fan DS, et al. Microsatellite instability and MLH1 promoter methylation in human retinoblastoma. Invest Ophthalmol Vis Sci 2004;45: 3404–3409.

52. Bawa S, Xiao W. A single amino acid substitution in MSH5 results in DNA alkylation tolerance. Gene 2003;315:177–182.

53. Calmann MA, Evans JE, Marinus MG. MutS inhibits RecA-mediated strand transfer with methylated DNA substrates. Nucleic Acids Res 2005;33:3591–3597.

54. Kohya N, Miyazaki K, Matsukura S, et al. Deficient expression of O(6)-methylguanine-DNA methyltransferase combined with mismatch-repair proteins hMLH1 and hMSH2 is related to poor prognosis in human biliary tract carcinoma. Ann Surg Oncol 2002;9:371–379.

55. Kruger S, Bier A, Plaschke J, et al. Ten novel MSH2 and MLH1 germline mutations in families with HNPCC. Hum Mutat 2004;24:351–352.

56. Liu B, Parsons RE, Hamilton SR, et al. hMSH2 mutations in hereditary nonpolyposis colorectal cancer kindreds. Cancer Res 1994;54:4590–4594.

57. Suter CM, Martin DI, Ward RL. Germline epimutation of MLH1 in individuals with multiple cancers. Nat Genet 2004;36:497–501.

58. Weissman AM. Themes and variations on ubiquitylation. Nat Rev Mol Cell Biol 2001;2:169–178.

59. Ciechanover A. Ubiquitin-mediated proteolysis and male sterility. Nat Med 1996; 2:1188–1190.

60. Dover J, Schneider J, Tawiah-Boateng MA, et al. Methylation of histone H3 by COMPASS requires ubiquitination of histone H2B by Rad6. J Biol Chem 2002;277:28,368–28,371.

61. Wilkinson KD. Ubiquitination and deubiquitination: targeting of proteins for degradation by the proteasome. Semin Cell Dev Biol 2000;11:141–148.

62. Rajapurohitam V, Bedard N, Wing SS. Control of ubiquitination of proteins in rat tissues by ubiquitin conjugating enzymes and isopeptidases. Am J Physiol Endocrinol Metab 2002;282:E739–E745.

63. Baarends WM, Wassenaar E, Hoogerbrugge JW, et al. Loss of HR6B ubiquitin-conjugating activity results in damaged synaptonemal complex structure and increased crossing-over frequency during the male meiotic prophase. Mol Cell Biol 2003;23:1151–1162.

64. Escalier D, Bai XY, Silvius D, Xu PX, Xu X. Spermatid nuclear and sperm periaxonemal anomalies in the mouse Ube2b null mutant. Mol Reprod Dev 2003;65:298–308.

65. Lyakhovich A, Shekhar MP. RAD6B overexpression confers chemoresistance: RAD6 expression during cell cycle and its redistribution to chromatin during DNA damage-induced response. Oncogene 2004;23:3097–3106.

66. Tateishi S, Niwa H, Miyazaki J, Fujimoto S, Inoue H, Yamaizumi M. Enhanced genomic instability and defective postreplication repair in RAD18 knockout mouse embryonic stem cells. Mol Cell Biol 2003;23:474–481.

67. Broomfield S, Hryciw T, Xiao W. DNA postreplication repair and mutagenesis in Saccharomyces cerevisiae. Mutat Res 2001;486:167–184.

68. Cheng NC, van de Vrugt HJ, van der Valk MA, et al. Mice with a targeted disruption of the Fanconi anemia homolog Fanca. Hum Mol Genet 2000;9:1805–1811.

69. van der Valk MA, Cheng NC, de Vries Y, et al. Cloning and characterization of murine fanconi anemia group A gene: Fanca protein is expressed in lymphoid tissues, testis, and ovary. Mamm Genome 2000;11:326–331.

70. Meetei AR, de Winter JP, Medhurst AL, et al. A novel ubiquitin ligase is deficient in Fanconi anemia. Nat Genet 2003;35:165–170.

71. Yang Y, Kuang Y, De Oca RM, et al. Targeted disruption of the murine Fanconi anemia gene, Fancg/Xrcc9. Blood 2001;98:3435–3440.

72. Nadler JJ, Braun RE. Fanconi anemia complementation group C is required for proliferation of murine primordial germ cells. Genesis 2000;27:117–123.
73. Whitney MA, Royle G, Low MJ, et al. Germ cell defects and hematopoietic hypersensitivity to gamma-interferon in mice with a targeted disruption of the Fanconi anemia C gene. Blood 1996;88:49–58.
74. Chen M, Tomkins DJ, Auerbach W, et al. Inactivation of Fac in mice produces inducible chromosomal instability and reduced fertility reminiscent of Fanconi anaemia. Nat Genet 1996;12:448–451.
75. Agoulnik AI, Lu B, Zhu Q, et al. A novel gene, Pog, is necessary for primordial germ cell proliferation in the mouse and underlies the germ cell deficient mutation, gcd. Hum Mol Genet 2002;11:3047–3053.
76. Xu Y, Baltimore D. Dual roles of ATM in the cellular response to radiation and in cell growth control. Genes Dev 1996;10:2401–2410.
77. Hamer G, Kal HB, Westphal CH, Ashley T, de Rooij DG. Ataxia telangiectasia mutated expression and activation in the testis. Biol Reprod 2004;70:1206–1212.
78. Shiloh Y. ATM and related protein kinases: safeguarding genome integrity. Nat Rev Cancer 2003;3:155–168.
79. Scherthan H, Jerratsch M, Dhar S, Wang YA, Goff SP, Pandita TK. Meiotic telomere distribution and Sertoli cell nuclear architecture are altered in Atm- and Atm-p53-deficient mice. Mol Cell Biol 2000;20:7773–7783.
80. Petrini JH. The Mre11 complex and ATM: collaborating to navigate S phase. Curr Opin Cell Biol 2000;12:293–296.
81. Li S, Ting NS, Zheng L, et al. Functional link of BRCA1 and ataxia telangiectasia gene product in DNA damage response. Nature 2000;406:210–215.
82. Brown TA. Genomes, 2nd Edition. 2002.

III

The Y Chromosome, Development, Spermatogenesis, and Sperm Maturation

10 Germ Cell-Specific Genes and Posttranscriptional Regulation in the Testis

Mark S. Fox, PhD,
and Renee A. Reijo Pera, PhD

Summary

Ten to 15% of couples are infertile. One of the most common causes of infertility is defective spermatogenesis characterized by the production of few or no sperm (oligospermia and azoospermia, respectively). However, little is known of the molecular causes of spermatogenic failure. Current assessment of infertility is based on sperm counts and testicular biopsies with little molecular analysis, apart from Y chromosome analysis in some cases. Thus, we sought to examine whether microarray technology might enable us to profile gene expression in infertile men and define subclasses of spermatogenic failure with a biological basis. We performed microarray analysis on a small group of infertile men and then focused further on analysis of a subset of genes that encode RNA-binding proteins in the *DAZ* gene family and/or interact with proteins encoded by this family. In this chapter, we review these experiments and also discuss the target RNAs of these RNA-binding proteins in more detail.

Key Words: Microarray; Sertoli cell only; azoospermia; oligospermia; germ cell; DAZ; DAZL; PUM1; PUM2.

1. INTRODUCTION

The birth of a healthy child begins with the fusion of functional gametes, the egg and sperm, resulting in the propagation of a functional embryo. The development of male gametes through spermatogenesis is characterized by mitotic replication of the spermatogonial stem cell population, meiotic differentiation, and spermiogenesis.

In 10–15% of couples, fertility is severely compromised *(1)*. One of the most common causes of infertility is poor sperm production, oligozoospermia, or azoospermia (the production of few or no sperm,

From: *The Genetics of Male Infertility*
Edited by: D.T. Carrell © Humana Press Inc., Totowa, NJ

respectively). Further, the testicular histology associated with severe oligozoospermic or azoospermic men can be categorized as nonobstructive azoospermia, Sertoli cell-only (SCO) syndrome, maturation arrest (pre- or postmeiotic arrest), and hypospermatogenesis. Recently, there has been much interest in using modern technologies to further define the causes of infertility, including microarray analysis (2). Indeed, such analysis may both identify new candidate genes and confirm the role of many genes in spermatogenesis, including genes such as transition protein 1, and protamines 1 and 2; proteins involved in the sequential replacement of histones by transition protein and finally by protamines during nuclear compaction of the sperm nucleus; deleted azoopsermia (DAZ) and deleted azoospermia-like (DAZL; refs. 3–18). Nonetheless, studies from model organisms suggest that perhaps several thousand genes may be required for germ cell development, thus the vast majority of genes that might be mutated or deleted in men with spermatogenic defects remain to be identified.

2. GENE EXPRESSION PROFILES OF HUMAN SPERMATOGENIC GERM CELLS

Recent technical and analytical advances have made it practical to examine and quantify expression of thousands of genes in parallel using microarrays from tissue samples with as few as 1000 cells (2). We tested whether these advances would allow us to compare gene expression in testis biopsies from infertile men. We began by comparing the transcriptional profiles of biopsy samples from three patients diagnosed with SCO syndrome to those with hypospermatogenesis (Fig. 1). The samples were hybridized to a microarray containing probes for 21,618 cDNAs. Initially, a hierarchical clustering algorithm identified distinct groups comprised of genes expressed primarily in Sertoli cells or germ cells within testicular tissue and those genes ubiquitously expressed between tissue types (Fig. 2; ref. 2). We examined a list of the 689 genes that had the greatest differential in expression to identify candidate genes whose expression are specific to germ cells within testicular tissue (3). We then used several methods of gene selection to create a more limited set of genes for further exploration. Moreover, when we searched gene and clone reports for information regarding expression and function in humans and/or model organisms, we found that 239 genes had previously been shown to be either significantly or primarily expressed in the testis. This list of significant genes was then further reduced to 177 genes by removal of false-positives through a number of algorithms (3).

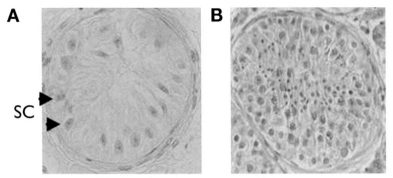

Fig. 1. Testiclar biopsies from (**A**) a patient diagnosed as Sertoli cell only with somatic cells, Sertoli cells, and interstitial cells but no germ cells and (**B**) a patient with normal spermatogenesis with seminferous tubules containing all stages of spermatogenesis.

If the individual microarray data points are an accurate reflection of germ cell transcription, then it would be expected that clones demonstrating a large variance in expression between SCO and normal samples would include genes previously known to have testis/germ cell function, as suggested previously. Examples of such genes included those that have been shown to be expressed during specific stages of spermatogenesis and sperm function, such as primordial germ cell development and migration (*DAZ, TSPY*), spermatogonial proliferation and survival (*DAZL, zona pellucida binding protein, basonuclin, T-STAR*; refs. *4–9*), various stages of meiosis (*cdc25c, TBP-like, serine/ threonine kinase 13 [aurora/IPL1-like]*; refs. *10–12*), and spermiogenesis (*protamine 2, mitochondrial capsule selenoprotein, acrosomal vesicle protein SP-10, AKAP-associated sperm protein, testis-specific protein TPX-1, calmegin*; refs. *13–17*). Another group of genes has more limited data that also suggested a role in spermatogenesis including *testis-specific bromodomain, testis-specific ankyrin motif protein,* and *testis-specific expressed transmembrane 4 protein,* as well as others *(18–26)*. Finally, perhaps the most interesting subset of genes identified was that which also included genes highly enriched or specific to female germ cells/ovary. Twenty genes were identified in this category, including six genes that encode hypothetical proteins, four encoded by expressed sequence tags, a gene involved in calcium modulation, another involved in apoptosis, and several that bind DNA or RNA or encode membrane proteins *(4,6,8,9,27–32)*.

To further establish a correlation between the microarray data and gene expression during spermatogenesis, nine genes spanning all stages of the spermatogenic differentiation and a control gene were

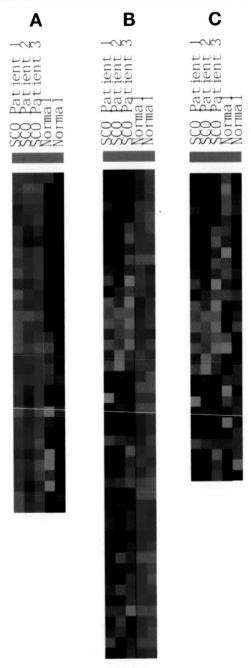

Fig. 2. Diagnosis of spermatogenic defects via molecular analysis. **(A)** Expression pattern of gene upregulated in biopsies containing Sertoli cells, **(B)** those upregulated in normal testis, and **(C)** those genes expressed ubiquitously expressed between tissue types.

selected for conformational experimentation. Eight of the nine genes were selected for their known association with spermatogenesis as described in the literature. *DAZ (4)* and *TSP (5)* genes are expressed in primordial germs cells and expression of these genes has been observed until the secondary spermatocyte stage of spermatogenesis. Expression of *zona pellucida-binding protein (7)* has been detected as early as primary spermatocyte continuing until maturation of the sperm. Replacement of histones by protamines begins with the expression of the transition proteins, specifically *transition protein 1 (33)*, whose expression can be detected after the first meiotic division. Both *synaptojanin (34)* and *protamine 2 (13)* genes are transcribed postmeiotically in the round spermatid stage of spermatogenesis. Three other genes were also selected for further analysis: the *neural polypyrimidine tract-binding protein (35), testis-specific bromodomain (18)*, and *testis-specific ankyrin motif-containing protein (19)*. Expression of these genes during spermatogenesis has as yet not been specifically detailed. The *glucuronidase* β gene was used as a positive control because expression is found in somatic and germ cells.

cDNAs were initially synthesized from RNA from normal testis, biopsy samples from SCO patients and subjected to polymerase chain reaction (PCR) amplification with respective gene-specific primers. This strategy allowed for a rapid preliminary evaluation of expression on a number of specific genes on a panel of tissue samples. In the three patients with SCO syndrome, as predicted by biopsy and microarray analysis, we found specific PCR products were only detect for the control *GUS*, except for the unexpected detection of *transition protein 1* in SCO patient 1 (Fig. 3). Reverse transcriptase-PCR enabled the detection of extremely few germ cells, suggesting that SCO patient 1 may have a very few number of spermatogenic cells that were not detected by the original histological method.

3. PRESENCE OR ABSENCE OF GERM CELLS: VALIDATION

Expression analysis using DNA microarrays has provided an overview of the genes that comprise a set of instructions for a complex developmental process, germ cell development. This list can now be searched for genes of interest in future experimental efforts (such as mouse genetic studies) or for genes that may be implicated in human male infertility. In particular, it is hoped that future studies may correlate gene expression with testicular biopsies in a large population of infertile men. Then, by combining expression analysis and clinical data, analysis might be extended toward the goal of predicting outcomes

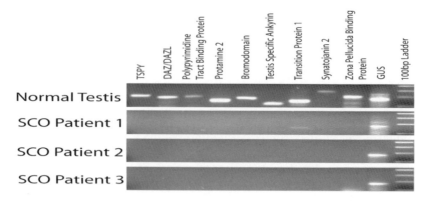

Fig. 3. Gene expression validation. Reverse transcriptase-PCR products of *TSPY*, *DAZ/DAZL*, *polypyrimidine tract-binding protein gene, protamine 2, bromodomain, ankyrin motif protein, transition protein 1, synaptojanin 2, zona pelucida-binding protein*, and *GUS* in normal adult testicular tissue and testicular tissue from Sertoli cell-only patients.

of assisted reproductive techniques, such as intracytoplasmic sperm injection.

4. IDENTIFICATION OF GERM CELLS-ENRICHED RNA-BINDING PROTEINS

Analysis of global gene expression in the normal testis identified many genes that are implicated in spermatogenesis with reported functions in cell envelope and membranes, cellular processes, metabolism, nucleotides, proteases and proteins modifications, replication and repair, transcription and regulation, transport, and in the regulation of RNA. Eight transcripts were identified that encoded proteins that could bind RNA (Table 1), two ribonuclease proteins, two members of the DEAD-box family, a polypyrimidine tract-binding protein, and two members of the *DAZ* gene family, DAZ and DAZL proteins.

The essential role of RNA–protein interactions for normal germ cell development is highlighted by the severity of the defects that result when this system is perturbed. Chromosomal deletions of the Y chromosome that encompass a cluster of *DAZ* genes that encode proteins with ribonucleoprotein motifs cause oligospermia and azoospermia (the production of few or no sperm, respectively) in men *(36–39)*. The *DAZ* genes arose via transposition of a germ cell-specific autosomal gene, *DAZL,* during primate evolution *(40–43)*. *DAZ* and *DAZL* are 90% identical; homologs are found in diverse organisms and are required for germ cell allocation or maintenance early in development

Table 1
RNA-Binding Proteins Enriched for in Male Adult Germ Cells

Name	*Accession number*
Ribonuclease, RNase A family, 11	AA609760
Three prime histone mRNA exonuclease 1	AA682626
Deleted in azoospermia 4	AA133797
Deleted in azoospermia-like	AA774538
KH domain-containing, RNA-binding, signal transduction-associated 3	AA456299
DEAH (Asp-Glu-Ala-His) box polypeptide 36	AA430052
DEAD (Asp-Glu-Ala-Asp) box polypeptide 20	AA460305
Polypyrimidine tract-binding protein 2	NM 021190

and/or meiosis *(44–47)*. To further define the function of the DAZ and DAZL proteins, additional studies have focused on localization of DAZ/DAZL and on defining proteins that interact with DAZ/DAZL *(4,48,49)*. *DAZ* and *DAZL* are expressed prenatally in gonocytes or primordial germ cells *(4,48)*. In the adult, the DAZ protein is restricted to multiple stages of male germ cells, whereas DAZL is expressed in adult germ cells of both sexes *(4,48)*. These results suggest that proteins encoded by the *DAZ* family may function at multiple points in human germ cell development. They may act during meiosis and during the establishment of stem cell populations.

5. IDENTIFICATION OF DAZ/DAZL INTERACTING PROTEINS AND RNAS

Within germline stem cells it has been established that multiple proteins containing RNA-binding motifs interact with DAZ and DAZL proteins (Fig. 4; refs. *49–53*). One of these proteins is the human homolog of *Drosophila* Pumilio, called PUMILIO-2 (PUM2). Human PUM2 shares 80% identity with *Drosophila* Pumilio over more than 280 amino acids that define the RNA-binding domain *(49,54)*. The homology of human PUM2 to *Drosophila* Pumilio is of particular interest given the well defined role of *Drosophila* Pumilio as a translational repressor that is required for both anterior–posterior patterning and germ cell development in the fly embryo and adult *(55–60)*. In addition, data from the evolutionarily distant roundworm, *Caenorhabditis elegans*, indicates that two members of the Pumilio family, fem-binding factor-1 and -2, act together to regulate germline stem cell maintenance by interacting with the 3′-untranslated region (UTR) of *gld-1* messenger

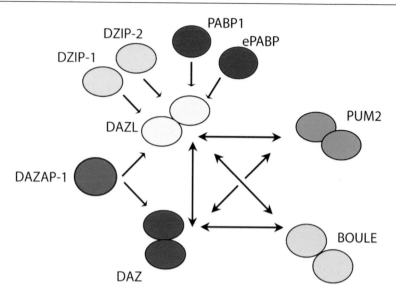

Fig. 4. Diagram illustrating protein–protein interactions with DAZ/DAZL *(49,50,52,53).*

RNAs (mRNAs; ref. *61*). A third Pumilio family member in *C. elegans*, PUF-8, also acts during germ cell development to regulate completion of meiosis *(62)*. Thus, the interaction of the human DAZ, DAZL, and PUM2 proteins allows us to hypothesize that DAZ/DAZL and PUM2 proteins interact to regulate RNA ligands necessary for early development of the germ cell lineage: allocation, maintenance, and differentiation of primordial germ cells and germline stem cells.

In model organisms, Pumilio binds to two different mRNAs, the *hunchback* mRNA (specifically, the nanos regulatory element [NRE] sequences) during embryonic abdominal patterning in *Drosophila* and *cyclin B* mRNA during embryonic germ cell migration in *Xenopus* *(56,63)*. Similarly, the mouse Dazl may bind to the 3'-UTRs of several mRNAs, including *Cdc25A* and *Tpx-1 (64)*. However, it is unlikely that these genes are the major targets of Dazl protein given the observations that Cdc25A is not essential for germ cell development and Tpx-1 is only expressed in the testis, whereas Dazl is essential for both male and female germ cell development *(65,66)*. Thus, we sought to identity mammalian target mRNAs that are regulated by these RNA-binding proteins by taking advantage of the observation that the PUM2 and DAZ/DAZL proteins can form a stable complex and colocalize in the germ cell lineage *(49,51)*. We immobilized PUM2 or DAZL fusion proteins to beads to co-immuoprecipitate human testis mRNAs. Messenger ribonucleoprotein complexes bound by each fusion protein were extracted and mRNAs were subjected to amplification via reverse transcriptase-PCR and the products were cloned. To enhance the specificity of the products obtained, serial copurifications were performed for each protein and resulting mRNAs were reverse-transcribed, radiolabeled, and used to screen colonies identified in the first screen. mRNAs specifically bound by both the DAZL and PUM2 fusions were identified as positives in at least two rounds of screening. This resulted in the identification of potential candidate target mRNAs of which three transcripts overlapped with those of Jiao et al. *(64)*, with both groups pulling down transcripts for *transition protein 1*, *XAGE*, and *GAGE*.

6. IDENTIFICATION OF PUM2 RESPONSE ELEMENT

Given the high conservation between *Drosophila* and human Pumilio homologs, we sought additional information regarding PUM2 RNA binding by examining its interaction with the *Drosophila* NRE. Using the methodology described in Moore et al. *(49)*, we cloned the minimal NRE-binding site into a plasmid, which allows the expression of a hybrid RNA molecule, and mutagenized 11 nt, 5 nt within Box A and 6 nt within Box B, sequences described by Zamore et al. *(67)*. The interaction between the RNA targets and PUM2 was assayed for via the three-hybrid system. This allowed us to define a minimal sequence that is required by PUM2 to bind to the NRE as "GNNNNN NNNNNNUGUA," as shown in Fig. 5. In previous studies *(67)*, mutations within a region defined as "Box A" of the NRE had no effect on binding of human PUM1 to the NRE sequence; likewise, mutation of the first two nucleotides of Box A and a second region, Box B, had no effect on *Drosophila* Pumilio binding. In contrast, when we compared binding of PUM2 to the NRE within Box A, PUM2 required only the first nucleotide. Similarly to PUM1 and *Drosophila* Pumilio, however, the sequence UGUA in Box B is essential for binding, confirming the assumption that the three proteins have different sequence similarities in vivo.

We next analyzed the sequences of the clones identified in the original screen to identify mRNAs that contained the 17-nt binding sequence. Twenty elements were identified in 14 transcripts (Tables 2 and 3), which were then screened for binding with PUM2. Two of the identified mRNAs for *Hypothetical protein FLJ10498* (SDA1 domain containing 1) and *Bullous Pemphigoid Antigen 1 (BPAG1)* recruited PUM2, as shown in Fig. 6. No interaction by either member of the DAZL gene family or by the pACT plasmid expressing only the GAL4 activation

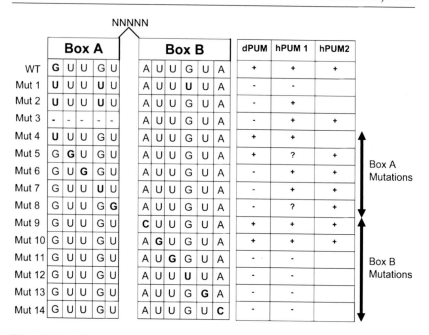

	Box A						Box B						dPUM	hPUM 1	hPUM2
WT	G	U	U	G	U		A	U	U	G	U	A	+	+	+
Mut 1	U	U	U	U	U		A	U	U	U	U	A	-	-	
Mut 2	U	U	U	U	U		A	U	U	G	U	A	-	+	
Mut 3	-	-	-	-	-		A	U	U	G	U	A	-	+	+
Mut 4	U	U	U	G	U		A	U	U	G	U	A	+	+	
Mut 5	G	G	U	G	U		A	U	U	G	U	A	+	?	+
Mut 6	G	U	G	G	U		A	U	U	G	U	A	-	+	+
Mut 7	G	U	U	U	U		A	U	U	G	U	A	-	+	+
Mut 8	G	U	U	G	G		A	U	U	G	U	A	-	?	+
Mut 9	G	U	U	G	U		C	U	U	G	U	A	+	+	+
Mut 10	G	U	U	G	U		A	G	U	G	U	A	+	+	+
Mut 11	G	U	U	G	U		A	U	G	G	U	A	-	-	
Mut 12	G	U	U	G	U		A	U	U	U	U	A	-	-	
Mut 13	G	U	U	G	U		A	U	U	G	G	A	-	-	
Mut 14	G	U	U	G	U		A	U	U	G	U	C	-	-	

NNNNN

Box A Mutations

Box B Mutations

Fig. 5. Pumilio and homologs bind to nanos regulatory elements (NREs).
Drosophila Pumilio (dPUM), human PUM1 (hPUM1), and PUM2 (hPum2)
proteins specifically recognize the NRE sequence. Several mutant messenger
RNAs with single-nucleotide changes abolish binding of Pumilio proteins to the
NRE sequences.

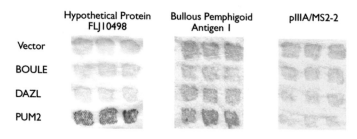

	Hypothetical Protein FLJ10498	Bullous Pemphigoid Antigen I	pIIIA/MS2-2
Vector			
BOULE			
DAZL			
PUM2			

Bullous Pemphigoid Antigen I	atcctggatattagacctattatactgtaagaatata
Hypothetical Protein FLJ10498	gttacaagagtaagaggttcttacttgtacataggct
Consensus from NRE	gnnnnnnnnnnntgta
Drosophila NRE sequence	gttgtccagaattgta

Fig. 6. RNA–PUM2 interactions in yeast. Of the 21 potential PUM2 *cis*-elements
screened, only two were positive for binding in a yeast three-hybrid assay. These
sequences are located in the 3′-untranslated regions of transcripts for *hypothetical
protein FLJ10498* (SDAD1) and *bullous pemphigold antigen 1*. RNA-binding proteins DAZL and BOULE did not recognize either sequence. No interactions were
detected with the vector alone or PUM2 in the absence of the nanos regulatory
element-related sequence.

Table 2
Potential Sequences Recognized by PUM2 Within the 3′-Untranslated Region of Each Gene

Name	Accession number
Hypothetical protein FLJ12910	BC011348
Triosephosphate isomerase 1 (TPI1)	NM 000365
Fatty acid desaturase 1 (FADS1)	NP 037534
Hamartin (tuberous sclerosis)	NM 000368
F-box-only protein 21 (FBXO21)	NM 015002
HSPB-associated protein 1 (HSPBAP1)	NM 024610
Stromal membrane-associated protein 1 (SMAP1)	NM 021940

Table 3
Potential Sequences Recognized by PUM2 Within the 3′-UTR of Each Gene

Name	Accession number
Integrin alpha 6 precursor (VLA-6) (CD49f)	NM 000210
Trytophenyl tRNA synthetase (WARS)	NM 004184
Diablo homolog	NM 019887
SDA1 domain-containing 1 (SDAD1)	BC063797
Hypothetical protein LOC57821	AK223354
Bullous pemphigoid antigen 1 (BPAG1)	NM 183380
Enhancer of rudimentary (*Drosophila*) homolog	NM004450

domain was detected, thus confirming that the RNA–protein interaction was specific to PUM2. FLJ10498 (SDAD1) is a protein of 86.6 kDa located on chromosome 4 that was first identified as a transcript in teratocarcinomas, whereas BPAG1 is a 230/240 kDa protein located on chromosome 6 that serves as an autoantigen in the blistering disease bullous pephigiod (*68–70*).

7. IDENTIFICATION OF DAZL AND PUM2 RESPONSE ELEMENT

To define whether DAZL in conjunction with PUM2 could bind to the *SDAD1* transcript, overlapping 90-bp fragments were constructed and analyzed for their ability to support binding of DAZL and PUM2. RNA–PUM2 interactions were detected for fragments 0–90, 128–218, 530–620, and 666–756, whereas DAZL was found to only bind two regions of the 3′-UTR, next to the stop codon in fragment 0–90 and in fragment 666–756, a sequence that also binds PUM2 (Fig. 7). A series

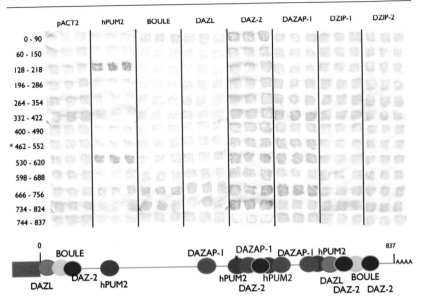

Fig. 7. Binding of proteins to the 3′-untranslated region (UTR) of the SDAD1 messenger RNA (mRNA). The 3′-UTR of the *SDAD1* transcript was subcloned into a vector and screened for protein binding via the yeast three-hybrid system. The fragments are numbered from 0 (corresponding to the stop codon of the predicted open reading frame of *SDAD1*) to 837 (the start of the polyadenylated tail of the transcript). Blue color indicates interaction between the RNA sequence and fusion proteins in the yeast three-hybrid assay. Multiple RNA-binding proteins bind the *SDAD1* mRNA.

of 5′ and 3′ deletion constructs were generated using annealed oligonucleotides and analyzed for the ability of these constructs to recruit binding of PUM2 and DAZL. In this way we were able to map two distinct PUM2-binding elements whose binding constraints were confirmed by gel shift assays competition experiments: PBE1–UNUUANUGUA (spacing between UNUUA and UGUA elements can differ up to three bases) and PBE2–UAUANNUAGU). Furthermore, comparison of sequences that DAZL binds in our analysis with those obtained by Jiao et al. yields a consensus sequence (UAUGUAGUUAUUAAAAAUUU-UUAAAUCA; ref. *64*). In addition, we identified sequences in the SDAD1 3′-UTR that may also be bound by conserved RNA-binding proteins that are known to interact with DAZ and DAZL (Fig. 4). Analysis of BOULE binding indicated that this protein can bind three regions of the 3′-UTR, a fragment near the stop codon (0–90), fragment 666–756, and fragment 734–824. DAZ-2 binds to fragments 0–90, 530–620, 666–756, and 734-824, whereas DAZAP-1 recognizes fragments

Table 4
Consensus Pumilio Regulatory Elements in the 3′-Untranslated Region of Genes Whose Expression Is Specific to Germ Cells Within Testicular Tissue

Name	Accession number
Zona pellucida-binding protein (ZPBP)	NM 007009
Homo sapiens acrosomal vesicle protein 1 (ACRV1)	NM 001612
GDNF family receptor alpha 2 (GFRA2)	NM 001495
Guanine nucleotide-binding protein (G protein), alpha-activating activity polypeptide, olfactory type (GNAL)	NM 182978
cDNA DKFZp434G1726	AL162052
Chromosome 13 open reading frame 23 (C13orf23)	NM 170719
MLF1-interacting protein (MLF1IP)	NM 024629
Chromosome 6 open reading frame 64 (C6orf64)	NM 018322
Protein-O-mannosyltransferase 1 (POMT1)	NM 007171
Casein kinase 2, alpha prime polypeptide (CSNK2A2)	NM 001896
Glycerol kinase 2 (GK2)	NM 033214
Aurora kinase C (AURKC)	NM 003160
PDZ-binding kinase (PBK)	NM 018492
Serine/threonine/tyrosine interacting protein (STYX)	NM 145251
BUB1 budding uninhibited by benzimidazoles 1 homolog	NM 004336
Nucleoporin 155kDa (NUP155)	NM 004298
DEAH (Asp-Glu-Ala-His) box polypeptide 36 (DHX36)	NM 020865
Bromodomain, testis-specific (BRDT)	NM 001726
cAMP responsive element modulator (CREM)	NM 001881
Suppressor of hairy wing homolog 2 (SUHW2)	NM 080764
ADP-ribosylation factor 1 (ARF1)	NM 001658
DnaJ (Hsp40) homolog, subfamily A	NM 005147
Lysozyme-like 6 (LYZL6)	NM 020426
Hypothetical LOC197387	BC038761.1
Solute carrier family 36 (proton/amino acid symporter)	NM 181774
Spermatogenesis-associated 4 (SPATA4)	NM 144644
Ribonuclease, RNase A family, 11	NM 145250

332–422, 462–552, 530–620, and 666–756 (Fig. 7). We were unable to detect any interactions between the 3′-UTR of the *SDAD1* gene and DZIP-1 or DZIP-2. A schematic of RNA–protein interactions suggest the potential for coordinate regulation of RNAs and the presence of a complex of proteins and RNAs that are definitive of germ cells.

8. PUM2 REGULATORY ELEMENTS WITHIN GERM CELL-ENRICHED TRANSCRIPTS

Sequence analysis of the clones identified by the co-immunoprecipitation screen demonstrated that five transcripts possess a putative PUM2 RNA-binding site (hPBE1; ref. *71*). Using the yeast three assay, we identified RNA–protein interactions for four out of the five transcripts, suggesting that this PUM2-binding sequence had been characterized in sufficient detail to be used in database searches *(71)*. Previously, we proposed that major targets of DAZL, that are essential for germ cell development, have not yet been identified. However, the constraints of the DAZL-binding element have not been fully elucidated to allow for an effective search of the germ cell profile. Another possibility would be to search the germ cell transcription profile using a *cis*-element of a protein known to interact with DAZL, in this case PUM2. A search through the 3′-UTRs of the 177 human genes either significantly or previously expressed in germ cells identified 27 possible targets of PUM2 (Table 4). Future analysis of these transcripts will identify those genes that are also bound by DAZL *(3)*.

9. CONCLUSION

The male germline has the unique ability to pass genetic information to the next generation via a highly organized differentiation process called spermatogenesis. In this chapter, we describe 177 potential transcripts that can be explored as prognostic markers for spermatogenic failure. Moreover, we propose that gene expression profiling may also be a useful tool to explore the relationship between gene expression and in vitro fertilization outcome. In addition to its clinical potential, gene profiling may also assist in design of experiments to uncover genetic requirements in spermatogenesis. This may be achieved by comparing gene profiles from patients suffering from different syndromes or from data mining, as in the case of discovering genes important in germ cell development that are posttranscriptionally regulated.

REFERENCES

1. Hull MG, Glazener CM, Kelly NJ, et al. Population study of causes, treatment, and outcome of infertility. Br Med J (Clin Res Ed) 1985;291:1693–1697.
2. Eisen MB, Spellman PT, Brown PO, Botstein D. Cluster analysis and display of genome-wide expression patterns. Proc Natl Acad Sci USA 1998;95: 14,863–14,868.
3. Fox MS, Ares VX, Turek PJ, Haqq C, Reijo Pera RA. Feasibility of global gene expression analysis in testicular biopsies from infertile men. Mol Reprod Dev 2003;66:403–421.

4. Reijo RA, Dorfman DM, Slee R, et al. DAZ family proteins exist throughout male germ cell development and transit from nucleus to cytoplasm at meiosis in humans and mice. Biol Reprod 2000;63:1490–1496.
5. Manz E, Schnieders F, Brechlin AM, Schmidtke J. TSPY-related sequences represent a microheterogeneous gene family organized as constitutive elements in DYZ5 tandem repeat units on the human Y chromosome. Genomics 1993;17:726–731.
6. Reijo R, Seligman J, Dinulos MB, et al. Mouse autosomal homolog of DAZ, a candidate male sterility gene in humans, is expressed in male germ cells before and after puberty. Genomics 1996;35:346–352.
7. Burks DJ, Carballada R, Moore HD, Saling PM. Interaction of a tyrosine kinase from human sperm with the zona pellucida at fertilization. Science 1995;269:83–86.
8. Iuchi S, Green H. Basonuclin, a zinc finger protein of keratinocytes and reproductive germ cells, binds to the rRNA gene promoter. Proc Natl Acad Sci USA 1999;96:9628–9632.
9. Venables JP, Vernet C, Chew SL, et al. T-STAR/ETOILE: a novel relative of SAM68 that interacts with an RNA-binding protein implicated in spermatogenesis. Hum Mol Genet 1999;8:959–969.
10. Maines JZ, Wasserman SA. Post-transcriptional regulation of the meiotic Cdc25 protein Twine by the Dazl orthologue Boule. Nat Cell Biol 1999;1:171–174.
11. Martianov I, Brancorsini S, Gansmuller A, Parvinen M, Davidson I, Sassone-Corsi P. Distinct functions of TBP and TLF/TRF2 during spermatogenesis: requirement of TLF for heterochromatic chromocenter formation in haploid round spermatids. Development 2002;129:945–955.
12. Kimura M, Matsuda Y, Yoshioka T, Okano Y. Cell cycle-dependent expression and centrosome localization of a third human aurora/Ipl1-related protein kinase, AIK3. J Biol Chem 1999;274:7334–7340.
13. Bunick D, Johnson PA, Johnson TR, Hecht NB. Transcription of the testis-specific mouse protamine 2 gene in a homologous in vitro transcription system. Proc Natl Acad Sci USA 1990;87:891–895.
14. Aho H, Schwemmer M, Tessman D, et al. Isolation, expression, and chromosomal localization of the human mitochondrial capsule selenoprotein gene (MCSP). Genomics 1996;32:184–190.
15. Turner RM, Musse MP, Mandal A, et al. Molecular genetic analysis of two human sperm fibrous sheath proteins, AKAP4 and AKAP3, in men with dysplasia of the fibrous sheath. J Androl 2001;22:302–315.
16. O'Bryan MK, Sebire K, Meinhardt A, et al. Tpx-1 is a component of the outer dense fibers and acrosome of rat spermatozoa. Mol Reprod Dev 2001;58:116–125.
17. Watanabe D, Okabe M, Hamajima N, Morita T, Nishina Y, Nishimune Y. Characterization of the testis-specific gene 'calmegin' promoter sequence and its activity defined by transgenic mouse experiments. FEBS Lett 1995;368:509–512.
18. Jones MH, Numata M, Shimane M. Identification and characterization of BRDT: A testis-specific gene related to the bromodomain genes RING3 and Drosophila fsh. Genomics 1997;45:529–534.
19. Ozaki K, Kuroki T, Hayashi S, Nakamura Y. Isolation of three testis-specific genes (TSA303, TSA806, TSA903) by a differential mRNA display method. Genomics 1996;36:316–319.
20. Ishibashi K, Suzuki M, Sasaki S, Imai M. Identification of a new multigene four-transmembrane family (MS4A) related to CD20, HTm4 and beta subunit of the high-affinity IgE receptor. Gene 2001;264:87–93.

21. Schultz SJ, Fry AM, Sutterlin C, Ried T, Nigg EA. Cell cycle-dependent expression of Nek2, a novel human protein kinase related to the NIMA mitotic regulator of Aspergillus nidulans. Cell Growth Differ 1994;5:625–635.

22. Gaudet S, Branton D, Lue RA. Characterization of PDZ-binding kinase, a mitotic kinase. Proc Natl Acad Sci USA 2000;97:5167–5172.

23. Liby K, Wu H, Ouyang B, Wu S, Chen J, Dai W. Identification of the human homologue of the early-growth response gene Snk, encoding a serum-inducible kinase. DNA Seq 2001;11:527–533.

24. Zariwala M, Liu J, Xiong Y. Cyclin E2, a novel human G1 cyclin and activating partner of CDK2 and CDK3, is induced by viral oncoproteins. Oncogene 1998;17:2787–2798.

25. Long KR, Trofatter JA, Ramesh V, McCormick MK, Buckler AJ. Cloning and characterization of a novel human clathrin heavy chain gene (CLTCL). Genomics 1996;35:466–472.

26. Jacquemin P, Martial JA, Davidson I. Human TEF-5 is preferentially expressed in placenta and binds to multiple functional elements of the human chorionic somatomammotropin-B gene enhancer. J Biol Chem 1997;272:12,928–12,937.

27. Bram RJ, Valentine V, Shapiro DN, Jenkins NA, Gilbert DJ, Copeland NG. The gene for calcium-modulating cyclophilin ligand (CAMLG) is located on human chromosome 5q23 and a syntenic region of mouse chromosome 13. Genomics 1996;31:257–260.

28. Scanlan MJ, Chen YT, Williamson B, et al. Characterization of human colon cancer antigens recognized by autologous antibodies. Int J Cancer 1998;76:652–658.

29. Wiemann S, Weil B, Wellenreuther R, et al. Toward a catalog of human genes and proteins: sequencing and analysis of 500 novel complete protein coding human cDNAs. Genome Res 2001;11:422–435.

30. Wysocka J, Myers MP, Laherty CD, Eisenman RN, Herr W. Human Sin3 deacetylase and trithorax-related Set1/Ash2 histone H3-K4 methyltransferase are tethered together selectively by the cell-proliferation factor HCF-1. Genes Dev 2003;17:896–911.

31. Kobayashi A, Ito E, Toki T, et al. Molecular cloning and functional characterization of a new Cap'n' collar family transcription factor Nrf3. J Biol Chem 1999;274:6443–6452.

32. Siess DC, Vedder CT, Merkens LS, et al. A human gene coding for a membrane-associated nucleic acid-binding protein. J Biol Chem 2000;275:33,655–33,662.

33. Steger K, Pauls K, Klonisch T, Franke FE, Bergmann M. Expression of protamine-1 and -2 mRNA during human spermiogenesis. Mol Hum Reprod 2000;6:219–225.

34. Nemoto Y, Wenk MR, Watanabe M, et al. Identification and characterization of a synaptojanin 2 splice isoform predominantly expressed in nerve terminals. J Biol Chem 2001;276:41,133–41,142.

35. Markovtsov V, Nikolic JM, Goldman JA, Turck CW, Chou MY, Black DL. Cooperative assembly of an hnRNP complex induced by a tissue-specific homolog of polypyrimidine tract binding protein. Mol Cell Biol 2000;20:7463–7479.

36. Reijo R, Lee TY, Salo P, et al. Diverse spermatogenic defects in humans caused by Y chromosome deletions encompassing a novel RNA-binding protein gene. Nat Genet 1995;10:383–393.

37. Reijo R, Alagappan RK, Patrizio P, Page DC. Severe oligozoospermia resulting from deletions of azoospermia factor gene on Y chromosome. Lancet 1996;347:1290–1293.

38. Simoni M, Gromoll J, Dworniczak B, et al. Screening for deletions of the Y chromosome involving the DAZ (Deleted in AZoospermia) gene in azoospermia and severe oligozoospermia. Fertil Steril 1997;67:542–547.

39. Pryor JL, Kent-First M, Muallem A, et al. Microdeletions in the Y chromosome of infertile men. N Engl J Med 1997;336:534–539.
40. Saxena R, Brown LG, Hawkins T, et al. The DAZ gene cluster on the human Y chromosome arose from an autosomal gene that was transposed, repeatedly amplified and pruned. Nat Genet 1996;14:292–299.
41. Chai NN, Phillips A, Fernandez A, Yen PH. A putative human male infertility gene DAZLA: genomic structure and methylation status. Mol Hum Reprod 1997;3:705–708.
42. Seboun E, Barbaux S, Bourgeron T, et al. Gene sequence, localization, and evolutionary conservation of DAZLA, a candidate male sterility gene. Genomics 1997;41:227–235.
43. Shan Z, Hirschmann P, Seebacher T, et al. A SPGY copy homologous to the mouse gene Dazla and the Drosophila gene boule is autosomal and expressed only in the human male gonad. Hum Mol Genet 1996;5:2005–2011.
44. Eberhart CG, Maines JZ, Wasserman SA. Meiotic cell cycle requirement for a fly homologue of human Deleted in Azoospermia. Nature 1996;381:783–785.
45. Karashima T, Sugimoto A, Yamamoto M. Caenorhabditis elegans homologue of the human azoospermia factor DAZ is required for oogenesis but not for spermatogenesis. Development 2000;127:1069–1079.
46. Houston DW, King ML. A critical role for Xdazl, a germ plasm-localized RNA, in the differentiation of primordial germ cells in Xenopus. Development 2000;127:447–456.
47. Maegawa S, Yasuda K, Inoue K. Maternal mRNA localization of zebrafish DAZ-like gene. Mech Dev 1999;81:223–226.
48. Dorfman DM, Genest DR, Reijo Pera RA. Human DAZL1 encodes a candidate fertility factor in women that localizes to the prenatal and postnatal germ cells. Hum Reprod 1999;14:2531–2536.
49. Moore FL, Jaruzelska J, Fox MS, et al. Human Pumilio-2 is expressed in embryonic stem cells and germ cells and interacts with DAZ (Deleted in AZoospermia) and DAZ-like proteins. Proc Natl Acad Sci USA 2003;100:538–543.
50. Xu EY, Moore FL, Pera RA. A gene family required for human germ cell development evolved from an ancient meiotic gene conserved in metazoans. Proc Natl Acad Sci USA 2001;98:7414–7419.
51. Moore FL, Jaruzelska J, Dorfman DM, Reijo-Pera RA. Identification of a novel gene, DZIP (DAZ-interacting protein), that encodes a protein that interacts with DAZ (deleted in azoospermia) and is expressed in embryonic stem cells and germ cells. Genomics 2004;83:834–843.
52. Dai T, Vera Y, Salido EC, Yen PH. Characterization of the mouse Dazap1 gene encoding an RNA-binding protein that interacts with infertility factors DAZ and DAZL. BMC Genomics 2001;2:6.
53. Collier B, Gorgoni B, Loveridge C, Cooke HJ, Gray NK. The DAZL family proteins are PABP-binding proteins that regulate translation in germ cells. EMBO J 2005;24:2656–2666.
54. Jaruzelska J, Kotecki M, Kusz K, Spik A, Firpo M, Reijo Pera RA. Conservation of a Pumilio-Nanos complex from Drosophila germ plasm to human germ cells. Dev Genes Evol 2003;213:120–126.
55. Lehmann R, Nusslein-Volhard L. Involvement of the Pumilio gene in the transport of an abdominal signal in the Drosophilia embryo. Nature 1987;329:167–170.
56. Murata Y, Wharton RP. Binding of pumilio to maternal hunchback mRNA is required for posterior patterning in Drosophila embryos. Cell 1995;80:747–756.

57. Asaoka-Taguchi M, Yamada M, Nakamura A, Hanyu K, Kobayashi S. Maternal Pumilio acts together with Nanos in germline development in Drosophila embryos. Nat Cell Biol 1999;1:431–437.

58. Parisi M, Lin H. The Drosophila pumilio gene encodes two functional protein isoforms that play multiple roles in germline development, gonadogenesis, oogenesis and embryogenesis. Genetics 1999;153:235–250.

59. Lin H, Spradling AC. A novel group of pumilio mutations affects the asymmetric division of germline stem cells in the Drosophila ovary. Development 1997;124:2463–2476.

60. Forbes A, Lehmann R. Nanos and Pumilio have critical roles in the development and function of Drosophila germline stem cells. Development 1998;125:679–690.

61. Crittenden SL, Bernstein DS, Bachorik JL, et al. A conserved RNA-binding protein controls germline stem cells in Caenorhabditis elegans. Nature 2002;417: 660–663.

62. Subramaniam K, Seydoux G. Dedifferentiation of primary spermatocytes into germ cell tumors in C. elegans lacking the pumilio-like protein PUF-8. Curr Biol 2003;13:134–139.

63. Nakahata S, Katsu Y, Mita K, Inoue K, Nagahama Y, Yamashita M. Biochemical identification of Xenopus Pumilio as a sequence-specific cyclin B1 mRNA-binding protein that physically interacts with a Nanos homolog, Xcat-2, and a cytoplasmic polyadenylation element-binding protein. J Biol Chem 2001;276:20,945–20,953.

64. Jiao X, Trifillis P, Kiledjian M. Identification of target messenger RNA substrates for the murine deleted in azoospermia-like RNA-binding protein. Biol Reprod 2002;66:475–485.

65. Aknin-Seifer IE, Touraine RL, Lejeune H, Laurent JL, Lauras B, Levy R. A simple, low cost and non-invasive method for screening Y-chromosome microdeletions in infertile men. Hum Reprod 2003;18:257–261.

66. Ruggiu M, Speed R, Taggart M, et al. The mouse Dazla gene encodes a cytoplasmic protein essential for gametogenesis. Nature 1997;389:73–77.

67. Zamore PD, Williamson JR, Lehmann R. The Pumilio protein binds RNA through a conserved domain that defines a new class of RNA-binding proteins. Rna 1997;3:1421–1433.

68. Yu Y, Zhang C, Zhou G, et al. Gene expression profiling in human fetal liver and identification of tissue- and developmental-stage-specific genes through compiled expression profiles and efficient cloning of full-length cDNAs. Genome Res 2001;11:1392–1403.

69. Minoshima S, Amagai M, Kudoh J, et al. Localization of the human gene for 230-kDal bullous pemphigoid autoantigen (BPAG1) to chromosome 6pter-q15. Cytogenet Cell Genet 1991;57:30–32.

70. Guo L, Degenstein L, Dowling J, et al. Gene targeting of BPAG1: abnormalities in mechanical strength and cell migration in stratified epithelia and neurologic degeneration. Cell 1995;81:233–243.

71. Fox M, Urano J, Reijo Pera RA. Identification and characterization of RNA sequences to which human PUMILIO-2 (PUM2) and deleted in Azoospermia-like (DAZL) bind. Genomics 2005;85:92–105.

11 The Genetics of Cryptorchidism

Alexander I. Agoulnik, PhD and Shu Feng, PhD

Summary

Cryptorchidism is one of the most frequent congenital abnormalities, with a recorded frequency of 3–4% among newborn males. Before sex determination, both female and male embryonic gonads are located in the same high intra-abdominal position. The developing testes migrate through a multiphase process of testicular descent (TD), first into a low abdominal position and then into the developing scrotum. A critical role in TD belongs to the gubernacular ligaments. Analysis of mouse mutants revealed a number of genes involved in this process. Insulin-like factor 3 (Insl3) controls the first abdominal phase of TD through its receptor, leucine-rich-containing repeats G protein-coupled receptor (Lgr8). The inguinoscrotal stage of TD is believed to be controlled by the hypothalamic–pituitary–gonadal axis, and specifically by androgens. Additionally, the targeted ablation of several transcription factors, such as Hoxa10, Hoxa11, and Desrt, causes cryptorchidism in mice, suggesting an involvement of multiple signaling pathways in TD. In this chapter, we review the mutation analysis and allele association studies for the candidate genes in human patients with cryptorchidism.

Key Words: Cryptorchidism; testicular descent; INSL3; LGR8; Steroid hormones.

1. CLINICAL CONSEQUENCES OF CRYPTORCHIDISM

Cryptorchidism, which will be used as a synonym to the undescended testes in this chapter, is one of the most common maladies in newborn males. The reported frequency of cryptorchidism is as high as 3–4%; however, among premature infants the rate cryptorchidism at birth is about 30% *(1,2)*. At 1 yr of age and later, when surgical intervention is recommended, the incidence of cryptorchidism in the general population is 0.8–1% *(2)*. In the last 30–40 yr, the frequency of cryptorchidism at 1 yr of age appears to have increased in some countries by 60% *(3,4)*, however, it is not clear whether such an

From: *The Genetics of Male Infertility*
Edited by: D.T. Carrell © Humana Press Inc., Totowa, NJ

increase reflects better recording methods, diagnostics, or the actual events *(2)*. The effect of the environmental endocrine disruptors affecting embryonic development and the role of hereditary factors in susceptibility to teratogens should be considered *(2,5)*. The most common form of cryptorchidism in humans is inguinoscrotal and retractable testes, which can affect one or both gonads. Although familial cases of cryptorchidism have been reported, most human occurrences are sporadic.

Testis exposure to the relatively high body temperature was shown to lead to germ cell degeneration. Consequently, patients with intraabdominal or intracanalicular testes manifest rapid decline in germ cell population *(6,7)*. Men with a history of testicular maldescent account for 5–10% of infertile couples *(2)*. Germ cell degeneration and dysplasia are thought to be the causes of an increased risk of testicular cancer in individuals with a history of cryptorchidism. About 10% of all patients with testis tumors have a history of cryptorchidism. On the other hand, men with testicular tumors have more than a 30-fold increase in the rate of bilateral cryptorchidism and a 15-fold higher incidence of unilateral cryptorchidism in their history *(2,8,9)*. However, it remains unclear whether cryptorchidism, infertility, and testicular cancer share a common cause, such as an intrinsic developmental/genetic defect, or if the latter two abnormalities are the result of the anomalous testis position *(6,7)*.

Testis descent follows the stage of testis determination, and is a part of the male sexual differentiation pathway. It is clear that the etiology of cryptorchidism is multifactorial, because several anatomical, neurological, and endocrine anomalies in human patients are associated with undescended testes *(7)*. Early surgical intervention (orchiopexy) is recognized as the most reliable treatment of cryptorchidism. With the use of recent advances in treatment, including the use of advanced reproductive technology methods, such as testicular sperm extraction and intracytoplasmic sperm injection, cryptorchidism-associated infertility can be effectively treated *(10)*. One should consider, however, that such treatment might facilitate the propagation of putative inherent abnormalities in the progeny of the affected fathers.

2. MAJOR DEVELOPMENTAL STEPS IN TESTICULAR DESCENT

The two-stage model of testicular descent (TD) in mammals separates two major phases, transabdominal and inguinoscrotal descent (Fig. 1; ref. *7*). It should be pointed out, however, that up to five anatomically recognized stages of TD were defined based on the

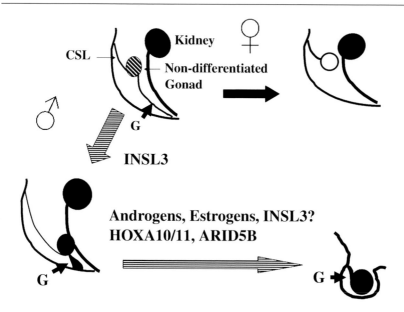

Fig. 1. The nondifferentiated gonad is located near the attached kidney with two mesenteric ligaments, cranial suspensory ligament (CSL) and the gubernaculum (G). Abdominal position of the ovary in females is provided by the persistence of CSL in the absence of gubernacular differentiation. INSL3-induced differentiation of gubernacula directs the first, transabdominal phase of testicular descent. The second, inguinoscrotal descent is controlled by androgens, estrogens, and transcription factors HOXA10, HOXA11, ARID5B, and possibly INSL3.

detailed histological analysis of human embryos *(11)*. The cranial suspensory and gubernacular ligaments are believed to play a major role in TD *(7)*. During the transabdominal phase, which occurs between weeks 10 and 23 of gestation in human embryos (in mouse between 15.5 and 17.5 d postcoitum), the testes move from their original position to the inguinal region, and by birth to the bladder neck. The high position of the ovary, attached to the abdominal wall through cranial ligament, seems to follow a default pathway. The process of transabdominal descent occurs in parallel with a shortening of the gubernacular ligament cord, outgrowth of the gubernacular bulb, and differentiation and eversion of the cremaster muscle. The human gubernaculum deposits a significant amount of the extracellular matrix rich in hyaluronic acid to form a cone-like structure at the caudal end of the male gonad *(7,12)*. In the human fetus, the second phase occurs before birth at weeks 24–34 of gestation, whereas in mice it is completed within 20 d after birth. This stage is characterized by the caudal extension of the gubernaculum, its involution and protrusion into the scrotal sac, development of the processus vaginalis, dilation of the inguinal canal by the gubernacular bulb, and some intraabdominal pressure to force the testis through the canal. In mice, TD is mediated by the contractions of the cremasteric muscle *(7)*. Human gubernacular histology evolves from a hydrated structure with a loose extracellular matrix and poorly differentiated fibroblasts into an essentially fibrous structure rich in collagen and elastic fibers. In rodents, however, the adult gubernaculum is differentiated into the cremaster muscle component of the spermatic cord *(13)*. Such differences in development, anatomy, and histology of this and other male organs should be taken into consideration when using model organisms *(14)*.

3. TRANSABDOMINAL TESTICULAR DESCENT AND INSULIN-LIKE 3 FACTOR

Insulin-like 3 factor (INSL3) is a secretary peptide hormone, structurally similar to the insulin and relaxin peptides *(15,16)*. The expression of INSL3 is limited to testicular fetal and adult Leydig cells in males. There is a differentiation-dependent increase in the level of INSL3 in the blood, and the expression of the gene coincides with the time of TD. It was shown that the INSL3 promoter is strongly regulated by steroidogenic factor 1 (SF1), a transcription factor and an important player in male differentiation *(17,18)*. The involvement of SF1 in *INSL3* gene expression provides the direct link between the sex determination pathway and TD mechanism.

In mice, the mutation of Insl3 results in high intraabdominal cryptorchidism and male sterility *(19,20)*. The mutant gubernaculum fails to differentiate, directly implying a regulatory role for this hormone in TD. Notably, surgical correction of cryptorchidism in young males fully restores fertility, indicating that spermatogenic arrest is secondary to cryptorchidism in these mutants. Remarkably, the transgenic overexpression of Insl3 in female mice causes male-like differentiation of gubernacula and descent of the ovaries *(21)*. Thus, INSL3 alone in the absence of androgens is capable of inducing first stage of TD. Insl3-transgenic females also develop inguinal hernia. The latter fact indicates that INSL3 might also play some role in the second stage of TD, specifically in the development of the processus vaginalis.

Through positional cloning of the crsp mouse mutant, our group isolated the GREAT receptor, later renamed as leucine-rich-containing repeats G protein-coupled receptor (LGR8; ref. *22*). Specific targeting of this gene results in the same phenotype as in Insl3-mutant mice *(23)*. Based on the similarity of the phenotypes and biochemical characteristics

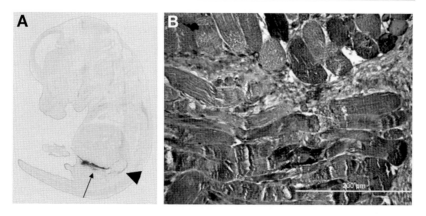

Fig. 2. Expression of mouse Lgr8 receptor in embryonic and adult gubernacula. **(A)** *In situ* hybridization of *Lgr8*-specific RNA probe to gubernacular ligaments (arrow). Testis is marked with an arrowhead. Hybridization was performed by GenePaint *(52)*. **(B)** Immunohistochemical localization of Lgr8 protein in the muscle cells of adult mouse gubernaculum.

of the receptor, we have suggested that INSL3 is in fact a cognate receptor for LGR8 *(22)*. This was confirmed both in experiments in vitro and in vivo *(24,25)*. It was shown that the INSL3 stimulation of cells transfected with LGR8 leads to an increase in the intracellular cyclic adenosince monophosphate concentration. The ligand binds to the receptor with a Kd in the low nanomolar range *(24)*. To address the question of whether Lgr8 is the only receptor for Insl3 in vivo, we have produced transgenic mice overexpressing Insl3 and deficient for Lgr8 *(25)*. Analysis of the gonadal position in such females revealed that Insl3 did not stimulate male-like differentiation of gubernaculae in the absence of the Lgr8 receptor. Transgenic females overexpressing Insl3 with the Lgr8 deletion, had a wild-type phenotype with ovaries in the normal, high abdominal position. Males of the same genotype developed cryptorchidism. Thus, the deletion of the *Lgr8* gene completely abrogated the abnormal phenotype associated with the overexpression of Insl3, providing a direct proof that Lgr8 is the only receptor for Insl3 *(25)*. During embryonic development, Lgr8 is expressed exclusively in the gubernaculum, thus confirming its direct involvement in gubernacular differentiation (Fig. 2). In adult mouse gubernacula Lgr8 is expressed mainly in striated muscles, indicating a role for Insl3 in myogenesis (Fig. 2). No specific targets of the INSL3 signaling are currently known. It was shown, however, that the treatment of the organ culture of the embryonic gubernaculum caused cell proliferation in vitro, suggesting a role of INSL3 in cell growth or survival *(26,27)*.

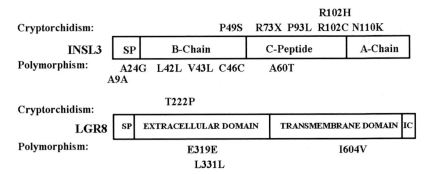

Fig. 3. Mutations of the human INSL3 and LGR8 proteins detected in human. The mutations shown above the protein were identified only in patients with testicular maldescent; the mutations shown below the protein were identified both in patients and control samples. SP, signal peptide; IC, intracellular domain.

Based on the specific involvement of the *INSL3/LGR8* pathway in TD in rodents, extensive mutation screening of these genes was undertaken in human cryptorchid patients at several laboratories *(15,16)*. The analysis of both sporadic and familial cases indeed revealed several mutant alleles. Most of them represented common polymorphisms, found both in controls and in affected patients. Some of them, however, were detected exclusively in the latter group. Surprisingly, all the patients with the *INSL3/LGR8* mutations were heterozygous for the wild-type allele (Fig. 3), implying that the mutation-dependent mechanism of testicular maldescent may be related to gene haploinsufficiency. In support of this conclusion, it was shown recently that in Leydig cells the *Insl3* gene is expressed constitutively *(28)*, and thus any decrease in its expression or an expression of INSL3 receptor in gubernaculae might be responsible for testicular maldescent.

As with other members of insulin-relaxin family of peptides, INSL3 is translated as a preprohormone and contains signal peptide, B-chain, C-peptide, and A-chain. Upon hormone maturation, signal peptide and C-peptide are excised, while the A and B chains are assembled with two interchain and one intrachain disulfide bonds. The majority of the INSL3 mutations led to a single amino acid substitution (missense mutations; Fig. 3; refs. *15* and *16*). The only exception is the R73X mutation, resulting in the termination of translation and most probably rendering a physiologically inactive hormone. The R73X mutation was found in one patient with unilateral cryptorchidism. However, the mutation does not seem to be explicitly associated with the abnormal phenotype, because at least one male relative with the same mutation did not have cryptorchidism at the time of examination

(29). The other cryptorchidism-specific mutations include R102H and R102C substitutions in C-peptide, described in patients with bi- or unilateral cryptorchidism, and P93L, found in two patients with unilateral cryptorchidism *(30)*. A mutation in the A-chain of INSL3 (N110K) was identified in a patient with the right testis located in the inguinal canal. N110 represents a highly conservative residue, therefore a suggestion was made that N110K substitution would be deleterious for the function of INSL3 *(31)*. Another study reported a B-chain mutation (P49S) in a patient with bilateral intraabdominal testes and under-masculinized genitalia. This patient had a 46XY karyotype, female external genitalia, but no uterus *(32)*. Functional analysis of the recombinant INSL3 peptides, containing all aforementioned substitutions, revealed that only P49S mutation affects the ability of INSL3 to activate its cognate receptor *(25)*. The region of INSL3 B-chain surrounding P49 is involved in the interaction with the receptor *(33)*, which might explain the compromised properties of the mutant peptide. Further functional, population, and if possible, hereditary analysis of other INSL3 alleles are needed to ascertain the role of these mutations in the etiology of cryptorchidism.

The INSL3 receptor, LGR8, is a G protein-coupled receptor with a large extracellular N-terminus, intracellular C-terminus, and a central part composed of seven transmembrane domains. The extracellular domain of LGR8 includes 10 leucine-rich repeats, believed to form highly organized structure participating in the ligand binding. T222P represents the only LGR8 mutation found so far, specific for the cryptorchid phenotype (Fig. 3; refs. *23* and *34*). The mutation was described in five patients with uni- and bilateral cryptorchidism, although some of the patients experienced spontaneous TD at puberty. Again, all patients contained this mutation in the heterozygous condition, which may explain the variability in the severity of the disease. At the amino acid level, the mutation affects one of the leucine-rich repeats and, according to functional analysis, renders the protein unable to be expressed on the cell surface membrane *(23,35)*.

Out of 730 patients analyzed to date for INSL3 variations, unique cryptorchidism-specific mutations were found in eight cases. Out of 184 patients analyzed for LGR8 variations, the cryptorchidism-specific mutation T222P was found in five cases. Thus, even if one assumes that all these mutations are deleterious for INSL3/LGR8 signaling and may lead to the testicular maldescent, this would explain only a small portion of all of the disease cases. An analysis of patients with a family history of undescended testes failed to reveal any of the INSL3/LGR8 mutations *(35)*. The fact that individuals with similar deleterious mutations are presented with different clinical phenotypes suggests that the other genetic and/or endocrine factors might affect the severity of INSL3-related deficiency.

4. THE ROLE OF STEROID HORMONES IN INGUINOSCROTAL DESCENT

A critical role in the second phase of TD was attributed to the hormonal status of the developing embryo *(7)*. It has been shown that androgen antagonists can produce cryptorchidism. This is consistent with the phenotype of testicular feminized *(Tfm)* mice and human patients lacking androgen receptors. In both cases, intraabdominal testes are situated at the level of the bladder neck with no eversion of the scrotal sac *(36,37)*. It is well known that testosterone regulates development of derivatives of the Wolffian duct, such as the epididymis, vas deferens, and seminal vesicles, as well as the development of the external male sex organs. During TD, testosterone fails to cause full differentiation of the gubernacula in *Tfm* and in *Gnrh (hpg)* or *Gnrh* receptor-mutant mice. Males of these two mutant genotypes, as well as mice with mutations of the LH receptor *(38)*, show low intraabdominal cryptorchidism. Additionally, androgens are involved in proper development of the processus vaginalis and differentiation of the inguinal canal.

It was proposed that in addition to the direct effect on gubernacular differentiation, androgens might act indirectly through the genitofemoral nerve (GFN) releasing its principal neurotransmitter calcitonin gene-related peptide. Disruption of the GFN in pathological cases or experimental animals leads to cryptorchidism. In the latter situation, it can be at least partially corrected by calcitonin gene-related peptide *(39)*. It has been suggested that in addition to the direct androgen action on the gubernaculum, the GFN mediates androgen effects on early postnatal gubernacular DNA synthesis and growth, especially in differentiating muscle cells of the gubernacular bulb and cremaster muscles.

The link between cryptorchidism and hormone deficiencies is also evident in human congenital disorders that cause hypogonadism or androgen resistance, such as functional prepubertal castrate syndrome, Noonan's syndrome, Klinefelter's syndrome, Reifenstein's syndrome, and hypogonadotropic eunuchoidism. All these conditions share a common theme of inadequate androgen function. At the same time, the significance of the hypothalamic–pituitary–gonadal (HPG) axis on the transabdominal stage of TD and its effect on gubernaculum differentiation is less clear.

The relation between INSL3 and the hormones of the HPG axis is not clear. The hpg and Gnrhr–/– mice apparently express Insl3 hormone, although the mutant males are cryptorchid *(40)*. Androgens synergize the effect of INSL3 on gubernaculum growth in vitro. On the other hand, as indicated previously, in tfm animals, the testes descend to the low abdominal position; the cranial suspensory ligaments remain in these mutants. Recently, we have shown that the overexpression of transgenic Insl3 on the Gnrhr-deficient background is sufficient for gubernacular differentiation and transabdominal descent of the gonads, both in male and female mice. However, the androgens are apparently required for the second stage of TD *(40)*. From the clinical standpoint, cryptorchidism in humans in most cases is not associated with abnormalities of androgen signaling. No specific mutations in the genes affecting androgen signaling were reported in patients with isolated cryptorchidism, although, as indicated previously, cryptorchidism is a common feature of different syndromes affecting hormonal balance in the developing embryos.

5. ENVIRONMENTAL FACTORS AND GENETICS SUSCEPTIBILITY

The modulation of hormonal homeostasis during development is another potential cause of testicular maldescent. It has been shown that the uterine exposure to environmental endocrine disruptors (EEDs) has deleterious effects on male reproductive tract development *(2,5,6)*. Experiments with laboratory animals clearly show that male progeny of pregnant females treated with various EEDs develop with the cryptorchid phenotype. TD was significantly inhibited by estradiol or the nonsteroidal estrogenic substance diethylstilbestrol *(2,5)*. The estrogen effect might be mediated through suppression of fetal Leydig cell development *(41)*, with a resulting decrease of androgen and INSL3 production. Alternatively, estrogens can directly target development of the cranial gonadal ligament and the gubernaculum, which both express estrogen receptors *(42)*. The failure of gonadotropin and testosterone injections to reverse estrogen-induced cryptorchidism in fetal mice *(43)* suggests that the second scenario may be true. It has been reported that the incidence of cryptorchidism in human populations seems to be on the rise, at least in industrial countries *(2)*. In farming communities, an increase risk of cryptorchidism was associated with exposure to EEDs *(6)*. From a genetic standpoint, the question arises whether there are specific alleles of the genes involved in TD that may have an increased sensitivity to EEDs.

Recently, an association was reported between a homozygosity for a specific haplotype (AGATA) of the estrogen receptor 1 (ESR1) gene and cryptorchidism *(44)*. It was shown that the homozygosity for one of the single-nucleotide polymorphism-defined haplotype of ESR1 variant was found only among Japanese patients with undescended testes. Significantly, no deviations from the normal range of basal serum gonadotropin and testosterone were detected in the patients, and there were no mutations in the androgen receptor gene, 5α-reductase-2, INSL3, or other genes, as well as no karyotype or Y-chromosome abnormalities. Based on these results, the authors suggested that a specific ESR1 allele might be responsible for cryptorchidism. Surprisingly, no mutations were found in the exons of ESR1 allele associated with these haplotype. We have recently screened 44 patients with idiopathic cryptorchidism from the United States and Europe for the presence of the AGATA haplotype. Although we have detected five patients heterozygous for this haplotype, no homozygous patients were found in our samples, thus indicating that the ESR1 link with cryptorchidism might be population-specific.

6. TRANSCRIPTIONAL FACTORS INVOLVED IN TESTICULAR DESCENT

Genetic targeting of *Hoxa10* and *Hoxa11* homeobox genes resulted in uni- and bilateral low abdominal cryptorchidism *(45–47)*. Both the gubernacular cord and bulb are sites of strong *Hoxa10* expression at day 15.5 postcoitum and postnatally, indicating that the abnormality is directly affected this organ. It was also shown that the spinal nerves undergo transformation, which might affect the GFN innervation of gubernacular and cremaster muscles. Shortening of the gubernacular cord and outgrowth of the bulb failed to occur in mutant mice. Cremasteric myocytes are disorganized and reduced in number. In addition to cryptorchidism, the mutant mice display homeotic transformation of vertebrae and lumbar spinal nerves. In our experiments, an overexpression of transgenic Insl3 in mice deficient for the *Hoxa10* gene does not correct the cryptorchid phenotype in males. These results suggest that although Insl3 is sufficient to direct the first transabdominal phase of TD in the absence of HPG axis signaling or Hoxa10, their presence is important for the inguinoscrotal phase of TD.

Mice deficient for Desrt, also known as AT-rich interactive domain 5B (Arid5b), manifest growth retardation, defects in male reproductive organs, and a cryptorchid phenotype *(48)*. A recent study showed an induction of smooth muscle marker genes, including smooth muscle α-actin and smooth muscle 22α, and retarded cellular proliferation in cells overexpressing Arid5b *(49)*. These data implicate Arid5b as a novel regulator of smooth muscle cell differentiation and proliferation. It should pointed out that although Hoxa10, Hoxa11, and Desrt mutant mice exhibit the cryptorchid phenotype, they also display an array of abnormalities not related to male development, complicating the assessment of their role in TD.

Mutation analysis of human *HOXA10* gene has been conducted in patients with cryptorchidism *(50,51)*. The first paper described several mutations and a 24 bp deletion in *HOXA10*, some of them found exclusively in affected patients *(50)*. However, no cryptorchidism-specific variants were detected in another population *(51)*. Thus, the significance of the detected mutations for the functional properties of the mutant proteins as well as their cause–effect role in cryptorchidism remains to be proven.

7. CONCLUSIONS

Progress in genome sequencing and analysis of transgenic mouse mutants has uncovered a number of genes involved in TD. The analysis of the *INSL3/LGR8* signaling revealed its function in the transabdominal phase of TD. Several mutant alleles of these two genes were associated with human cryptorchidism, and it was demonstrated that the function of some of the mutant ligands and receptors was compromised. However, direct evidence of the involvement of these genes in human disease is still missing. Similarly, some specific alleles of *HOXA10* and the homozygosity for the ESR1 haplotype were associated in some populations with cryptorchidism. It is clear, however, that mutations in these genes are unlikely to explain the majority of the abnormalities observed in human populations.

The question arises, "what is the basis for the failure to detect human mutations in the candidate genes identified from mouse mutant studies?" Several possible reasons can be pointed out. First, TD is a complex process, which occurs during a significant time period in embryonic development and involves a number of different phases. Each step may be controlled by a number of factors, and thus the resulted cryptorchid phenotype can be caused by a failure of multiple genetic and hormonal signaling pathways. Second, the cryptorchidism-causing mutations directly affect male fertility, and therefore are under constant negative selective pressure in the population. Third, the candidate genes identified based on the rodent studies may play a lesser role in the etiology of the human disease as a result of the significant differences in the development of reproductive organs between these species. With completion of the genome sequencing of other mammalian species, such as dog and pig, new genetic animal models and phenotype-driven cloning of the cryptorchidism causative genes may provide new clues to the mechanisms of the testicular maldescent in human population.

REFERENCES

1. Morley R, Lucas A. Undescended testes in low birthweight infants. Br Med J (Clin Res Ed) 1987;295:753.
2. Thonneau PF, Gandia P, Mieusset R. Cryptorchidism: incidence, risk factors, and potential role of environment; an update. J Androl 2003;24:155–162.
3. Giwercman A, Carlsen E, Keiding N, Skakkebaek NE. Evidence for increasing incidence of abnormalities of the human testis: a review. Environ Health Perspect 1993;101:65–71.
4. Jensen TK, Toppari J, Keiding N, Skakkebaek NE. Do environmental estrogens contribute to the decline in male reproductive health? Clin Chem 1995;41:1896–1901.
5. Vidaeff A, Sever LE. In utero exposure to environmental estrogens and male reproductive health: a systematic review of biological and epidemiologic evidence. Reprod Toxicol 2005;20:5–20.
6. Toppari J, Kaleva M. Maldescendus testis. Horm Res 1999;51:261–269.
7. Hutson JM, Hasthorpe S, Heyns CF. Anatomical and functional aspects of testicular descent and cryptorchidism. Endocr Rev 1997;18:259–280.
8. Ong C, Hasthorpe S, Hutson JM. Germ cell development in the descended and cryptorchid testis and the effects of hormonal manipulation. Pediatr Surg Int 2005;21:240–254.
9. Husmann DA. Cryptorchidism and its relationship to testicular neoplasia and microlithiasis. Urology 2005;66:424–426.
10. Raman JD, Schlegel PN. Testicular sperm extraction with intracytoplasmic sperm injection is successful for the treatment of nonobstructive azoospermia associated with cryptorchidism. J Urol 2003;170:1287–1290.
11. Barteczko KJ, Jacob MI. The testicular descent in human. Origin, development and fate of the gubernaculum Hunteri, processus vaginalis peritonei, and gonadal ligaments. Adv Anat Embryol Cell Biol 2000;156:1–98.
12. Tanyel FC, Talim B, Atilla P, Muftuoglu S, Kale G. Myogenesis within the human gubernaculum: histological and immunohistochemical evaluation. Eur J Pediatr Surg 2005;15:175–179.
13. Hrabovszky Z, Di Pilla N, Yap T, Farmer PJ, Hutson JM, Carlin JB. Role of the gubernacular bulb in cremaster muscle development of the rat. Anat Rec 2002;267:159–165.
14. Wensing CJ. The embryology of testicular descent. Horm Res 1988;30:144–152.
15. Adham IM, Agoulnik AI. Insulin-like 3 signalling in testicular descent. Int J Androl 2004;27:257–265.
16. Bogatcheva NV, Agoulnik AI. INSL3/LGR8 role in testicular descent and cryptorchidism. Reprod Biomed Online 2005;10:49–54.

17. Zimmermann S, Schwarzler A, Buth S, Engel W, Adham IM. Transcription of the Leydig insulin-like gene is mediated by steroidogenic factor-1. Mol Endocrinol 1998;12:706–713.

18. Truong A, Bogatcheva NV, Schelling C, Dolf G, Agoulnik AI. Isolation and expression analysis of the canine insulin-like factor 3 gene. Biol Reprod 2003;69:1658–1664.

19. Zimmermann S, Steding G, Emmen JM, et al. Targeted disruption of the Insl3 gene causes bilateral cryptorchidism. Mol Endocrinol 1999;13:681–691.

20. Nef S, Parada LF. Cryptorchidism in mice mutant for Insl3. Nat Genet 1999;22:295–299.

21. Adham IM, Steding G, Thamm T, et al. The overexpression of the insl3 in female mice causes descent of the ovaries. Mol Endocrinol 2002;16:244–252.

22. Overbeek PA, Gorlov IP, Sutherland RW, et al. A transgenic insertion causing cryptorchidism in mice. Genesis 2001;30:26–35.

23. Gorlov IP, Kamat A, Bogatcheva NV, et al. Mutations of the GREAT gene cause cryptorchidism. Hum Mol Genet 2002;11:2309–2318.

24. Kumagai J, Hsu SY, Matsumi H, et al. INSL3/Leydig insulin-like peptide activates the LGR8 receptor important in testis descent. J Biol Chem 2002;277: 31,283–31,286.

25. Bogatcheva NV, Truong A, Feng S, Engel W, Adham IM, Agoulnik AI. GREAT/LGR8 is the only receptor for insulin-like 3 peptide. Mol Endocrinol 2003;17:2639–2646.

26. Emmen JM, McLuskey A, Adham IM, Engel W, Grootegoed JA, Brinkmann AO. Hormonal control of gubernaculum development during testis descent: gubernaculum outgrowth in vitro requires both insulin-like factor and androgen. Endocrinology 2000;141:4720–4727.

27. Kubota Y, Temelcos C, Bathgate RA, et al. The role of insulin 3, testosterone, Mullerian inhibiting substance and relaxin in rat gubernacular growth Mol Hum Reprod 2002;8:900–905.

28. Sadeghian H, Anand-Ivell R, Balvers M, Relan V, Ivell R. Constitutive regulation of the Insl3 gene in rat Leydig cells. Mol Cell Endocrinol 2005;241:10–20.

29. Tomboc M, Lee PA, Mitwally MF, Schneck FX, Bellinger M, Witchel SF. Insulin-like 3/relaxin-like factor gene mutations are associated with cryptorchidism. J Clin Endocrinol Metab 2000;85:4013–4018.

30. Foresta C, Ferlin A. Role of INSL3 and LGR8 in cryptorchidism and testicular functions. Reproductive BioMedicine Online 2004;9:294–298.

31. Canto P, Escudero I, Soderlund D, et al. A novel mutation of the insulin-like 3 gene in patients with cryptorchidism. J Hum Genet 2003;48:86–90.

32. Lim HN, Raipert-de Meyts E, Skakkebaek NE, Hawkins JR, Hughes IA. Genetic analysis of the INSL3 gene in patients with maldescent of the testis. Eur J Endocrinol 2001;144:129–137.

33. Bullesbach EE, Schwabe C. Tryptophan B27 in the relaxin-like factor (RLF) is crucial for RLF receptor-binding. Biochemistry 1999;38:3073–3078.

34. Ferlin A, Simonato M, Bartoloni L, et al. The INSL3-LGR8/GREAT ligand–receptor pair in human cryptorchidism. J Clin Endocrinol Metab 2003;88:4273–4279.

35. Feng S, Cortessis VK, Hwang A, et al. Mutation analysis of INSL3 and GREAT/LGR8 genes in familial cryptorchidism. Urology 2004;64:1032–1036.

36. Lyon MF, Glenister PH. Reduced reproductive performance in androgen-resistant Tfm/Tfm female mice. Proc R Soc Lond (Biol) 1980;208:1–12.

37. Sultan C, Paris F, Terouanne B, et al. Disorders linked to insufficient androgen action in male children. Hum Reprod Update 2001;7:314–322.

38. Zhang FP, Poutanen M, Wilbertz J, Huhtaniemi I. Normal prenatal but arrested postnatal sexual development of luteinizing hormone receptor knockout (LuRKO) mice. Mol Endocrinol 2001;15:172–183.
39. Ng SL, Bidarkar SS, Sourial M, Farmer PJ, Donath S, Hutson JM. Gubernacular cell division in different rodent models of cryptorchidism supports indirect androgenic action via the genitofemoral nerve. J Pediatr Surg 2005;40:434–441.
40. Feng S, Bogatcheva NV, Truong A, Engel W, Adham IM, Agoulnik AI. Overexpression of insulin-like 3 does not prevent cryptorchidism in Gnrhr or Hoxa10 deficient mice. J Urol 2006;176:399–404.
41. Delbes G, Levacher C, Duquenne C, Racine C, Pakarinen P, Habert R. Endogenous estrogens inhibit mouse fetal Leydig cell development via estrogen receptor alpha. Endocrinology 2005;146:2454–2461.
42. Agoulnik AI. Cryptorchidism—an estrogen spoil? J Clin Endocrinol Metab 2005; 90:4975–4977.
43. Hutson JM, Watts LM. Both gonadotropin and testosterone fail to reverse estrogen-induced cryptorchidism in fetal mice: further evidence for nonandrogenic control of testicular descent in the fetus. Pediatr Surg Int 1990;5:13–18.
44. Yoshida R, Fukami M, Sasagawa I, Hasegawa T, Kamatani N, Ogata T. Association of cryptorchidism with a specific haplotype of the estrogen receptor alpha gene: implication for the susceptibility to estrogenic environmental endocrine disruptors. J Clin Endocrinol Metab 2005;90:4716–4721.
45. Rijli FM, Matyas R, Pellegrini M, et al. Cryptorchidism and homeotic transformations of spinal nerves and vertebrae in Hoxa-10 mutant mice. Proc Natl Acad Sci USA 1995;92:8185–8189.
46. Satokata I, Benson G, Maas R. Sexually dimorphic sterility phenotypes in Hoxa10-deficient mice. Nature 1995;374:460–463.
47. Hsieh-Li HM, Witte DP, Weinstein M, et al. Hoxa 11 structure, extensive antisense transcription, and function in male and female fertility. Development 1995;121:1373–1385.
48. Lahoud MH, Ristevski S, Venter DJ, et al. Gene targeting of Desrt, a novel ARID class DNA-binding protein, causes growth retardation and abnormal development of reproductive organs. Genome Res 2001;11:1327–1334.
49. Watanabe M, Layne MD, Hsieh CM, et al. Regulation of smooth muscle cell differentiation by AT-rich interaction domain transcription factors Mrf2alpha and Mrf2beta. Circ Res 2002;91:382–389.
50. Kolon TF, Wiener JS, Lewitton M, Roth DR, Gonzales ET Jr, Lamb DJ. Analysis of homeobox gene HOXA10 mutations in cryptorchidism. J Urol 1999; 161:275–280.
51. Bertini V, Bertelloni S, Valetto A, Lala R, Foresta C, Simi P. Homeobox HOXA10 gene analysis in cryptorchidism. J Pediatr Endocrinol Metab 2004;17:41–45.
52. Visel A, Thaller C, Eichele G. GenePaint.org: an atlas of gene expression patterns in the mouse embryo. Nucleic Acids Res 2004;32:D552–D556.

12 The Chromatoid Body and microRNA Pathways in Male Germ Cells

Martti Parvinen, MD, PhD,
Noora Kotaja, PhD,
Durga Prasad Mishra, PhD,
and Paolo Sassone-Corsi, PhD

Summary

The chromatoid body (CB) is a finely filamentous, lobulated perinuclear granule located in the cytoplasm of male germ cells. The role of the CB in the mouse has remained elusive, although it was proposed to be involved in RNA storing and metabolism. We have found that the CB is related to the RNA processing body of somatic cells and that it seems to operate as an intracellular nerve center of the microRNA (miRNA) pathway. Our findings underscore the importance of posttranscriptional gene regulation and of the miRNA pathway in the control of postmeiotic male germ cell differentiation.

Key Words: Transcription; translation; VASA; MIWI; argonaute; RISC; Dicer.

1. INTRODUCTION

The program of gene expression during spermatogenesis is based on unique rules. A very special feature concerns the process of chromatin remodeling, which involves various unconventional steps with respect to somatic cells. In addition, many genes use alternative promoters and splice isoforms specific for the male germline. Transcription in germ cells during spermatogenesis follows a highly specialized program corresponding to a series of differentiation steps occurring in spermatogonial cells, spermatocytes, and haploid spermatids *(1,2)*. In the testis, specific gene expression is in part achieved through transcription factor cyclic adenosine monophosphate response element modulator (CREM)

From: *The Genetics of Male Infertility*
Edited by: D.T. Carrell © Humana Press Inc., Totowa, NJ

and its cofactors, which demonstrate that a testis-specialized transcription machinery has evolved. This germ cell-specific program of activation and silencing of gene expression is essential for the coordination of postmeiotic events required for sperm development and function. One characteristic event is the arrest of transcription in spermiogenesis, which coincides with changes in the acquisition of the transcriptional machinery and chromatin compaction. Indeed, at the transition from round to elongating spermatids there is accumulation of a remarkable amount of transcripts whose translation is repressed for various days. Although this process constitutes an essential regulatory step, the molecular mechanisms involved in translational repression are not fully understood.

2. UNIQUE CHROMATIN REMODELING AND TRANSCRIPTIONAL REGULATION IN MALE GERM CELLS

Spermatogenesis follows a program finely regulated by the hypothalamic–pituitary axis that features the transformation of an undifferentiated diploid stem cell into highly differentiated haploid spermatozoa. Differentiation of germ cells into spermatozoa occurs in the seminiferous epithelium, and relies on a complex paracrine dialog with Sertoli cells. Testosterone secreted by Leydig cells under the influence of pituitary-secreted luteinizing hormone and follicle-stimulating hormone acting on Sertoli cells stimulates gene transcription and the secretion of peptides that promote germ cell differentiation. Biochemical stimulation of germ cells is thought to occur via the secretion of regulatory molecules from Sertoli cells, such as growth factors and proteases. Although evidence exists for the control of gene transcription from the hypothalamic–pituitary axis *(3)*, how these highly specialized endocrine regulations are involved in the control of chromatin remodeling is still unclear.

The postmeiotic developmental phase of spermiogenesis involves the differentiation of spermatids into spermatozoa. It constitutes a remarkable process as germ cells undergo an enormous morphogenetic transformation involving acrosome and flagellar formation, DNA compaction, and cytoplasmic ejection. Male germ cell-specific nuclear proteins, the transition proteins and protamines, sequentially replace histones to allow for DNA compaction and permit reshaping of the round spermatid nucleus. In addition to the histone-to-protamine transition process, a remarkable number of histone variants are present in germ cells, whose expression follows a highly dynamic program *(4)*. Many of the histone variants are testis-specific, underscoring the importance of highly specialized epigenetic events in the structuring and regulation of chromatin.

A significant number of gene promoters display a highly restricted activity to male germ cells. This notion provides evidence for the presence in these cells of a unique balance of common regulators and germ cell-specific factors. Following meiosis, the beginning of spermiogenesis is characterized by a massive wave of transcriptional activity *(5)*, which results in the activation of a number of essential postmeiotic genes in early haploid cells. To insure this efficient and timely transcription, various general transcription factors, such as TATA binding protein (TBP) and Transcription Factor IIB (TFIIB), are differentially regulated in germ cells *(6)*. In addition, some testis-specific examples of transcriptional regulatory complexes have been reported. One of these includes CREM and its co-activator, activator of CREM in testis (ACT; ref. *7*). The targeted ablation of both *crem* and *act* genes by homologous recombination in the mouse germline results in impaired spermatogenesis *(8,9)*. The activity of the CREM–ACT complex is modulated by a special regulatory system: a testis-specific kinesin, KIF17b, is responsible for the nuclear export of ACT, determining the interruption of CREM-dependent postmeiotic gene transcription *(10)*.

One aspect of gene regulation that is not fully explored in male germ cells concerns the regulation of RNA function, stability, and translation by the microRNA (miRNA) pathway. Because of the previously mentioned translational repression of postmeiotic transcripts, it is reasonable to assume that miRNAs are indeed likely to play an essential role during spermatogenesis. Interestingly, MIWI, a member of the PIWI subfamily of Argonaute proteins, associates with ribohomopolymers and specifically with transcripts of CREM-target genes, suggesting a functional connection of MIWI to RNA processing *(11)*.

Argonaute proteins are widely expressed in many tissues. In contrast, all members of the PIWI family are expressed mainly in testis *(12,13)*, although their role in the RNA interference (RNAi) pathway is still obscure. It is tempting to speculate that MIWI may operate as a male germ cell-specific miRNA pathway component involved in functional messenger RNA (mRNA) regulation in testis.

3. THE CHROMATOID BODY

The remarkable history of the chromatoid body (CB) began more than 100 yr ago, when it was first described by Benda *(14)*. For many years, its presence remained unappreciated and then its origin was debated, as being nuclear *(15)*, nucleolar *(16)*, or a derivation from intermitochondrial dense

material during the late pachytene stage of the prophase of the first meiotic division *(17,18)*. The CB appears to be a very conserved feature of
germ cells throughout the animal kingdom *(19)*. These contain cytoplasmic cloud-like accumulations of material-denominated nuage. In
Drosophila, the polar bodies present in the oocytes are also identified as
nuage. In mammalian spermatogenic cells, the equivalent of nuage corre-
sponds to the CB. In early spermatids of the rat, it has a diameter of
1–1.5 µm and a finely filamentous lobular structure (Fig. 1). Typically, it
is found associated with a multitude of vesicles. The CB is first seen in
mid- and late-pachytene spermatocytes as an intermitochondrial dense
material. During early spermiogenesis, the CB is seen near the Golgi complex and frequently connected by material continuities through nuclear
pore complexes with intranuclear particles *(20)*.

The varying localization of the CB during successive stages of spermatogenesis is one of its primary features. It appears at the nuclear
envelope in association with nuclear pore complexes during early
spermiogenesis and associates with the annulus later in spermiogenesis
(17,21). In living cells, the CB moves around the Golgi complex and
has frequent contacts with it. The CB also moves perpendicularly to the
nuclear envelope and even through cytoplasmic bridges to the neighbor
spermatids *(20)*.

The presence of RNA *(22)* and ribonucleoprotein *(23)* in the CB as
well as in all nuage material in spermatogenic cells *(24)* was first suggested by histochemical studies, whereas the presence of DNA has been
excluded *(25)*. There are indications that the CB may function as a source
of mRNA and/or of its partially processed precursors during the late
stages of spermiogenesis, when the spermatid nucleus becomes gradually
inactive *(25,26)*. In support of this hypothesis, it was found that TP2
mRNA and mRNA-binding proteins p48/52 localize in the CB *(27,28)*.

Interestingly, a major CB component is the DEAD-box RNA helicase, VASA. This protein is thought to act as an RNA chaperone and is
a general marker of all germ cells. The mouse VASA homolog, MVH,
was recently used as a marker of sperm formation from embryonic stem
cells *(29)*. The features described previously and the presence of MVH
indicate that the CB could constitute a structure underlying the mechanisms of posttranscriptional processing and storage of several mRNA
species in germ cells.

4. THE miRNA PATHWAY

RNAi and miRNA pathways are evolutionarily conserved control
mechanisms that use RNA molecules to inhibit gene expression at the

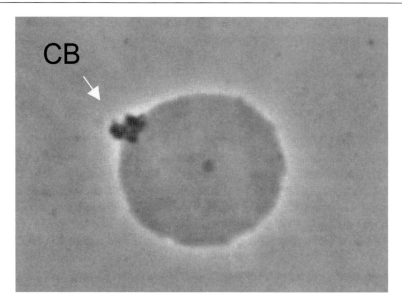

Fig. 1. The chromatoid body (CB) appears as a cloud-like, dense structure in the cytoplasm of male germ cells. Its perinuclear localization is evident in this phase contrast image. For a comprehensive review article on the CB, *see* ref. *20.*

level of mRNA degradation, translational repression, or chromatin modification and silencing *(30–32)*. RNAi has been shown to be present throughout spermatogenesis in mice *(33)*, but its function and cellular control during germ cell development remain uncertain.

Two classes of 21- to 25-nucleotide small RNAs, small-interfering RNAs (siRNAs) and miRNAs, act as sequence-specific regulators of gene expression *(31)*. siRNAs mediate degradation of mRNAs, having sequences fully complementary to their sequence, whereas miRNAs are proposed to regulate gene expression by inhibiting protein synthesis through imperfect basepairing to the 3′-untranslated region of target mRNAs *(30,31)*. Both siRNA and miRNA precursors are processed to mature small RNAs in the cytoplasm of cells by the large endonuclease Dicer *(30,34)*. Mature miRNAs and siRNAs are assembled into miRNA- and siRNA-induced silencing complexes (miRISC and siRISC, respectively), which subsequently act on their targets by translational repression or mRNA cleavage (Fig. 2). Essential components of RISC complexes are the members of the Argonaute family of proteins *(13)*. These proteins share the so-called PAZ and PIWI domains and are classified into two subfamilies depending on sequence similarity to either *Arabidopsis argonaute1* or *Drosophila piwi (12,13)*. In mammals, argonaute1 subfamily members, Ago1 to Ago4, have been

dsRNA

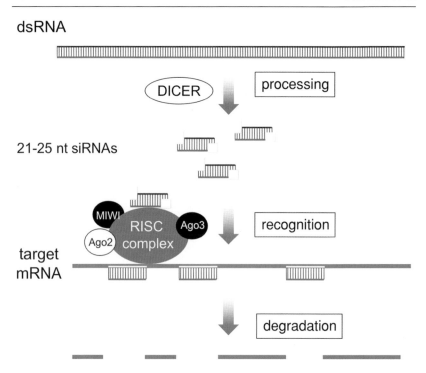

Fig. 2. Schematic representation of the silencing pathway of gene expression induced by small RNAs. The RNA interference machinery converts the sequence-specific information of long double-stranded RNAs (dsRNAs) into small, 21- to 25-nt long dsRNAs (small interfering RNAs, microRNAs), which assemble into an effector complex, the RNA-induced silencing complex. For the role of Dicer and the Argonaute proteins, *see* Subheading 4, and refs. *30–34*.

shown to be involved in the RNAi/miRNA pathway *(35,36)*. All four members of the PIWI subfamily are mainly expressed in testis *(12)*, and two of them, MIWI and MILI, are crucial for progression through spermatogenesis in mouse *(11,37)*.

5. FUNCTIONAL LINK OF THE RISC PATHWAY WITH THE CB

The highly restricted localizaton of MVH in the CB has been used as specific marker for this structure *(38)*. We analyzed the formation of the CB along the differentiation of postmeiotic germ cells and found that MVH is expressed throughout the development of round spermatids. Strikingly, this pattern correlates with MIWI distribution, which indeed colocalizes with MVH. In addition, other members of the Argonaute family of proteins, including Ago2 and Ago3, were found in the CB *(39)*. As it has been recently shown that in somatic cells Ago proteins localize in cytoplasmic processing bodies (P-bodies; refs. *40* and *41*), these findings suggested a possible functional similarity between P-bodies and the CB. This similarity included also other important components, such as the decapping enzyme component Dcp1a *(42)*, the 5′ to 3′ exonuclease Xrn1, and the RNA-binding protein GW182, all present in P-bodies and found in the CB. Thus, the P-bodies of somatic cells and the CB of male germ cells share a number of significant similarities.

The coordinate presence of various components of the RISC pathway in the CB was strongly suggestive of miRNAs production in this site. Indeed, *in situ* hybridizations using probes specific for various miRNAs known to be expressed in testis demonstrated their localization with Ago proteins in CBs. The analysis revealed high concentration of miR-21, miR-122a, and let-7a, which all colocalized with MVH in CB *(39)*. Interestingly, the use of *in situ* hybridization using oligo dT probes for mRNA molecules, the natural targets for miRNA-mediated regulation, demonstrated accumulation of mRNAs in CBs. Thus, the CB seems to concentrate important elements of the RISC complex and of the miRNA pathway.

The role of the protein Dicer in the miRNA pathway is central (Fig. 2). Dicer processes miRNA precursor molecules folded into double-stranded RNA-like hairpins to mature miRNAs. These are subsequently transferred to the miRISC complex where the effector phase of the process takes place *(30,34)*. A direct interaction between Dicer and Ago proteins may be required for the transfer of miRNAs to the effector complex *(34)*. Importantly, Dicer is present in both meiotic spermatocytes and postmeiotic round spermatids, but not in elongated spermatids. We have found that the Dicer protein in testis is enzymatically active and that it concentrates in CBs, coordinately with the other elements of the miRNA machinery *(39)*.

One additional finding that could be highly relevant for understanding the role played by the CB is the physical interaction of Dicer with MVH *(39)*. Although the role of this DEAD-box RNA helicase with respect to the enzymatic activity of the Dicer protein still needs to be established, it would appear that MVH constitutes a male germ cell-specific component of the miRNA pathway.

6. CONCLUSIONS

The functional role and the molecular nature of the CB in germ cells has been elusive and debated for many years *(20)*. Our results indicate

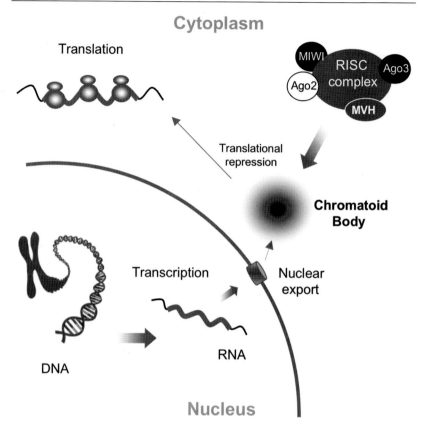

Fig. 3. Model of chromatoid body (CB) function in postmeiotic male germ cells. After transcription, haploid gene transcripts are assembled in the ribonucleoprotein particles containing RNA-binding proteins and transported through nuclear pore complexes into the cytoplasm where they are loaded to the CB. Argonaute family members, including MIWI, Ago2, and Ago3, and the RNA-induced silencing complex are also located in the CB. CBs contain RNA-binding and -processing proteins, such as the adenosine triphosphate-dependent RNA helicase of the DEAD-box protein family, mammalian VASA homolog, and the components of miRNA pathway that associate with mRNAs and direct them to storage or degradation.

that the CB would function as an RNA storing and processing structure. Specifically, the presence of Dicer/Argonaute and miRNAs reveals that the CB occupies a privileged position in posttranscriptional control of gene expression through the small RNAs pathway (Fig. 3).

The expression and localization of components of the siRNA and miRNA pathways during spermatogenesis has not been fully explored. RNAi has been shown to be active during the whole spermatogenesis program *(33)*, and many miRNAs whose expression is enriched in testis have been identified *(43,44)*. Our findings importantly expand our knowledge and link these pathways to a cytoplasmic, structural organelle: the CB *(39)*. Interestingly, the CB is endowed of the remarkable property of moving very actively and three dimensionally in the cytoplasm of round spermatids. During these movements, CBs make frequent contacts with the nuclear envelope. Continuity in electron-dense material between the nucleus and the CB through nuclear pore complexes has been observed *(20)*. One hypothesis suggests that rapidly moving CBs collect mRNA leaving the nucleus. Interestingly, miRNA precursors processed in the nucleus are exported to the cytoplasm through nuclear pore complexes *(45)*. Based on our findings, we suggest a model in which pre-miRNAs transported to the cytoplasm are loaded through nuclear pores to the CB. Thus, the CB functions as a subcellular concentration site for components of the miRNA pathway, centralizing the miRNA posttranscriptional control system in the cytoplasm of haploid male germ cells.

7. ACKNOWLEDGMENTS

The authors thank W. Filipowicz, H. Lin, T. Noce, S. Kimmins, T. Hobman, J. Lykke-Andersen, M. J. Fritzler, M. Kiledjian, J. Steitz, and all members of the Sassone-Corsi laboratory for help, reagents, and discussions. N. K. was supported by the European Molecular Biology Organization. Our studies are supported by grants from Centre National de la Recherche Scientifique, Institut National de la Santé et de la Recherche Médicale, Fondation de la Recherche Médicale, and Université Louis Pasteur. The P. S.-C. laboratory is an "Equipe Labelisée" of La Ligue contre le Cancer.

REFERENCES

1. Sassone-Corsi P. Transcriptional checkpoints determining the fate of the male germcells. Cell 1997;88:163–166.
2. Sassone-Corsi P. Unique chromatin remodelling and transcriptional regulation in spermatogenesis. Science 2002;296:2176–2178.
3. Foulkes NS, Schlotter F, Pevet P, Sassone-Corsi P. Pituitary hormone FSH directs the CREM functional switch during spermatogenesis. Nature 1993;362: 264–267.
4. Kimmins S, Sassone-Corsi P. Chromatin remodelling and epigenetic features of germ cells. Nature 2005;434:583–589.
5. Penttila TL, Yuan L, Mali P, Hoog C, Parvinen M. Haploid gene expression: temporal onset and storage patterns of 13 novel transcripts during rat and mouse spermiogenesis. Biol Reprod 1995;53:499–510.
6. Schmidt EE, Schibler U. High accumulation of componenets of RNA polymerase II transcription machinery in rodent spermatid. Development 1995;121:2373–2383.

7. Fimia GM, De Cesare D, Sassone-Corsi P. CBP independent activation of CREM and CREB by the LIM only protein ACT. Nature 1999;398:165–169.
8. Nantel F, Monaco L, Foulkes NS, et al. Spermiogenesis deficiency and germ cell apoptosis in CREM mutant mice. Nature 1996;380:159–162.
9. Kotaja N, De Cesare D, Macho B, et al. Abnormal sperm in mice with targeted deletion of the act (activator of cAMP-responsive element modulator in testis) gene. Proc Natl Acad Sci USA 2004;101:10,620–10,625.
10. Macho B, Brancorsini S, Fimia GM, Setou M, Hirokawa N, Sassone-Corsi P. CREM-dependent transcription in male germ cells controlled by a kinesin. Science 2002;298:2388–2390.
11. Deng W, Lin H. miwi, a murine homolog of piwi, encodes a cytoplasmic protein essential for spermatogenesis. Dev Cell 2002;2:819–830.
12. Sasaki T, Shiohama A, Minoshima S, Shimizu N. Identification of eight members of the Argonaute family in the human genome small star, filled. Genomics 2003; 82:323–330.
13. Carmell MA, Xuan Z, Zhang MQ, Hannon GJ. The Argonaute family: tentacles that reach into RNAi, developmental control, stem cell maintenance, and tumorigenesis. Genes Dev 2002;16:2733–2742.
14. Benda C. Neue Mitteilungen über die Entwickelung der Genitaldrüsen und die Metamorphose der Samenzellen (Histogenese der Spermatozoen). Verhandlungen der Berliner Physiologischen Gesellschaft. Arch Anat Physiol 1891;549–552.
15. Sud BN. The chromatoid body in spermatogenesis. QJ Micros Sci 1961;102: 273–292.
16. Comings DE, Okada TA. The chromatoid body in mouse spermatogenesis: evidence that it may be formed by the extrusion of nucleolar components. J Ultrastruct Res 1972;39:15–23.
17. Fawcett DW, Eddy EM, Phillips DM. Observations on the fine structure and relationships of the chromatoid body in mammalian spermatogenesis. Biol Reprod 1970;2:129–153.
18. Söderström KO. Formation of chromatoid body during rat spermatogenesis. Z Mikrosk Anat Forsch 1978;92:417–430.
19. Ikenishi, K. Germ plasm in Caenorhabditis elegans, Drosophila and Xenopus. Dev Growth Differ 1998;40:1–10.
20. Parvinen M. The chromatoid body in spermatogenesis Int J Androl 2005;28: 189–201.
21. Setchell BP. The Mammalian Testis. Paul Elek, London; 1978, pp. 193–199.
22. Sud, BN. Morphological and histochemical studies of the chromatoid body and related elements in the spermatogenesis of the rat. QJ Micros Sci 1961;102:495–505.
23. Paniagua R, Nistal M, Amat P, Rodriguez MC. Presence of ribonucleoproteins and basic proteins in the nuage and intermitochondrial bars of human spermatogonia. J Anat 1985;143:201–206.
24. Paniagua R, Nistal M, Amat P, Rodriguez MC. Ultrastructural observations on nucleoli and related structures during human spermatogenesis. Anat Embryol (Berl) 1986;174:301–306.
25. Biggiogera M, Fakan S, Leser G, Martin TE, Gordon J. Immunoelectron microscopical visualization of ribonucleoproteins in the chromatoid body of mouse spermatids. Mol Reprod Dev 1990;26:150–158.
26. Moussa F, Oko R, Hermo L. The immunolocalization of small nuclear ribonucleoprotein particles in testicular cells during the cycle of the seminiferous epithelium of the adult rat. Cell Tissue Res 1994;278:363–378.

27. Saunders PT, Millar MR, Maguire SM, Sharpe RM. Stage-specific expression of rat transition protein 2 mRNA and possible localization to the chromatoid body of step 7 spermatids by in situ hybridization using a nonradioactive riboprobe. Mol Reprod Dev 1992;33:385–391.

28. Oko R, Korley R, Murray MT, Hecht NB, Hermo L. Germ cell-specific DNA and RNA binding proteins p48/52 are expressed at specific stages of male germ cell development and are present in the chromatoid body. Mol Reprod Dev 1996;44:1–13.

29. Toyooka Y, Tsunekawa N, Akasu R, Noce T. Ebryonic stem cells can form germ cells in vitro. Proc Natl Acad Sci USA 2003;100:11,457–11,462.

30. Filipowicz W, Jaskiewicz L, Kolb FA, Pillai RS. Post-transcriptional gene silencing by siRNAs and miRNAs. Curr Opin Struct Biol 2005;15:331–341.

31. Zamore PD, Haley B. Ribo-gnome: the big world of small RNAs. Science 2005;309:1519–1524.

32. Bernstein E, Allis CD. RNA meets chromatin. Genes Dev 2005;19:1635–1655.

33. Shoji M, Chuma S, Yoshida K, Morita T, Natatsuji N. RNA interference during spermatogenesis in mice. Dev Biol 2005;282:524–534.

34. Sontheimer EJ. Assembly and function of RNA silencing complexes. Nat Rev Mol Cell Biol 2005;6:127–138.

35. Meister G, Landthaler M, Patkaniowska A, Dorsett Y, Teng G, Tuschl T. Human Argonaute2 mediates RNA cleavage targeted by miRNAs and siRNAs Mol Cell 2004;15:185–197.

36. Liu J, Carmell MA, Rivas FV, et al. Argonaute2 is the catalytic engine of mammalian RNAi. Science 2004;305:1437–1441.

37. Kuramochi-Miyagawa S, Kimura T, Ijiri TW, et al. Mili, a mammalian member of piwi family gene, is essential for spermatogenesis. Development 2004;131:839–849.

38. Toyooka Y, Tsunekawa N, Takahashi Y, Matsui Y, Satoh M, Noce T. Expression and intracellular localization of mouse Vasa-homologue protein during germ cell development. Mech Dev 2000;93:139–149.

39. Kotaja N, Bhattacharyya SN, Jaskiewicz L, et al. The chromatoid body of male germ cells: similarity with P-bodies and presence of Dicer and microRNA pathway components. Proc Natl Acad Sci USA 2006;103:2647–2652.

40. Liu L, Valencia-Sanchez MA, Hannon GJ, Parker R. MicroRNA-dependent localization of targeted mRNAs to mammalian P-bodies. Nat Cell Biol 2005;7:719–723.

41. Pillai RS, Bhattacharyya SN, Artus CG, et al. Inhibition of translational initiation by Let-7 MicroRNA in human cells. Science 2005;309:1573–1576.

42. Cougot N, Babajko S, Séraphin B. Cytoplasmic foci are sites of mRNA decay in human cells. J Cell Biol 2004;165:31–40.

43. Barad O, Meiri E, Avniel A, et al. MicroRNA expression detected by oligonucleotide microarrays: system establishment and expression profiling in human tissues. Genome Res 2004;14:2486–2494.

44. Yu Z, Raabe T, Hecht NB. MicroRNA Mirn122a reduces expression of the post-transcriptionally regulated germ cell transition protein 2 (Tnp2) messenger RNA (mRNA) by mRNA cleavage. Biol Reprod 2005;73:427–433.

45. Cullen BR. Transcription and processing of human microRNA precursors. Mol Cell 2004;16:861–865.

13 Sperm Maturation in the Epididymis

Role of Segment-Specific Microenvironments

Gail A. Cornwall, PhD and Hans H. von Horsten, PhD

Summary

Spermatozoa undergo a maturation process and acquire motility and fertility as they migrate from the proximal to the distal end of the long convoluted tubule known as the epididymis. Regions of the epididymis are subdivided into discrete segments defined structurally and functionally by connective tissue septa. Each segment is a unique microenvironment that together allows maturation to occur. This chapter focuses on how these distinct microenvironments are created, including the involvement of segment-specific expression of secretory proteins and cellular proteins allowing each segment to respond uniquely to external stimuli and novel mechanisms the epididymis uses to deliver and remove proteins from the epididymal lumen.

Key Words: Epididymis; sperm maturation; CRES; fertilization; lumacrine.

1. WHY STUDY THE EPIDIDYMIS?

Although it is well known that the development of germ cells occurs in the testis in a process known as spematogenesis, it is often overlooked that testicular sperm are nonfunctional gametes and lack the ability to naturally fertilize an egg. It is only after sperm migrate through the epididymis and undergo a maturation process that they acquire progressive motility and the ability to fertilize. Although significant progress has been made over the past years, we still have yet to identify the critical molecular and biochemical pathways that allow maturation to occur.

From: *The Genetics of Male Infertility*
Edited by: D.T. Carrell © Humana Press Inc., Totowa, NJ

The necessity of understanding the normal processes of epididymal sperm maturation is emphasized by the fact that up to 40% of infertile men exhibit idiopathic infertility, which in many cases can reflect maturational disorders. Assisted reproductive technologies, such as intracytoplasmic sperm injection, are effective treatments for ididopathic infertility, because one only needs access to spermatozoa regardless of functional maturity. However, intracytoplasmic sperm injection seems to have become the end to all treatments, such that the basic investigation of epididymal function has, to some degree, fallen by the wayside. This is indeed a frightening observation because common sense would dictate that most couples trying to conceive would prefer the least invasive method possible to circumvent their fertility problem and, if the processes of sperm maturation were defined, approaches to maturing sperm in vitro could be developed.

The importance of epididymal study is also underscored by the continued lack of development of a male contraceptive. Although considerable emphasis has been placed on developing male contraceptives, the focus has primarily been on using a hormonal approach (a combination of testosterone and progestin) to disrupt spermatogenesis. Although this approach should work in theory, currently there are profound limitations, including the requirement of repeated injections, long periods of time to achieve an effect as well as to reverse the contraceptive effect, and the possibility of undesirable side effects including changes in libido. Unless these disadvantages can be improved, the worldwide acceptance of a hormone-based male contraceptive comes into question. Indeed, although oral hormonal contraceptives for women have been in place for decades and are considered to be relatively safe, the worldwide acceptance rate is only 20%, whereas in the United States the acceptance is only 10% (1). Thus, alternatives are needed for a male contraceptive. Targeting specific molecules in the epididymis would be a more attractive approach than disrupting spermatogenesis because the contraceptive effects would be rapid and more readily reversible and side effects associated with alterations in hormones would be avoided.

With these priorities in mind, epididymal biologists have identified key areas of epididymal research that need further emphasis, including studying spermatozoa and associated maturational changes during epididymal transit, the specifics of sperm–protein interactions as well as sperm interactions with nonprotein molecules in the epididymal lumen, studies of the cytoplasmic droplet and its role in maturation, the development of better in vitro systems to facilitate study of sperm maturation, understanding the mechanisms of sperm storage and maintenance of sperm activity, examination of interstitial–epithelial cell interactions, as well as identifying functions for the vast number of epididymal secretory proteins that are part of the epididymal luminal microenvironment *(2)*. From studies thus far it is becoming apparent that sperm maturation is not only the secretion and binding of a select group of proteins to the sperm surface, but rather involves an incredibly sophisticated and finely tuned relationship between the epididymal epithelium and spermatozoa. Further studies in the many areas described previously are needed to provide a sound knowledge of the epididymis from which new therapies and contraceptive targets can be developed.

The goal of this chapter is to summarize in brief the recent progress in the field of epididymal biology with particular focus on regionalized gene expression and study of epididymal secretory proteins and their putative functions in sperm maturation, novel mechanisms for the delivery of proteins to spermatozoa during epididymal transit, as well as unique mechanisms for the functional control and removal of secretory proteins from the epididymal lumen. It is hoped that the reader will become as intrigued as the authors are by the incredible complexities of this organ including the distinctive mechanisms the epididymis uses to achieve its primary goal, namely the maturation of spermatozoa and thus perpetuation of the species.

2. SPERM MATURATION IN THE EPIDIDYMIS: SEGMENT-SPECIFIC MICROENVIRONMENTS

In brief, spermatozoa exiting the testis and entering the single, long, convoluted tubule known as the epididymis are nonfunctional in that they lack progressive motility and the ability to fertilize an egg. As sperm migrate from the proximal to the distal epididymis, they undergo a maturation process and acquire motility and fertility. It is generally accepted that epididymal sperm are, for the most part, synthetically inactive and thus maturation requires the interaction of sperm with proteins that are synthesized and secreted by the epididymal epithelium. The epididymis is grossly divided into three regions: the caput (head), corpus (body), and cauda (tail). The most proximal caput region, in some species, is also known as the initial segment. Each epididymal region carries out distinctive functions, with the caput and corpus carrying out early and late sperm maturational events, respectively, while the cauda region primarily serves as a storage site for functionally mature spermatozoa.

Although the primary cell type along the epididymal tubule remains the same from the proximal to the distal epididymis, of considerable interest to epididymal biologists is the highly regionalized gene expression within these epithelial cells. Neighboring cells can express quite different subsets of genes, which contribute to the ever-changing luminal environment that spermatozoa encounter as they move from the proximal to the distal epididymis and which ultimately allow sperm maturation to occur. Although previously it was thought that varying patterns of gene expression along the tubule were loosely associated with different epididymal regions, work by Turner et al. in 2003 demonstrated that the presence of connective tissue septa further subdivides the caput, corpus, and cauda epididymis into discrete intraregional segments and that region-specific gene expression may in fact be highly ordered and compartmentalized within these precise segments (3). Indeed, examination of β-galactosidase activity by immersion of whole mouse epididymis in X-gal solution revealed a precise staining in the initial segment, no staining in the remainder of the caput, and intense staining in the corpus epididymis. Furthermore, the β-galactosidase activity was precisely contained with discrete segments delineated by the connective tissue septa with changes in expression occurring as the tubule passed through the septa (3). By using size exclusion dyes and radiolabeled molecules, these authors further demonstrated that the connective tissue septa may also act as barriers, restricting the movement of molecules from the interstitial space of one segment to the next. This would allow segment-specific paracrine signaling to occur between stromal and epithelial cells, which could regulate the tightly controlled segment-specific expression of genes (3).

Thus the epididymal tubule is a highly ordered and segmented organ, with each segment representing a unique physiological compartment. Each compartment possesses distinctive gene expression profiles within the epithelium that dictate segment-specific secretion of proteins into the luminal fluid, directly or indirectly affecting sperm maturation. Segment-specific expression of genes encoding signaling molecules, regulatory proteins, transporters, and receptors also contribute to the formation of unique microenvironments by allowing the epithelium to respond uniquely to different stimuli, such as hormones and other regulatory factors (Fig. 1). Identifying and determining the function of segment-specific proteins is of paramount importance for understanding epididymal sperm maturation.

2.1. Segment-Specific Gene Expression

Space limitations preclude a thorough discussion of the many genes that exhibit regionalized gene expression in the epididymis. Therefore, we mention only briefly groups of genes based on their putative functions. Although much of the earlier data was drawn from published

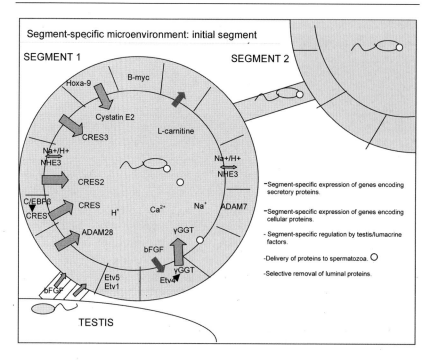

Fig. 1. Schematic representation of factors contributing to the formation of a segment-specific microenvironment in the epididymal initial segment of the mouse. Examples of secreted and cellular proteins are noted.

reports of expression levels determined by reverse transcriptase-polymerase chain reaction or Northern analysis of epididymal regions *(4)*, most recently the application of gene profiling technology to the epididymis has yielded volumes of information of segment-specific gene expression that is available to the public. In particular, our laboratory screened 15K expressed sequence tags from the National Institute of Aging that were derived from pre- and peri-implantation embryos, embryonic day 12.5 female gonad/mesonephros, and newborn ovary comparing the mouse initial segment with the remainder of the epididymis *(5)*. Because the gene chips used in these studies represented sequences derived from early-stage embryos, the microarray analysis was biased toward identifying new subsets of genes expressed in the adult epididymis. This information is available at http://www.ttuhsc.edu/cbb/faculty/cornwall/nelson/supplemental.xls. Subsequent to our studies, Johnston et al. examined the varying expression profiles of genes from all segments of the mouse epididymis using Affymetrix mouse gene chips *(6)*. This information is available in a searchable website at the Mammalian Reproductive Genetics database (http://mrg.

genetics.washington.edu). Because each study used different sources of sequences, a broad representation of sequences is presented. Following is a brief summary of genes and gene products exhibiting regionalized expression in the epididymis, including proteases and protease inhibitors, modifying enzymes, signaling molecules, and transcription factors.

During epididymal transit, sperm-associated proteins including ADAM2 (fertilinβ), ADAM3 (cyritestin), ADAM24 (testase), CE9, and others are proteolytically processed to their mature and presumably functionally active forms *(7–10)*. Although the identity of the proteases involved in the activation of these proteins is not known, furin-like proteases have been implicated for several of these processing events *(7)*. Recent studies by our laboratory show that several members of the prohormone convertase family of proprotein processing enzymes including furin, PC7, PC4, and PACE4 are expressed in the epididymis in a regionalized manner and several are present in epididymal fluid suggesting a possible role for these proteases in sperm maturational events (Cormier and Cornwall, unpublished data). Indeed, PC4 knockout male mice are infertile despite normal spermatogenesis and motility, suggesting that critical fertilization molecules may not be processed correctly *(11)*. Other proteases expressed in a segment-specific manner in the epididymis include several of the matrix metalloproteases, MMP2, MMP3, MMP9 *(12)*, ADAM28 *(13)*, and procathepsin L *(14)*.

Several protease inhibitors that show segment-specific expression have also been identified. Several members of the cystatin-related epididymal spermatogenic (CRES) subgroup of family 2 cystatins of cysteine protease inhibitors including CRES, CRES2, CRES3, and cystatin E2 are highly restricted to the initial segment region of the mouse epididymis *(15–18)*. Although the function of these secretory proteins in vivo is not known, in vitro CRES is an inhibitor of several members of the prohormone convertases *(19)*, suggesting CRES may regulate proprotein processing events in the epididymis. Other protease inhibitors expressed in the epididymis include Eppin, a member of the whey acidic protein type four–disulfide core gene family. In the human, Eppin associates with semenogelin on the surface of ejaculated spermatozoa and may provide antimicrobial activity for spermatozoa *(20)*. Studies in which primates were immunized with Eppin resulted in a contraceptive effect in 78% of the monkeys that was reversible in 71%, suggesting an important function for this protein in fertility and a possible role as a male contraceptive *(21)*.

Other gene and gene products expressed in a region-dependent manner in the epididymis include those encoding antioxidant enzymes such γ glutamyl transpeptidase, glutathione peroxidases, and superoxide dismutase *(22–25)*. Because the epididymal lumen is oxygen-rich, unsaturated fatty acids in sperm membranes may be susceptible to oxidative damage. The expression of these enzymes may protect spermatozoa from oxidative damage. Lysosomal enzymes such as β-hexosaminidase, α mannosidase, and β-galactosidase are secreted into the epididymal lumen, where they may affect sperm function either directly or indirectly by modifying carbohydrate moieties *(4,26,27)*.

A variety of signaling molecules are also expressed in a region-dependent manner in the epididymal epithelium. It is likely that these proteins respond to various external stimuli in the luminal environment, ultimately affecting epithelial cell function. For example, in the caput, several members of the retinoid signaling pathway are expressed such as epididymis-specific extracellular retinoic acid-binding protein and the related MEP17, mMUP4-L, and mEP19, cellular retinoic acid-binding protein and retinoic acid α receptor *(28)*. It is likely that these proteins participate in the delivery and trafficking of retinoids to and within the epididymal cells.

The bone morphogenetic proteins belong to the transforming growth factor-β superfamily of growth factors and function as signaling molecules. Bone morphogenetic protein (BMP) 7 and BMP8a are both expressed in the epididymis and the loss of *Bmp8a* gene function leads to epididymal degeneration that ultimately results in infertility *(29)*. Interestingly, although both BMPs are expressed in the initial segment, the degenerative effects observed in the *Bmp8a* knockout are observed in more distal epididymal regions, suggesting a possible paracrine role for BMP8a in the epididymis. Several peptides such as proopiomelanocortin, β-endorphin, proenkephalin, and neuropeptide Y are expressed in the epididymis and may also function in paracrine signaling pathways *(4)*.

The region-dependent expression of genes implies that there are region-dependent transcription factors. Perhaps the most well studied are the members of the *Etv4* subfamily including *Etv4*, *Etv5*, and *Etv1*. All family members are expressed in the initial segment, and their messenger RNAs (mRNAs) are profoundly reduced following the loss of signaling from the testis (*see* section 3.), suggesting these transcription factors may regulate a subset of genes dependent on testicular luminal fluid factors *(30)*. Other transcription factors expressed in the initial segment include the androgen receptor *(31)*, estrogen receptor α *(32)*, B-myc *(33)*, C/EBPβ *(34)*, and Pem *(35)*. Estrogen receptor α expression is important for normal fluid resorption by the epithelium and specifically is necessary for expression of a critical transporter NA+/H+ exchanger 3 as evidenced by examination of the knockout mouse *(32,36)*. C/EBPβ function is necessary for transactivation of the CRES gene *(34)*. Although the epididymal gene targets for B-myc are not known, cell culture studies suggest that it is involved in the regulation of cell growth *(37)*.

Although the regional or segment-specific expression of genes has been well-documented in the epididymis, the biological roles their gene products carry out is for the most part unknown. However, recent generation of knockout mouse models have revealed the critical roles some of these epididymal expressed genes play. The loss of several genes that are involved in fluid transport or signaling in the initial segment region including that for apolipoprotein E receptor 2 *(38)*, estrogen receptor α*(Esr1)* *(32,36)*, HE6 *(Gpr64)* *(41)*, or the complete loss of the initial segment region resulting from the loss of the c-ros tyrosine kinase receptor *(Ros1)* *(42)* leads to an inability of sperm to regulate their cell volume, resulting in a characteristic hairpin loop of the sperm flagella (Table 1). Other epididymal expressed genes, including those for lysosomal proteins, such as β-hexosaminidase and cathepsin A *(ctsa)* or follicle-stimulating hormone receptor *(Fshr)*, exhibit an altered epithelium and/or changes in lysosomal size (Table 1; refs. *49–51*).

3. TESTIS/LUMACRINE REGULATION OF THE INITIAL SEGMENT

Studies have clearly established that the epididymis is an androgen-dependent organ. Indeed, following castration, epididymal weight decreases to 25% of intact after 2 wk. Restoration of circulating testosterone reverses the cellular changes in the caput, corpus, and cauda epididymis but not in the initial segment *(59)*. Supra-physiological levels of androgens also do not reverse these changes in the initial segment. Interestingly, ligation of the efferent ducts, which connect the testis to the epididymis and are the passageway for sperm and luminal components to enter the initial segment from the testis, results in a profound regression of the initial segment region *(59)*. Because ligation of the efferent ducts does not affect circulating androgen levels, these studies suggest that the maintenance of initial segment morphology requires components in the luminal fluid from the testis (i.e., lumacrine regulation; ref. *60*). Furthermore, gene expression studies revealed a subset of initial segment expressed genes that are down-regulated following efferent duct ligation, including CRES subgroup members, and others, suggesting that luminal factors are not only needed

Table 1
Gene Knockouts That Exhibit Epididymal Phenotypes

Gene	Function/expression/Phenotype	Reference
Apolipoprotein E receptor-2 (apoer2)	Member of the low-density lipoprotein (LDL)receptor gene family, functions in endocytosis and signal transduction. Expressed in initial segment. Cauda sperm exhibit flagellar angulation and impaired motility. Decreased level of phospholipid hydroperoxide glutathione peroxidase protein observed in epididymal sperm from knockout suggests altered ability of sperm to regulate cell volume decrease resulting in hairpin morphology of . sperm. Increased levels of clusterin in epididymal luminal fluid of the knockout suggests apoER2 also functions as a clusterin receptor.	38
Apolipoprotein B (Apob)	Lipid absorption and triglyceride homeostasis. Expressed in testis and epididymis. Heterozygous males show reduced fertility. Sperm do not fertilize in vivo or in vitro but fertilize eggs if zona pellucida is removed. Sperm counts and motility decreased.	39
Estrogen receptor-α (Esr1)	Transcription factor. Primarily expressed in efferent ducts and initial segment. Disruption of fluid reabsorption in the efferent ducts. Dilation of rete testis and efferent ducts with subsequent fluid accumulation in seminiferous tubules, dilution of sperm, and resulting infertility. Decreased expression and activity of the Na^+/H^+ exchanger 3 transporter affecting Na^+ reabsorption and passive water transport.	32,36
Anion exchanger 2 (Slc4a2)	Na^+-independent anion transporter that mediates exchange of Cl^- and HCO^-_3 across cell membranes. Expressed primarily in initial segment, caput, with less expression in the cauda. Squamous metaplasia of the epithelium.	40

(Continued)

Table 1 *(Continued)*

Gene	Function/expression/Phenotype	Reference
HE6 *(Gpr64)*	Orphan member of the LNB-7TM (B_2) subfamily of G protein-coupled receptors. Expressed in efferent ducts and initial segment. Heterozygous males showed a dysregulation of fluid reabsorption within efferent ducts leading to fluid accumulation in testis . Sperm exhibit flagellar angularity, decreased motility, and decreasing fertility with age. Sperm accumulate in efferent ducts.	*41*
c-ros tyrosine kinase receptor *(Ros1)*	Tyrosine kinase receptor. Expressed in initial segment. Failure of initial segment to develop. Male mice are infertile. Sperm exhibit flagellar angulation attributed to inability to regulate cell volume, some decreased motility. Increased luminal pH in cauda epididymidis.	*42–44*
Nuclear oxysterol receptor LXR α and β *(lxr)*	Transcription factor, activated by oxysterols, oxidized derivatives of cholesterol. LXR proteins highest in caput, less expression in cauda. In double knockout, regression of proximal caput epithelium, amorphous substance in lumen, cauda spermatozoa exhibited detached heads, flagellar angulation. Late onset of defects at 6 months of age.	*45*
Prosaposin *(psap)*	Secreted protein targeted to lysosomal compartment, lysosomal activator of hydrolases, trophic factor. Decreased epididymal weight, smaller tubular diameter, shorter undifferentiated epithelial cells.	*46*
Nuclear phospholipid hydroperoxide glutathione *(Gpx4)*	Selenoenzyme, member of the glutathione peroxidase family. Expressed in germ cells. Decreased thiol oxidation in cauda spermatozoa of the knockout.	*47*

(Continued)

Table 1 *(Continued)*

Gene	Function/expression/Phenotype	Reference
Inositol polyphosphate 5-phosphatase *(Inpp5b)*	Signaling protein in IP3 pathway. Expressed in Sertoli cells, germ cells, epididymis. Sperm from knockout mice exhibit decreased fertility, reduced motility. Conditional germ cell knockouts are fertile suggesting phenotype is a result of defects in Sertoli cell and/or epididymal function. Reduced levels of fertilin beta protein processing in the knockout sperm.	*48*
FSH receptor *(Fshr)*	Follicle-stimulating hormone receptor involved in maintenance of spermatogenesis. Expressed in Sertoli cells. Decreased caput and corpus epithelium, decreased sperm motility.	*49*
Cathepsin A *(Ctsa)*	Lysosomal carboxypeptidase. Lysosomal abnormalities, vacuolated, expanded epithelium in caput and corpus. Abnormal halo cells.	*50*
β-hexo-saminidase A and B *(Hexa,b)*	Lysosomal enzyme. Increased number and size of lysosomes in initial segment and intermediate zone.	*51*
Mononuclear phagocytic growth factor stimulating colony factor *(Csf1)*	Decreased density of macrophages in testis, caput, and cauda epididymis. Macrophages do not exhibit normal localization in caput.	*52*
Somatic- and testis-specific angiotensin-converting enzyme *(Ace)*	Regulator of the renin-angiotensin system. Reduced fertility in male mice. Impaired sperm transport in oviducts and zona binding. Mice lack the somatic ACE but have the testis-specific ACE are fertile. Conflicting data on whether dipeptidase or glycosylphosphatidylinositol releasing activity of testicular ACE is critical for fertility.	*53–55*

(Continued)

Table 1 *(Continued)*

Gene	Function/expression/Phenotype	Reference
Bone morphogenetic protein 8A *(Bmp8A)*	Degeneration of epididymal epithelium.	*29*
γ- Glutamyl transpeptidase *(Ggtp)*	Hypoplasia of the epididymis.	*56*
Hoxa-10, Hoxa-11	Transcription factors. Hoxa-10 knockout results in homeotic transformation of corpus to caput epididymidis and proximal vas deferens to cauda epididymidis, whereas hoxa-11 knockout knockout results in homeotic transformation of proximalvas deferens to cauda epididymis.	*57–58*

for the maintenance of initial segment morphology but for function as well *(15,16,60)*.

Although it is not known if one or many testis factors are required to maintain initial segment function, studies by Lan et al. suggest that basic fibroblast growth factor may be one such factor. Administration of fibroblast growth factor-2 but not epidermal growth factor to efferent duct-ligated rats restored GGT mRNA, protein, and activity in the initial segment to control levels. Furthermore, these investigators proposed that fibroblast growth factor may elicit its effects on Ggt_pr4 gene expression via activation of the ras–raf–mitogen-activated protein kinase pathway and downstream activation of the ETV4 transcription factor *(60–62)*. Most recently, studies by these investigators suggest that, not surprisingly, not all testis-regulated genes respond the same to changes in ETV4 transcriptional activity. The administration of an ETV5-dominant negative plasmid by in vivo electroporation to the rat initial segment resulted in the downregulation of Etv5, Etv4, and Etv1 mRNAs in the initial segment as well as putative target genes γ-glutamyl transpeptidase (Ggt_pr4), steroid 5 α reductase (Srd5a1), and glutathione peroxidase (Gpx5; ref. *30*). However, although the testis-regulated genes CRES*(cst8)* and MEP17*(len8)* contain ETS-binding sites within their promoters, they did not respond to the dominant negative, suggesting that there either may be several testis factors, each differentially regulating specific subsets of genes, or that one or a few testis factors may mediate different downstream effects via the activation of multiple signaling pathways and subsequent effector molecules *(30)*.

4. NOVEL MECHANISMS FOR DELIVERY OF EPIDIDYMAL PROTEINS TO SPERMATOZOA

During epididymal transit, spermatozoa acquire new surface-associated proteins synthesized and secreted from the epididymal epithelium. Most of these proteins possess the typical signal sequences indicating trafficking through the Golgi and subsequent packaging and release from secretory granules (merocrine secretion). However, several studies have shown that epididymal sperm also acquire proteins that lack signal sequences, suggesting an unusual secretion pathway in the epithelium. Differential extraction of spermatozoa indicates these proteins act like integral membrane proteins and in fact, some of these proteins are thought to be anchored to the sperm plasma membrane by a glycosylphosphatidylinositol *(63,64)*. In the epididymal lumen, several of these proteins are associated with membranous vesicles known as epididymosomes. Although previously thought to be an artifact of fixation, these small, membrane-bound vesicles originate from the epididymal epithelial cells in a process known as apocrine secretion. This type of secretion involves the formation of apical blebs containing various-sized vesicles from the epithelial cells. Once the blebs have detached, they are thought to fragment and release the small vesicles *(65)*. Although similar types of vesicles have been known for some time to be secreted by the prostate (prostasomes) and are present in the semen, where they have proposed roles as protection for sperm against complement, enhancement of motility, and stabilization of the sperm membrane, Yanagimachi was the first to describe such vesicles in the epididymal lumen and show interaction of these vesicles with spermatozoa *(66)*. Analysis of proteins associated with the epididymosomes reveal protein profiles quite different from that of proteins in the lumen. Proteins associated with epididymosomes include P26h, believed to be involved in zona pellucida binding, HE5, macrophage migration inhibitory factor, ubiquitin, and glutathione peroxidase, all of which have been shown to be transferred to spermatozoa in the epididymis *(64,67–69)*. The studies examining the transfer of P26 from epididymosomes to spermatozoa demonstrated that transfer was pH-dependent and required high zinc concentrations (consistent with endogenous levels in the epididymal fluid). These investigators also observed that not all proteins present in the vesicles were transferred to spermatozoa, suggesting that only some proteins have the ability to be transferred or that complete fusion and transfer of vesicles to spermatozoa does not occur *(70)*. Other studies examining epididymosomes in the cauda fluid from the ram epididymis identified different subsets of proteins present in these vesicles, including dipeptidyl peptidase V, neprilysin, mannosidase, and actin, but observed no interactions of such vesicles with spermatozoa, also suggesting that transfer of proteins may be by a subtle exchange rather than complete fusion *(71)*. It is also possible that epididymosomes are heterogeneous with different protein compositions depending on downstream functions. The functional significance of epididymosomes in sperm maturation remains to be elucidated. It is possible that epididymosomes are designed to ensure the safe delivery of some proteins to the sperm cell and perhaps to particular sperm domains without possible damage by luminal proteases. Alternatively, given the complexities of sperm maturation and the vast multitude of cellular and extracellular events the epididymis must carry out for maturation to occur, it is possible the epididymis has developed new strategies to deliver cellular proteins and their associated functions to the sperm surface rather than synthesize a secretory protein that carries out the same function as its cellular form. Along this line of thinking, studies by Sutovsky et al. *(68)* showed that ubiquitin is associated with epididymosomes and that during epididymal transit these vesicles delivered ubiquitin to damaged or defective spermatozoa, thus flagging them for removal. Thus, by the mechanism of apocrine secretion, a cellular process, ubiquitination, is now carried out extracellularly.

5. SELECTIVE REMOVAL OF PROTEINS FROM THE EPIDIDYMAL LUMEN

Although much focus has been spent on studying secretory proteins within the epididymal lumen and how they may affect maturation, how these secretory proteins are removed from the lumen is quite overlooked. Although some proteins secreted by the proximal epididymis remain in the luminal fluid to the cauda, many proteins are highly segment-specific in their localization, suggesting that their continued presence in downstream segments may be detrimental and that selective mechanisms must be in place for their removal. Furthermore, many proteins are secreted into the epididymal lumen by default, because they function within the secretory pathway rather than extracellularly. If these proteins are not removed, they might interfere with proteins that do have extracellular roles, thus affecting sperm maturation. A recent conceptual paper has proposed the existence of an extracellular quality control system that is analogous to the intracellular machinery responsible for the removal of misfolded proteins from the endoplasmic reticulum and cytosol *(72)*. The extracellular quality control system has been proposed to consist of chaperones, proteolytic enzymes, and endocytosis mediators. Because of the active secretory functions of the epididymal epithelium and the critical nature of the maturation process occurring within the epididymal lumen, it is quite likely that such a mechanism is also active within the epididymal luminal compartment.

CRES is detected in the lumen of mouse segments 1 and 2 but abruptly disappears in segment 3 *(73)*. Protein analysis of epididymal fluid using Tricine gels to detect protein degradation products did not distinguish any smaller forms of CRES, rather only an abrupt disappearance of the majority of the protein from the lumen by suggesting proteolytic degradation within the lumen is likely not responsible for its turnover *(74)*. CRES may then be one of the proteins that could be potentially harmful if it is enriched beyond a critical threshold level within the extracellular compartment. Indeed, cystatins are amyloidogenic and, given the correct local environmental conditions, will oligomerize. In the worse situation, cystatin C will form large protein aggregates or amyloid fibers that are associated with the neurodegenerative disease amyloid angiopathy *(75)*. Based on its relationship with cystatins, we theorize that CRES may self-aggregate within the epididymal lumen, making it a target for removal by quality control machinery in the luminal fluid.

Biochemical analyses of caput luminal fluid demonstrated that CRES was part of high-molecular-weight soluble complexes in the lumen *(74)*. The formation of high-molecular-weight but soluble protein complexes in the lumen may be a means to control protein function before the removal of such complexes by endocytosis. Indeed, cystatin C dimers are not functional cysteine protease inhibitors *(76)*. Although the noncovalent aggregation of CRES seems to be a natural event, it bears the potential danger of amyloid fiber formation, particularly in light of the dramatic concentration of epididymal secretory proteins that occurs as a consequence of the active fluid reabsorption being carried out by the epididymal epithelium. Therefore, we hypothesized that the equilibrium of CRES aggregation and disaggregation needs to be tightly modulated by chaperones and other quality control proteins. Examination of fluid phase liquid chromatography fractionated caput luminal fluid by SDS-agarose gels, indentified CRES complexes that were resistant to denaturation by SDS *(74)*. Further studies revealed that CRES is a substrate for transglutaminase, a calcium-dependent enzyme that catalyzes isopeptide bond formation between glutamyl and lysinyl residues and thus can covalently crosslink proteins. The transglutaminases are known modulators of protein aggregation and may well be part of extracellular quality control machinery that is involved in the removal of proteins from the epididymal luminal fluid *(72)*. Our studies suggest that both properties inherent in CRES protein as well as the presence of transglutaminase participate in the formation of stable CRES protein complexes that may mediate CRES function and ultimately may target it for nonspecific adsorptive endocytosis.

In addition to our studies with CRES, other investigators have noted a different type of high-molecular-weight protein complex in epididymal fluid. Studies by Ecryod et al. identified prion protein in large-molecular-weight soluble complexes in ram luminal fluid *(78)*. Prion protein, unlike CRES which is a secretory protein, is typically attached to the cell plasma membrane by a glycosylphosphatidylinositol anchor, thus its presence in "soluble" form in epididymal fluid is perplexing. Further examination of prion protein complexes by these investigators identified the presence of five other proteins that copurified with prion protein, including clusterin, a known chaperone, bacterial permeability-increasing protein (BPI), α mannosidase, cauxin, and β-galactosidase. These proteins appeared to associate with one another by hydrophobic interactions rather than through protein–protein interactions *(78)* and as such form a lipoprotein-like vesicle. It was proposed that such a mechanism may allow clearance of hydrophobic proteins without precipitation. Taken together, it appears that the epididymis has developed highly specialized mechanisms for the removal of luminal proteins, whether it is via protein crosslinking or formation of stable lipid-like structures.

6. CONCLUSION

In summary, the maturation of spermatozoa in the epididymis is an incredibly complex process requiring the exposure of spermatozoa to a series of individual microenvironments created by the epididymal epithelium. Understanding the multifaceted nature of each microenvironment is required to fully define epididymal function in sperm maturation and provide new therapies for infertility as well targets for contraception.

REFERENCES

1. Habenicht UF. Industry's perspective on contraceptive development. In: Hinton BT, Turner TT, eds. The Third International Conference on the Epididymis, Van Doren Company, Charlottesville; 2003:203–207.
2. Turner TT. Which aspects of epididymal function require increased emphasis in future research? In: Hinton BT, Turner TT, eds. The Third International Conference on the Epididymis, Van Doren Company, Charlottesville; 277–282.

3. Turner TT, Bomgardner D, Jacobs JP, Nguyen QAT. Association of segmentation of the epididymal interstitium with segmented tubule function in rats and mice. Reproduction 2003;125:871–878.

4. Cornwall GA, Lareyre JJ, Matusik RJ, Hinton BT, Orgebin-Crist M-C. Gene expression and epididymal function. In: Robaire B, Hinton BT, eds. The Epididymis: From molecules to clinical practice, A comprehensive survey of the efferent ducts, the epididymis and the vas deferens. Kluwer Academic/Plenum Publishers, New York; 2002:169–199.

5. Hsia N, Cornwall GA. DNA microarray analysis of region-specific gene expression in the mouse epididymis. Biol Reprod 2004;70:448–457.

6. Johnston DS, Jelinsky SA, Bang HJ, et al. The mouse epididymal transcriptome: transcriptional profiling of segmental gene expression in the epididymis. Biol Reprod 2005;73:404–413.

7. Lum L, Blobel CP. Evidence for distinct serine protease activities with a potential role in processing the sperm protein fertilin. Dev Biol 1997;191:131–145.

8. Kim E, Nishimura H, Iwase S, Yamagata K, Kashiwabara S, Baba T. Synthesis, processing, and subcellular localization of mouse ADAM3 during spermatogenesis and epididymal sperm transport. J Reprod Dev 2004;50:571–578.

9. Zhu GZ, Myles DG, Primakoff P. Testase 1 (ADAM 24) a plasma membrane-anchored sperm protease implicated in sperm function during epididymal maturation or fertilization. J Cell Sci 2001;114:1787–1794.

10. Petruszak JAM, Nehme CL, Bartles JR. Endoproteolytic cleavage in the extracellular domain of the integral plasma membrane protein CE9 precedes its redistribution from the posterior to the anterior tail of the rat spermatozoon during epididymal maturation. J Cell Biol 1991;114:917–927.

11. Mbikay M, Tadros H, Ishida N, et al. Impaired fertility in mice deficient for the testicular germ cell protease PC4. Proc Natl Acad Sci USA 1997;94:6842–6846.

12. Metayer S, Dacheux F, Dacheux J-L, Gatti J-L. Comparison, characterization, and identification of proteases and protease inhibitors in epididymal fluids of domestic mammals. Matrix metalloproteinases are major fluid gelatinases. Biol Reprod 2002;66:1219–1229.

13. Oh J, Woo J-M, Choi E, Kim T, et al. Molecular, biochemical, and cellular characterization of epididymal ADAMs, ADAM7 and ADAM28. Biochem Biophys Res Comm 2005;331:1374–1383.

14. Okamura N, Tamba M, Uchiyama Y, et al. Direct evidence for the elevated synthesis and secretion of procathepsin L in the distal caput epididymis of boar. Biochim Biophys Acta 1995;1245:221–226.

15. Cornwall GA, Orgebin-Crist M-C, Hann SR. The CRES gene: a unique testis-regulated gene related to the cystatin family is highly restricted in its expression to the proximal region of the mouse epididymis. Mol Endocrinol 1992;6: 1653–1664.

16. Hsia N, Cornwall GA. Cres2 and Cres3: new members of the cystatin-related epididymal spermatogenic subgroup of family 2 cystatins. Endocrinology 2003; 144:909–915.

17. Cornwall GA, Hsia N. A new subgroup of the family 2 cystatins. Mol Cell Endocrinol 2003;200:1–8.

18. Li Y, Friel PJ, McLean DJ, Griswold MD. Cystatin E1 and E2, new members of male reproductive tract subgroup within cystatin type 2 family. Biol Reprod 2003;69:489–500.

19. Cornwall GA, Cameron A, Lindberg I, Hardy DM, Cormier N, Hsia N. The cystatin-related epididymal spermatogenic protein inhibits the serine protease prohormone convertase 2. Endocrinology 2003;144:901–908.

20. Wang Z, Widgren EE, Sivashanmugam P, O'Rand MG, Richardson RT. Association of eppin with semenogelin on human spermatozoa. Biol Reprod 2005;72:1064–1070.
21. O'Rand MG, Widgren EE, Sivashanmugam P, et al. Reversible immunocontraception in male monkeys immunized with eppin. Science 2004;306:1189–1190.
22. Palladino MA, Hinton BT. Expression of multiple gamma-glutamyl transpeptidase messenger ribonucleic acid transcripts in the adult rat epididymis is differentially regulated by androgens and testicular factors in a region–specific manner. Endocrinology 1994;135:1146–1156.
23. Ghyselinck NB, Jimenez C, Lefrancois AM, Dufaure J-P. Molecular cloning of a cDNA for androgen-regulated proteins secreted by the mouse epididymis. Mol Endocrinol 1990;4:5–12.
24. Schwaab V, Faure J, Dufaure J-P, Drevet JR. GPx3: the plasma-type glutathione peroxidase is expressed under androgenic control in the mouse epididymis and vas deferens. Mol Reprod Dev 1998;51:362–372.
25. Perry AC, Jones R, Hall L. Isolation and characterization of a rat cDNA clone encoding a secreted superoxide dismutase reveals the epididymis to be a major site of its expression. Biochem J 1993;293:21–25.
26. Hermo L, Adamali HI, Mahuran D, Gravel RA, Tralser JM. beta-Hexosaminidase immunolocalization and alpha- and beta-subunit gene expression in the rat testis and epididymis. Mol Reprod Dev 1997;46:227–242.
27. Okamura N, Tamba M, Liao H-J, et al. Cloning of complementary DNA encoding a 135-kilodalton protein secreted from porcine corpus epididymis and its identification as an epididymis-specific alpha-mannosidase. Mol Reprod Dev 1995;42: 141–148.
28. Orgebin-Crist M-C. The epididymis in a post-genome era. In: Hinton BT, Turner TT, eds. The Third International Conference on the Epididymis. Van Doren Company, Charlottesville; 2003:2–22.
29. Zhao GQ, Liaw L, Hogan BL. Bone morphogenetic protein 8A plays a role in the maintenance of spermatogenesis and the integrity of the epididymis. Development 1998;125:1103–1112.
30. Yang L, Fox SA, Kirby JL, Troan BV, Hinton BT. Putative regulation of expression of members of the ETS variant 4 transcription factor family and their downstream targets in the rat epididymis. Biol Reprod 2006;74:714–720.
31. Viger RS, Robaire B. Gene expression in the aging brown Norway rat epididymis. J Androl 1995;16:108–117.
32. Hess RA, Bunick D, Lee KH, et al. A role for oestrogens in the male reproductive system. Nature 1997;390:509–512.
33. Cornwall GA, Collis R, Xiao Q, Hsia N, Hann SR. B-Myc, a proximal caput epididymal protein, is dependent on androgens and testicular factors for expression. Biol Reprod 2001;64:1600–1607.
34. Hsia N, Cornwall GA. CCAAT/enhancer binding protein beta regulates expression of the cystatin-related epididymal spermatogenic (Cres) gene. Biol Reprod 2001;65: 1452–1461.
35. Pitman JL, Lin TP, Kleeman JE, Erickson GF, MacLeod CL. Normal reproductive and macrophage function in Pem homeobox gene-deficient mice. Dev Biol 1998;202:196–214.
36. Zhou Q, Clark L, Nie R, et al. Estrogen action and male fertility: roles of the sodium/hydrogen exchanger-3 and fluid reabsorption in reproductive tract function. Proc Natl Acad Sci USA 2001;98:14,132–14,137.

37. Gregory MA, Xiao Q, Cornwall GA, Lutterbach B, Hann SR. B-Myc is preferentially expressed in hormonally-controlled tissues and inhibits cellular proliferation. Oncogene 2000;19:4886–4895.

38. Andersen OM, Yeung C-H, Vorum H, et al. Essential role of the apolipoprotein E receptor-2 in sperm development. J Biol Chem 2003;278:23,989–23,995.

39. Huang LS, Voyiaziakis E, Chen HL, Rubin EM, Gordon JW. A novel functional role for apolipoprotein B in male infertility in heterozygous apolipoprotein B knockout mice. Proc Natl Acad Sci USA 1996;93:10,903–10,907.

40. Medina JF, Recalde S, Prieto J, et al. Anion exchanger 2 is essential for spermiogenesis in mice. Proc Natl Acad Sci USA 2003;100:15,847–15,852.

41. Davies B, Baumann C, Kirchhoff C, et al. Targeted deletion of the epididymal receptor HE6 results in fluid dysregulation and male infertility. Mol Cell Biol 2004;24:8642–8648.

42. Sonnenberg-Riethmacher E, Walter B, Riethmacher D, Godecke S, Birchmeier C. The c-ros tyrosine kinase receptor controls regionalization and differentiation of epithelial cells in the epididymis. Genes Dev 1996;10:1184–1193.

43. Yeung CH, Anapolski M, Sipila P, et al. Sperm volume regulation: maturational changes in fertile and infertile transgenic mice and association with kinematics and tail angulation. Biol Reprod 2002;67:269–275.

44. Yeung CH, Breton S, Setiawan I, Lang F, Cooper TG. Increased luminal pH in the epididymis of infertile c-ros knockout mice and the expression of sodium-hydrogen exchangers and vacuolar proton pump H+-ATPase. Mol Reprod Dev 2004;68: 159–168.

45. Frenoux JM, Vernet P, Volle DH, et al. Nuclear oxysterol receptors, LXRs, are involved in the maintenance of mouse caput epididymidis structure and functions. J Mol Endocrinol 2004;33:361–375.

46. Morales CR, Zhao Q, El-Alfy M, Suzuki K. Targeted disruption of the mouse prosaposin gene affects the development of the prostate gland and other male reproductive organs. J Androl 2000;21:765–775.

47. Conrad M, Moreno SG, Sinowatz F, et al. The nuclear form of phospholipid hydroperoxide glutathione peroxidase is a protein thiol peroxidase contributing to sperm chromatin stability. Mol Cell Biol 2005;25:7637–7644.

48. Hellsten E, Evans JP, Bernard DJ, Janne PA, Nussbaum RL. Disrupted sperm function and fertilinβ processing in mice deficient in the inositol polyphosphate 5-phosphatase Inpp5b. Develop Biol 2001;240:641–653.

49. Grover A, Smith CE, Gregory M, Cyr DG, Sairam MR, Hermo L. Effects of FSH receptor deletion on epididymal tubules and sperm morphology, numbers, and motility. Mol Reprod Dev 2005;72:135–144.

50. Korah N, Smith CE, D'Azzo A, Mui J, Hermo L. Characterization of cell- and region-specific abnormalities in the epididymis of cathepsin A deficient mice. Mol Reprod Dev 2003;66:358–373.

51. Adamali HI, Somani IH, Huang JQ, Gravel RA, Tralser JM, Hermo L. Characterization and development of the regional- and cellular-specific abnormalities in the epididymis of mice with beta-hexosaminidase A deficiency. J Androl 1999;20:803–824.

52. Pollard JW, Dominguez MG, Mocci S, Cohen PE, Stanley ER. Effect of the colony-stimulating factor-1 null mutation, osteopetrotic (csfm(op)), on the distribution of macrophages in the male mouse reproductive tract. Biol Reprod 1997;56:1290–1300.

53. Hagaman JR, Moyer JS, Bachman ES, et al. Angiotensin-converting enzyme and male fertility. Proc Natl Acad Sci USA 1998;95:2552–2557.
54. Fuchs S, Frenzel K, Hubert C, et al. Male fertility is dependent on dipeptidase activity of testis ACE. Nature Med 2005;11:1140–1142.
55. Kondoh G, Tojo H, Nakatani Y, et al. Angiotensin-converting enzyme is a GPI-anchored protein releasing factor crucial for fertilization. Nature Med 2005; 11:160–166.
56. Lieberman MW, Wiseman AL, Shi ZZ, et al. Growth retardation and cysteine deficiency in gamma-glutamyl transpeptidase-deficient mice. Proc Natl Acad Sci USA 1996;93:7923–7926.
57. Hsieh-Li HM, Witte DP, Weinstein M, et al. Hoxa 11 structure, extensive antisense transcription, and function in male and female fertility. Development 1995;121: 1373–1385.
58. Satokata I, Benson G, Mass R. Sexually dimorphic sterility phenotypes in Hoxa10-deficient mice. Nature 1995;374:460–463.
59. Ezer N, Robaire B. Androgenic regulation of the structure and functions of the epididymis. In: Robaire B, Hinton BT, eds. The Epididymis: from molecules to clinical practice. A comprehensive survey of the efferent ducts, the epididymis and the vas deferens. Kluwer Academic/Plenum Publishers, New York; 2002:297–316.
60. Hinton BT, Lan ZJ, Rudolph DB, Labus JC, Lye RJ. Testicular regulation of epididymal gene expression. J Reprod Fertil Suppl 1998;53:47–57.
61. Hinton BT, Kirby JL, Rodriguez CM, Lye RJ, Troan BV, Yang L. Signal transduction pathways to gene expression. In: Hinton BT, Turner TT, eds. The Third International Conference on the Epididymis. Van Doren Company, Charlottesville; 2003:103–113.
62. Lan ZJ, Labus JC, Hinton BT. Regulation of gamma-glutamyl transpeptidase catalytic activity and protein level in the initial segment of the rat epididymis by testicular factors: role of basic fibroblast growth factor. Biol Reprod 1998; 58:197–206.
63. Cooper TG. Interactions between epididymal secretions and spermatozoa. J Reprod Fertil Suppl 1998;53:119–136.
64. Kirchhoff C, Hale G. Cell-to-cell transfer of glycosylphosphatidylinositol-anchored proteins during sperm maturation. Mol Hum Reprod 1994;2:177–184.
65. Aumuller G, Wilhelm B, Seitz J. Apocrine secretion—fact or artifact? Ann Anat 1999;181:437–446.
66. Yanagimachi R, Kamiguchi Y, Mikamo K, Suzuki F, Yanagimachi H. Maturation of spermatozoa in the epididymis of the Chinese hamster. Am J Anat 1985;172: 317–330.
67. Frenette G, Lessard C, Madore E, Fortier MA, Sullivan R. Aldose reductase and macrophage migration inhibitory factor are associated with epididymosomes and spermatozoa in the bovine epididymis. Biol Reprod 2003;69:1586–1592.
68. Sutovsky P, Moreno R, Ramalho-Santos J, Dominko T, Thompson WE, Schatten G. A putative, ubiquitin-dependent mechanism for the recognition and elimination of defective spermatozoa in the mammalian epididymis. J Cell Sci 2001;114: 1665–1675.
69. Saez F, Frenette G, Sullivan R. Epididymosomes and prostasomes: their roles in posttesticular maturation of the sperm cell. 2003;24:149–154.
70. Sullivan R, Saez F, Girouard J, Frenette G. Role of exosomes in sperm maturation during the transit along the male reproductive tract. 2005;35:1–10.
71. Gatti J-L, Metayer S, Belghazi M, Dacheux F, Dacheux J-L. Identification, proteomic profiling, and origin of ram epididymal fluid exosome-like vesicles. Biol Reprod 2005;72:1452–1465.

72. Yerbury JJ, Stewart EM, Wyatt AR, Wilson MR. Quality control of protein folding in extracellular space. EMBO Rep 2005;6:1131–1136.
73. Cornwall GA, Hann SR. Transient appearance of CRES protein during spermatogenesis and caput epididymal sperm maturation. Mol Reprod Dev 1995;41:37–46.
74. von Horsten HH, SanFrancisco S, Whelly S, Cornwall GA. Cystatin-related epididymal spermatogenic (CRES) protein forms oligomers in epididymal fluid and is a substrate for a secreted tissue-type 2 transglutaminase. (In preparation.)
75. Staniforth RA, Giannini S, Higgins LD, et al. Three-dimensional domain swapping in the folded and molten-globule states of cystatins, an amyloid-forming structural superfamily. Embo J 2001;20:4774–4781.
76. Ekiel I, Abrahamson M. Folding-related dimerization of human cystatin C. J Biol Chem 1996;271:1314–1321.
77. Candi E, Tarcsa E, Idler WW, Kartasova T, Marekov LN, Steinert PM. Covalent blocking of fibril formation and aggregation of intracellular amyloidogenic proteins by transglutaminase-catalyzed intramolecular cross-linking. Biochemistry 2005;44:2072–2079.
78. Ecroyd H, Belghaz M, Dacheux J-L, Gatti J-L. The epididymal soluble prion protein forms a high-molecular-mass complex in association with hydrophobic proteins. Biochem J 2005;392:211–219.

14 The Structure of the Y Chromosome and Its Role in Male Infertility

Leslie Ayensu-Coker, MD,
Colin Bishop, PhD,
and Jan Rohozinski, PhD

Summary

Male infertility accounts for a significant proportion of reproductive failure. Although ejaculatory disorders and impotence can be successfully treated with medical therapy, disorders of genetic origin are more difficult to successfully overcome. Recent advances in our knowledge of Y chromosome structure and function have provided insight into many aspects of the genetic basis of spermatogenic failure and its possible inheritance when assisted reproductive technologies are used to produce offspring.

Key Words: Y chromosome; azoospermia; *AZF*; pseudo-autosomal region male infertility.

1. BACKGROUND

Infertility affects roughly 15% of reproductive aged couples. Although the background prevalence has not changed, changes in lifestyle and delayed childbearing have resulted in an increased number of couples seeking medical attention. Infertility can be categorized as 50% female in origin, 35% male, and 15% unexplained. Female factor infertility can be further separated into disorders of ovulation (20%), tubal disease (15%), cervical/uterine factors (5%), and endometriosis (10%; ref. *1*). Ovulation induction methods are used to treat cases of oligomenorrhea/ amenorrhea. Combined ovulation induction with intrauterine insemination and/or in vitro fertilization (IVF) is used to treat other ovulatory problems and unexplained infertility. Tubal damage associated with infection and endometriosis requires surgical interventions in combination with IVF.

From: *The Genetics of Male Infertility*
Edited by: D.T. Carrell © Humana Press Inc., Totowa, NJ

Sperm disorders are the single most common cause of male factor infertility (2). Ejaculatory disorders and impotence also result in infertility but are effectively treated with medical therapy. Sperm disorders may be separated into oligozoospermia and azoospermia; in cases of sperm dysfunction, the likelihood of natural conception is low.

Oligozoospermia (sperm density <20 million/mL) is sometimes caused by androgen deficiency and may associated with a decrease in motility, known as asthenozoospermia. Asthenozoospermia may be caused by sperm structural defects, prolonged periods of sexual abstinence, genital tact infection, antisperm antibodies, partial duct obstruction, and/or varicocele. Oligoasthenozoospermia is the most common identifiable anomaly found in the semen analysis (3). The most frequent causes are cryptorchidism, endocrinopathy, drugs, excessive heat, toxins, infection, autoimmunity, trauma, and varicocele (3). Drugs are ineffective for idiopathic oligozoospermia and the role of varicocele ligation is uncertain (4).

Azoospermia, the lack of sperm in the ejaculate, can be divided into obstructive and nonobstructive categories. Obstructive azoospermia is characterized by normal sperm production and is often caused by congenital absence or anomalies of the vas deferens. Nonobstructive azoospermia is characterized by a varying degree of spermatogenic failure and is likely to be associated with an increased number of chromosomal abnormalities (5,6).

With the development of intracytoplasmic sperm injection (ICSI), microsurgical epididymal sperm aspiration, and testicular sperm extraction more than a decade ago, men with sperm disorders are now able to father children. These techniques do not correct deficient spermatogenesis but provide a means of bypassing the problem. In standard IVF, human oocytes are harvested from hyperstimulated ovaries and incubated in a culture dish with sperm. Couples with severe male factor infertility reported poor results with standard IVF because approx 150,000 motile sperm per oocyte are required for proper fertilization. To overcome this requirement, micromanipulation techniques were developed. Zona drilling, partial zona dissection, and subzonal insertion of sperm, the microinjection of spermatozoa into the space between the zona pellucida and the plasma membrane, have been used to overcome severe male factor infertility. Typically only three to four sperm were inserted per oocyte; however, the high rate of polyspermy with partial zona dissection and subzonal insertion of sperm have proved lethal to the developing embryo. These problems are not encountered with ICSI, which requires the injection of only a single sperm per egg. ICSI is now the standard of care for treatment of severe male factor infertility, because it produces higher clinical pregnancy rates and has broader applicability.

2. THE STRUCTURE OF THE Y CHROMOSOME

It is believed that more than 60% of men with idiopathic male infertility may have a genetic basis for their subfertility *(2)*. This naturally turns attention to the Y chromosome. The human Y chromosome is one of the smallest chromosomes in the genome. It contains more than 60 million nucleotides, with the least number of genes compared with any other chromosome, and acts as a genetic determinant of male characteristic features. Approximately 95% of the sequence is nonrecombining, and is present only in males. This nonrecombining region, also known as the male-specific region, MSY, represents a mosaic of heterochromatic sequences and three classes of euchromatic (X-transposed, X degenerate, and amplionic) sequences *(7)*. The heterochromatic region contains about 30 Mb of sequence and the euchromatic region contains about 24 Mb of sequence *(8)*. There are two pseudoautosomal regions, PABY1 and PABY2, on the short (Yp) and long (Yq) arms of the Y chromosome, respectively, with homologs found on the X chromosome *(7)*. This comprises 5% of the chromosome and is the only region that participates in meiotic recombination.

Because of its haploid status and absence of recombination, sequence variations in the Y chromosome are largely to the result of accumulation of *de novo* mutations *(9)*. Variations also arise from polymorphisms detected as single-nucleotide polymorphisms (SNPs) or micro- and mini-satellites *(10)*.

There are several genes on the Y chromosome associated with genetic anomalies and linked to infertility (Table 1; ref. *11*). One gene controlling spermatogenesis is referred to as azoospermia factor (*AZF*), located in the Yq11.23 region. It was originally established by Tiepolo and Zuffardi in 1976 that deletions of the long arm of the Y chromosome are associated with spermatogenic failure *(7)*. Vogt et al. observed that Y-chromosome microdeletions follow a certain deletion pattern, with three recurrently deleted, presumably nonoverlapping, subregions in the proximal, middle, and distal Yq11. These are designated *AZFa*, *AZFb*, and *AZFc*, respectively. It has since been shown that *AZFb* and *AZFc* regions are not independent, but show overlap and that the *AZFa* region, which spans 0.8-Mb of sequence is independent of the other two regions *(13)*. Approximately 20% of men suffering from infertility of nonobstructive (curable) oligo- or azoospermia with normal chromosomes have been found to show microdeletions of *AZF* sequences *(12)*.

Table 1
Y Chromosome-Linked Genes Associated With Genetic Disorders *(11)*

Gene abbreviation	Gene	Locus	Disorder
AZF1	Azoospermia factor 1	Yq11	Possibly? Sertoli cell only syndrome
DAZ	Deleted in azoospermia	Yq11	Possibly? Sertoli cell only syndrome
SRY	Sex-determining region Y	Yq11.3	Gonadal dysgenesis, XY type
USP9y	Ubiquitin-specific protease 9, Y chromosome	Yq11.2	Azoospermia

Deletion of the *AZFc* is the most common known cause of spermatogenic failure *(14)*. This region was completely sequenced *(15)* and found to contain massive palindromes spanning as much as 3-Mb sequences. The expression of the *AZF* gene is found to be testis-specific in human and several other mammals. The identification of the palindromic complexes P1 to P5 encompassing azoospermia factors may lead to a better understanding of the biological roles of various repeat elements *(13)*.

The deleted azoospermia *(DAZ)* gene family was identified in a study in which 12 infertile men were found to have overlapping deletions on the Y chromosome *(5)*. *DAZ* is reported to have at least four copies, is transcribed in the adult testis, and encodes an RNA-binding protein *(16)*.

The sex-determining region on chromosome Y (*SRY*), also known as testis-determining factor, is involved in male sex determination and is one of the most highly characterized of the Y-chromosome genes. The gene encodes a transcription factor of about 204 amino acids from a single open reading frame (ORF) of about 669 basepairs *(17)*. *SRY* is a member of the high-mobility group DNA-binding protein with a highly conserved HMG-box domain. *SRY* was mapped to the human Y chromosome by molecular analysis of sex-reversed patients. Analysis of four XX males with testes were found to have a minute portion of the Y translocated to the X chromosome. This fragment was found to be critical in defining the sex-determining region on the human Y chromosome *(18)*.

Mutations within the gene *USP9Y* has been reported in two individuals with spermatogenic failure leading to infertility *(11)*. Four base pair deletions result in premature truncation of the encoded protein. The *USP9Y* gene has a homolog, *USP9X*, on the X chromosome and both are ubiquitously expressed.

3. CONCLUSION

Because many cases of male infertility have been shown to be of genetic origin, the potential risk of transmitting infertility to future generations is of concern. There has been no evidence currently that the physical health of children is affected by use of infertility treatment techniques. There have been studies, however, showing that the deletions involved in spermatogenesis disorders are transmitted to male offspring via ICSI. The fertility status of these children is not known because these children have not yet entered puberty *(19)*.

REFERENCES

1. Speroff L, Glass R, Kase N. Female infertility. In: Clinical Gynecologic Endocriniology and Infertility, 6th ed. Lippincott Williams & Wilkins, Hagerstown, MD 1999;1020–1021.
2. Razvi K, Chew S, Yong EL, Kumar J, Ng SC. The clinical management of male infertility. Singapore Med J 1999;4:291–297.
3. Rehman K, Grunbam A, Carrier S. Evaluation and treatment of oligoathenospermia in the era of assisted reproductive techniques. J Sex Reprod Med 2002;2:1–5.
4. Templeton A. Infertility—epidemiology, aetiology and effective management. Health Bulletin (Edinb) 1995;53:294–298.
5. Reijo R, Alagappan RK, Patrizio P, Page DC. Severe oligozoospermia resulting from deletions of azoospermia factor gene on Y chromosome. Lancet 1996;347:1290–1293.
6. Girardi SK, Mielnik A, Schlegel PN. Submicroscopic deletions in the Y chromosome of infertile men. Hum Reprod 1997;8:1635–1641.
7. Tiepolo L, Zuffardi O. Localization of factors controlling spermatogenesis in the nonfluorescent portion of the human chromosome long arm. Hum Genet 1976; 34:119–124.
8. Vollrath D, Foote S, Hilton A, et al. The human Y chromosome: a 43-interval map based on naturally occurring deletions. Science 1992;258:52–59.
9. Santos FR, Pandya A, Kayser M, et al. A polymorphic L1 retroposon insertion in the centromere of the human Y chromosome. Human Mol Genet 2000;9:421–430.
10. Mathias H, Bayes M, Tyler-Smith C. Highly informative compound haplotypes for the human Y chromosome. Human Mol Genet 1994;1:115–123.
11. Ali S, Hasnain SE. Molecular dissection of the human Y-chromosome. Gene 2002;283:1–10.
12. Vogt PH, Edelmann A, Kirsch S, Hengariu O, Hirschmann P, Kiesewater F. Human Y chromosome azoospermia factors (AZF) mapped to different subregions in YQ11. Hum Mol Genet 1996;5:933–943.

13. Repping S, Skaletsky H, Lange J, et al. Recombination between palindromes P5 and P1 on the human Y chromosome causes massive deletions and spermatogenic failure. Am J Human Genet 2002;71:906–922.

14. Briton-Jones C, Haines CJ. Microdeletions on the long arm of the Y chromosome and their association with male-factor infertility. Hong Kong Med J 2000;6:184–189.

15. Kuroda-Kawaguchi T, Skaletsky H, Brown LG, et al. The AZFc region of the Y chromosome features massive palindromes and uniform recurrent deletions in infertile men. Nat Genet 2001;29:279–286.

16. Saxena R, de Vries JW, Repping S, et al. Four DAZ genes in two clusters found in the AZFc region of the human Y chromosome. Genomics 2000;67:256–267.

17. Behlke MA, Bogan JS, Beer-Romero P, Page DC. Evidence that the SRY protein is encoded by a single exon on the human Y chromosome. Genomics 1993;17:736–739.

18. Sinclair AH, Berta P, Palmer MS, et al. A gene from the human sex-determining region encodes a protein with homology to a conserved DNA-binding motif. Nature 1990;346:240–244.

19. Sutcliffe AG. Intracytoplasmic sperm injection and other aspects of new reproductive technologies. Arch Dis Child 2000;83:98–101.

15 Y Chromosome Microdeletions and Haplotypes

Ken McElreavey, PhD,
Celia Ravel, MD,
Brahim El Houate, MSc,
Jacqueline Mandelbaum, MD, PhD,
Sandra Chantot-Bastaraud, MD,
and Jean-Pierre Siffroi, MD, PhD

Summary

The human Y chromosome contains a number of genes and gene families that are necessary for spermatogenesis. Many of these genes are embedded in repetitive elements that are subject to deletion events. Deletions of azoospermia factor (AZF) regions *AZFa*, *AZFb*, and *AZFc* are found in approx 10–15% of men with either unexplained severe oligozoospermia or azoospermia. These deletions fall on different Y chromosome backgrounds and there is no evidence for a link between a Y-chromosome lineage and the presence or absence of an *AZF* deletion. Several partial *AZFc* deletions have been described. One of these, which removes around half of all the genes within the *AZFc* region, appears to be present as in inconsequential polymorphism in populations of northern Eurasia. A second deletion, termed gr/gr, results in the absence of several *AZFc* genes and has been suggested to be a genetic risk factor for spermatogenic failure. However, the link between the gr/gr deletion and infertility is more complex. First, the gr/gr deletion is actually not a single type of deletion but a combination of deletions that vary in size and complexity and result in the absence of different members of the deleted azoospermia (*DAZ*) gene family as well as other *AZFc* genes, such as *CDY1*. Second, there are regional or ethnic differences in the frequency of gr/gr deletions. In some Y-chromosome lineages, these deletion appear to be fixed and may have little influence on spermatogenesis. Third, these observations have influenced a number of association studies aimed to determine the relationship between the gr/gr deletion and male infertility. Consequently, some studies suggest that the gr/gr

From: *The Genetics of Male Infertility*
Edited by: D.T. Carrell © Humana Press Inc., Totowa, NJ

deletion confers a strong genetic susceptibility to reduced sperm counts, whereas others suggest that the genetic susceptibility may not exist or be limited to specific Y-chromosome haplotypes.

Clearly there is need for additional studies that combine an analysis of a series of markers in the *AZFc* region together with the haplotype of the Y chromosome in well-defined case and control populations. Many of the genes in the *AZFc* region present in multiple copies and gr/gr deletions can be associated with reciprocal duplication events. Therefore, there is a need to determine gene dosage if the relationship between gr/gr deletions and infertility is to be completely understood.

Key Words: Y chromosome; haplotype; haplogroup; male infertility; spermatogenesis; microdeletion; gr/gr; DAZ.

1. Y-CHROMOSOME POLYMORPHISMS DEFINE DISTINCT LINEAGES

The vast majority (57 of 60 Mb) of the Y chromosome does not recombine with the X chromosome and is transmitted as a single block from father to son with all functional variants and neutral polymorphisms being linked. A Y-chromosome lineage or haplogroup (Hg) is a monophyletic group of Y chromosomes defined by stable binary markers, such as single-nucleotide variants or insertion/deletions. More than 200 binary markers have been characterized on the human Y chromosome *(1)* and it is likely that many others will be available in the near future that can be used to further refine Y lineages. Y-chromosome microsatellites are variable in all populations and a particular combination of allelic states can be used to define a Y-chromosome haplotype within a defined Hg. The population distribution of Y chromosome variation indicates that most lineages are largely confined to particular human populations, which has important implications for association studies *(2)*. A number of association studies have been published that measure the frequencies of Y-chromosome haplotypes in case and control groups of men with different male-specific phenotypes, including infertility. The distinct population affinities displayed by many Y-chromosome haplotypes and their high degree of geographical specificity means that an association between the Y-chromosome background and a phenotype in one population or country may not be relevant for another. Conversely, the absence of an association in one population does not imply its absence in other populations. However, these studies are useful because they may identify classes or lineages of the Y chromosome that may be at increased risk of developing infertility. Furthermore, an increased awareness of the physical structure and detailed organization of Y chromosomes within a lineage is essential to aid in the interpretation of data generated by association studies. This problem has been highlighted by attempts to correlate different types of microdeletions of the Y chromosome with reduced sperm counts and/or infertility. These studies will be the object of this chapter.

2. AZF DELETIONS ARE ASSOCIATED WITH MALE INFERTILITY

Three regions of the long arm of the Y chromosome, termed azoospermia factor (AZF)a, AZFb, and AZFc are associated with reduced or absent sperm counts *(3)*. Men presenting with AZF deletions appear to be otherwise healthy, although it should be stressed that there does not appear to be any longer-term studies to determine if these men are at risk from other health problems. All of the AZF microdeletions are the result of intrachromosomal exchange between regions containing highly repetitive sequences. Intrachromosomal exchange between repetitive elements derived from the HERV15 class of endogenous retroviruses cause deletions of the AZFa region *(4,5)*. Complete AZFb deletions are associated with recombination between palindromic sequences, are 6.23 Mb in length, and extend 1.5 Mb into the proximal portion of AZFc *(6)*. Likewise AZFb+AZFc deletions are also a consequence of recombination between palindromic sequences. These deletions are 7.66 Mb in size and do not include the distal portion of AZFc *(6)*. Deletions of the AZFc region are estimated to occur in 1 in 4000 males and are the most common class of deletion (~80% of the total) in men with a more severe phenotype (azoospermia or severe oligozoospermia [$<1 \times 10^6$/mL]) and are considered to be the consequence of homologous recombination between two direct repeats of 229 kb in length (termed b2/b4; ref. *7*) in a region of the Y chromosome that is made up almost entirely of long direct and inverted repeats termed amplicons. Within the AZFc region there are several candidate fertility genes, including three copies of basic protein on Y chromosome, 2 (*BPY2*), two copies of *CDY1a* and *CDY1b*; Chromodomain protein, Y chromosome 1 (*CDY1*), and four copies of the deleted in azoospermia (*DAZ*) gene *(3,7)*. It is still not clear if each of these factors contribute to infertility or if there is a key infertility gene. The different AZF deletions arise on various Y-chromosome lineages and there does not appear to be a Y Hg that either protects against deletion formation or is more sensitive to deletions *(8,9)*. However, it should be noted that studies to date have focused on AZFa or AZFb and AZFc deletions and it cannot be ruled out that AZFa deletions, although rare, may fall on specific Y-chromosome backgrounds.

3. PARTIAL AZFc DELETIONS AND Y-CHROMOSOME VARIANTS

The relationship between partial AZFc deletions and reduced sperm counts (or fertility) is unclear. Some of these deletions appear to have little effect on fertility, whereas others appear to be associated with significant risk for developing spermatogenic failure. However, the relationship is complex and, as indicated previously, data that may be applicable to one population may not be applicable to another. To understand the depth of this problem we must first consider the intricate sequence organisation of the AZFc region.

The entire AZFc region spans 4.5 Mb and consists of three palindromes with six distinct families of amplicons, which may have resulted from a complex series of tandem duplication and inversion events (7). These amplicons were termed turquoise, gray, yellow, green (g), blue (b), and red (r). Other sequences (u1, u2, and u3) occur once each in the region but share a high degree of sequence identity to other Y chromosome loci. The four *DAZ* genes on the human Y chromosome exist in two clusters and each cluster consists of an inverted pair of *DAZ* genes (*DAZ1/DAZ2* and *DAZ3/DAZ4 [10]*). Changes in *DAZ* gene copy number have been demonstrated using the techniques of fluorescence *in situ* hybridization, quantitative polymerase chain reaction and the analysis of sequence-family variants (SFVs) that can distinguish between *DAZ* copies and between *DAZ* clusters. SFVs are defined as subtle differences between closely related but nonallelic sequences. In particular, the SFV sY587 (also known as DAZ-SNV V) can distinguish between *DAZ1/2* gene pair and *DAZ3/4* gene pair and has proven to be particularly informative.

Yen 2001 *(11)* predicted that recombination could occur between any pair of amplicons that are present in the same orientation (resulting in the deletion of the intervening sequences) and that such deletions may have an effect on fertility. Using Southern blot-based techniques, Yen and colleagues have determined that most men have four *DAZ* copies (similar to the original individual used to determine the structure of the *DAZ* genes *[12]*). In the same study, a small number of men (6%) were observed to carry six copies of the *DAZ* gene on different Y chromosome Hgs. The significance of this observation will be discussed later.

A large partial deletion of the AZFc region has been reported and it is suggested that this deletion does not to affect fertility. Vogt and colleagues described a large deletion of the AZFc region that includes the sequences u3 and *DAZ3/4* (termed g1/g3; ref. *14*). This deletion occurs on haplogroup N3, a Y-chromosome lineage that is found at high frequencies in northern Europe (52% of Finns) and in other populations of northern Eurasia. Further work by Mitchell and colleagues indicated that this deletion also includes the *CDY1b* gene (they termed the deletion u3-gr/gr *[12]*). This deletion has been suggested to originate from an inversion of sequences mediated by the b2/b3 amplicons followed by recombination between the g1 and g3 sequences resulting in the loss of intervening sequences, including *DAZ3/4 (13)*. Repping et al. *(15)* suggested a second pathway by which this deletion could have arisen, namely a gr/rg inversion (g1, r1, r2 recombining with r3, r4, g3) followed by a b2/b3 deletion (Fig. 1). In reality, both mutational pathways are probably occurring and this can be tested in the general male population, because each pathway requires an intermediary step. In an analysis of interphase nuclei from men carrying Y chromosomes representing 44 different lineages, 4 of 44 individuals carried the predicted gr/rg inversion and 3 of 44 carried the b2/b3 inversion *(15)*. This deletion was also present in low frequencies in three other Y chromosome lineages (H*, O*, and O3*). Machev et al. *(14)* also found the deletion in the Y chromosome Hgs Y*(xD, E, J, K) and P. A large portion of AZFc, including 12 testis-specific genes or transcripts, is removed by this deletion, raising the important question of whether it contributes to infertility. However, presence of this deletion (referred to variously as u3-gr/gr, g1/g3, or b2/b3) at high frequencies in some populations suggests that it may be a polymorphism with limited or no effect on fertility.

A second partial AZFc deletion removes a 1.6-Mb proximal segment of AZFc including two copies of the *DAZ* gene cluster (*DAZ1/2*). Vogt and colleagues identified this deletion in 5 of 63 oligozoospermic samples and not in 107 fertile control samples and suggested that it may be responsible for reduced sperm numbers *(16)*. This deletion has subsequently been termed gr/gr (g1/g2, r1/r3, r2/r4) in reference to the resulting organization of the amplicons *(17)*. Gr/gr deletions were detected in 22 individuals following an initial screen of DNA samples from 689 men *(17)*. In a subsequent association study by the same group, gr/gr deletions were found in 9 of 237 (3.7%) men with spermatogenic failure of unknown origin. In 148 men with normal spermatogenesis, this deletion was not detected, suggesting that the gr/gr deletion correlates with decreased sperm production and that the gr/gr deletion is a significant risk factor for spermatogenic failure *(17)*. However, the association between gr/gr deletions and infertility is not so simple. In the same study *(17)*, the authors screened a human Y-chromosome biodiversity panel that

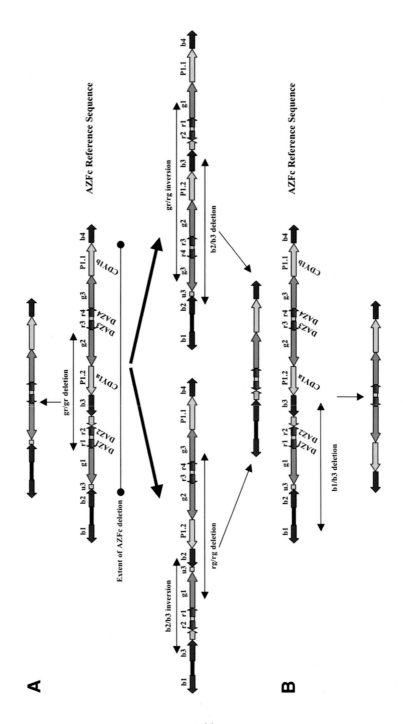

represented 43 different Y-chromosome lineages. Gr/gr-deleted Y chromosomes were found in 14 independent Y-chromosome lineages. This indicates that the deletion has occurred multiple times during human evolution. In one Y-chromosome lineage (D2b), all samples screened (12/12) carried the gr/gr deletion, suggesting that it may be fixed in this Y chromosome Hg *(17)*. The fertility status of the individuals contributing to this panel is unknown but it suggests that in some Y-chromosome lineages the gr/gr deletion may have a limited effect on fertility. The gr/gr-deleted D2b Y-chromosome lineage is present in about 30–40% of Japanese men and has been reported to be associated with reduced sperm counts *(18)*. It is important to note that the association with this Hg was not observed in a follow-up study. Although there may be a weak association between the D2b haplogroup and reduced sperm counts, the majority of the Japanese population with this lineage have sperm counts that are more than 40×10^6 *(13,18)*. Although some more recent association studies have indicated a strong association between gr/gr deletions and reduced sperm counts, others have questioned the validity of this link. de Llanos et al. detected gr/gr deletions in 12 of 283 (4.2%) consecutive intracytoplasmic sperm injection candidates with either azoospermia or oligozoospermia and deletions were not found in a control panel of 232 men *(19)*. Ferlin et al. *(20)* reported an increased frequency of not only *DAZ1/DAZ2* (gr/gr) deletions, but also *DAZ3/DAZ4* deletions in men with reduced sperm counts compared with normospermic individuals.

Fig. 1. *(Opposite page)* Models of the origins of the most frequent partial AZFc deletions. **(A)** The reference AZFc sequence is indicated and the organization of amplicons belonging to various families are shown in colors (b1 to b4 [blue], r1 to r4 [red], g1 to g3 [green]). Two small palindromes P1.1 and P1.2 (yellow) lie within a larger P1 palindrome. Sequences with the same color code exhibit more than 99.9% sequence identity. The relative position of the unique sequence u3 is also indicated. The relative location of *CDY1* and *DAZ* gene copies is indicated underneath their respective amplicons. The deletion of the entire AZFc region occurs as consequence of recombination between amplicons b2 and b4 and is indicated. The schematic representation of the gr/gr-deleted chromosome is indicated above the reference sequence. Under the reference sequence, two pathways are indicated that could give rise to the b2/b3 deletion (also referred to as u3-gr/gr and g1/g3 *[13,14]*). Both pathways predict an inversion–deletion model. In one scenario (right), homologous recombination generates a gr/rg inversion (g1, r1, r2 recombining with r3, r4, g3), which is followed by a deletion between b2 and b3 amplicons. In a second scenario (left), there is an inversion mediated by b2 and b3 amplicons followed by an rg/rg deletion. All of these events are a consequence of homologous recombination. **(B)** Schematic representation of the generation of a b1/b3 deletion. This deletion was predicted by Yen *(11)* and removes a proximal portion of AZFc. It has been observed in a very small number of normospermic and infertile individuals *(see refs. 15 and 21)* and consequently the relationship of the b1/b3 deletion to infertility is unknown.

However, several studies have not detected strong associations. Hucklenbroich et al. *(21)* observed that the incidence of gr/gr deletions in a population of ethnic Germans from Westphalia was not significantly different between a case population of 348 men (4% gr/gr-deleted) with nonobstructive oligospermia/azoospermia and a control population of 170 normospermic men (1.8% gr/gr-deleted). A lack of association between the gr/gr with reduced sperm counts was also observed by Mitchell and colleagues *(13)*. In our own studies, we have failed to find an association between the gr/gr deletion and reduced sperm counts in a study of patients attending a clinical center in Paris *(22)*.

In the light of this apparently conflicting data, how can we clarify the impact of partial AZFc deletions on human spermatogenesis? In some cases, partial deletions are associated with a secondary duplication. In their initial study, Repping et al. *(17)* screened 20 of the 22 men with gr/gr deletions using interphase fluorescence *in situ* hybridization and detected two men with a secondary duplication. Such a b2/b4 duplication, which has also been inferred from the data of Mitchell and colleagues *(13)*, could rescue the gr/gr-deleted phenotype. This idea is supported by the observations of Yen and colleagues that around 6% of men actually carry six copies of the *DAZ* gene *(12)*.

The key to solving these problems may lie in three important factors: the markers used in the screening process to identify partial AZFc deletions, the phenotype that is studied, and the Y-chromosome lineage on which the deletion has arisen.

It is important to emphasize that not all gr/gr deletions are the same. In the study by Machev et al. *(13)*, novel SFVs that differentiate between the two copies of the *CDY1* gene in AZFc were used as part of the screening panel. Although an association between partial AZFc deletions and reduced sperm counts was not observed when they screened samples using markers used by other groups, they did observe a weak association between the absence of markers defining *DAZ3/4* and *CDY1a* ($p = 0.042$) and infertility. A stronger association was observed between the loss of the *CDY1a* SFV alone and infertility ($p = 0.002$). It is important to emphasize that the loss of this SFV does not necessarily infer a deletion, because gene conversion events could also explain this observation. However, the data suggest that the use of additional informative markers within the AZFc region may unmask novel deletions that could be genuinely associated with reduced sperm counts. This has also been suggested by the study of Hucklenbroich et al. *(21)*, who found novel partial AZFc deletions in their infertile cohort but not in samples from normospermic men.

The second factor that needs to be explored is the phenotype that is under study. An interesting survey of gr/gr deletions in men seeking fertility treatment in Australia failed to detect an association between gr/gr deletions and reduced sperm counts *(23)*. However, the authors did note an increased incidence of gr/gr deletions in men who were normospermic and yet infertile. Most of the studies published to date have sought to determine an association between the gr/gr deletion and men with reduced sperm counts and obviously this type of association would not be detected. It also raises the possibility that the gr/gr deletions could be associated with defaults in sperm mobility or morphology rather than actual numbers.

The third confounding effect could be the Y-chromosome lineage on which the deletion arises. As mentioned previously, some Y lineages have partial AZFc deletions that appear to have little or limited effects on fertility and this may be to the result of compensatory alterations elsewhere on the Y, or perhaps on the X chromosome or autosomes. This concept is reinforced by the observations of Nathanson et al. *(24)* in a study of the frequency of gr/gr deletions in men with testicular cancer compared with the incidence of these deletions in various control groups. In this study, the difference in the incidence of gr/gr deletion between the control groups was statistically significant.

The definition of the Y-chromosome haplotype in cases of partial AZFc deletions is likely to play an essential role in understanding the contribution of the deletion to reduced sperm counts. There is a pressing need for large-scale studies on well-characterized normospermic and oligospermic/azoospermic individuals of different ethnic origins with multiple informative AZFc markers if the correlation between these deletions and the phenotype is finally to be resolved.

4. CONCLUSION

Different types of deletions on the Y chromosome have been reported that cause infertility. These include the deletions AZFa, AZFb, and AZFc. Several partial deletions of AZFc have been described that, in some cases, may be trivial polymorphisms that are present on specific Y-chromosome lineages and in other cases may be associated with a risk of infertility. The latter include the gr/gr deletions that have been proposed to be associated with reduced sperm counts. However, the relationship between the gr/gr deletions and infertility is not clear because there are several types of gr/gr deletions that show marked region/ethnic differences in frequency and in some cases may be associated with duplication events. There is a need for larger studies on well-defined populations that include a description of the Y chromosome lineages to fully understand the relationship of these deletions with fertility.

5. ACKNOWLEDGMENTS

The authors wish to thank Association pour la Recherche sur le Cancer for their financial support for our studies.

REFERENCES

1. Y Chromosome Consortium. A nomenclature system for the tree of human Y-chromosomal binary haplogroups. Genome Res 2002;12:339–348.
2. Rosser ZH, Zerjal T, Hurles ME, et al. Y-chromosomal diversity in Europe is clinal and influenced primarily by geography, rather than by language. Am J Hum Genet 2000;67:1526–1543.
3. McElreavey K, Krausz C, Bishop CE. The human Y chromosome and male infertility. Results Probl Cell Differ 2000;28:211–232.
4. Kamp C, Hirschmann P, Voss H, Huellen K, Vogt PH. Two long homologous retroviral sequence blocks in proximal Yq11 cause AZFa microdeletions as a result of intrachromosomal recombination events. Hum Mol Genet 2000;9: 2563–2572.
5. Sun C, Skaletsky H, Rozen S, et al. Deletion of azoospermia factor a (AZFa) region of human Y chromosome caused by recombination between HERV15 proviruses. Hum Mol Genet 2000;9:2291–2296.
6. Repping S, Skaletsky H, Lange J, et al. Recombination between palindromes P5 and P1 on the human Y chromosome causes massive deletions and spermatogenic failure. Am J Hum Genet 2002;71:906–922.
7. Kuroda-Kawaguchi T, Skaletsky H, Brown LG, et al. The AZFc region of the Y chromosome features massive palindromes and uniform recurrent deletions in infertile men. Nat Genet 2001;29:279–286.
8. Paracchini S, Stuppia L, Gatta V, et al. Y-chromosomal DNA haplotypes in infertile European males carrying Y-microdeletions. J Endocrinol Invest 2000;23: 671–676.
9. Quintana-Murci L, Krausz C, Heyer E, et al. The relationship between Y chromosome DNA haplotypes and Y chromosome deletions leading to male infertility. Hum Genet 2001;108:55–58.
10. Saxena R, de Vries JW, Repping S, et al. Four DAZ genes in two clusters found in the AZFc region of the human Y chromosome. Genomics 2000;67:256–267.
11. Yen P. The fragility of fertility. Nat Genet 2001;29:243–244.
12. Lin YW, Thi DA, Kuo PL, et al. Polymorphisms associated with the DAZ genes on the human Y chromosome. Genomics 2005;86:431–438.
13. Machev N, Saut N, Longepied G, et al. Sequence family variant loss from the AZFc interval of the human Y chromosome, but not gene copy loss, is strongly associated with male infertility. J Med Genet 2004;41:814–825.
14. Fernandes S, Paracchini S, Meyer LH, et al. A large AZFc deletion removes DAZ3/DAZ4 and nearby genes from men in Y haplogroup N. Am J Hum Genet 2004;74:180–187.
15. Repping S, van Daalen SK, Korver CM, et al. A family of human Y chromosomes has dispersed throughout northern Eurasia despite a 1.8-Mb deletion in the azoospermia factor c region. Genomics 2004;83:1046–1052.
16. Fernandes S, Huellen K, Goncalves J, et al. High frequency of DAZ1/DAZ2 gene deletions in patients with severe oligozoospermia. Mol Hum Reprod 2002;8: 286–298.

17. Repping S, Skaletsky H, Brown L, et al. Polymorphism for a 1.6-Mb deletion of the human Y chromosome persists through balance between recurrent mutation and haploid selection. Nat Genet 2003;35:247–251.

18. Kuroki Y, Iwamoto T, Lee J, et al. Spermatogenic ability is different among males in different Y chromosome lineage. J Hum Genet 1999;44:289–292.

19. de Llanos M, Ballesca JL, Gazquez C, Margarit E, Oliva R. High frequency of gr/gr chromosome Y deletions in consecutive oligospermic ICSI candidates. Hum Reprod 2005;20:216–220.

20. Ferlin A, Tessari A, Ganz F, et al. Association of partial AZFc region deletions with spermatogenic impairment and male infertility. J Med Genet 2005;42:209–213.

21. Hucklenbroich K, Gromoll J, Heinrich M, et al. Partial deletions in the AZFc region of the Y chromosome occur in men with impaired as well as normal spermatogenesis. Hum Reprod 2005;20:191–197.

22. Ravel C, Chantot-Bastaraud S, El Houate B, et al. GR/GR deletions within the azoospermia factor c region on the Y chromosome might not be associated with spermatogenic failure. Fertil Steril 2006;85:229–231.

23. Lynch M, Cram DS, Reilly A, et al. The Y chromosome gr/gr subdeletion is associated with male infertility. Mol Hum Reprod 2005;11:507–512.

24. Nathanson KL, Kanetsky PA, Hawes R, et al. The Y deletion gr/gr and susceptibility to testicular germ cell tumor. Am J Hum Genet 2005;77:1034–1043.

16 The Genetics of Male Infertility

From Bench to Clinic

David M. de Kretser, MD,
Moira K. O'Bryan, PhD,
Michael Lynch, PhD,
Anne Reilly, BScHons,
Claire Kennedy, PhD,
David Cram, PhD,
and Robert I. McLachlan, MD, PhD

Summary

This chapter provides an overview of the causes of male infertility and identifies the developments that have occurred in the identification of genetic causes of spermatogenic disorders. The approaches to the identification of new genetic causes of infertility are discussed, and provide an indication of the mechanisms that can be disrupted by targeted inactivation of genes in mice. The emerging genetic targets provide new directions for the development of tests to detect mutations in these genes in men with infertility.

Key Words: Male infertility; genetics; spermatogenesis; mutagenesis.

1. INTRODUCTION

For the clinician, the inability to define the cause of a spermatogenic defect and develop an evidenced-based treatment regime is a source of great frustration. In this chapter, a brief review of the defined causes of male infertility is undertaken to illustrate the lack of information concerning the cause of spermatogenic defects that form the

From: *The Genetics of Male Infertility*
Edited by: D.T. Carrell © Humana Press Inc., Totowa, NJ

Table 1
Classification of Causes of Male Infertility

Hormonal:
- Hypothalamic lesions:
  - Kallmann's syndrome
  - Opiate induced
- Pituitary lesions:
  - Tumors
  - Hemochromatosis
  - Luteinizing hormone and follicle-stimulating hormone suppression from androgen abuse, opiates
- Testicular:
  - Androgen biosynthetic defects
  - Androgen receptor mutations

Testicular:
- Anorchia, torsion
- Maldescent of testis
- Orchitis: nonspecific, mumps
- Irradiation, chemotherapy
- Drugs
- Heat exposure
- Varicocele
- Immunological: sperm antibodies
- Genetic
  - Klinefelter's syndrome
  - Y-chromosome deletions
  - Primary ciliary dyskinesia
- Metabolic
  - Renal failure
  - Liver failure
- Testicular tumors
- Idiopathic spermatogenic defects

Post-Testicular
- Obstructive
  - Congenital absence of vas
  - After sexually transmitted disease
  - Post-inguinal surgery
  - Vasectomy
  - Intraprostatic
- Epididymal maturational defects
- Accessory gland infection
- Sperm antibodies
- Coital
  - Infrequent intercourse
  - Erectile dysfunction
  - Ejaculatory disturbances
- Sperm–oocyte interactions

Table 2
Frequency of Causes of Male Infertility in Patients in a Tertiary Clinical Setting in Melbourne in 1986 (*n* = 1041)

Primary testicular	
• Klinefelter's syndrome	1.9%
• Past cryptorchidism	6.4%
• Past mumps orchitis	1.6%
• Past irradiation and chemotherapy	0.5%
• Varicocele	40%
• Idiopathic spermatogenic disorders	44.4%
Secondary testicular failure	
• Hypothalamic/pituitary disorders	0.5%
Genital tract obstructions	
• Vasal agenesis	0.6%
• Epididymal obstructions	3.5%
Coital disorders	0.5%

basis of infertility. This data will set the context in which the search for genetic causes of male infertility is proceeding.

Male infertility can be the result of abnormalities in hormonal control, spermatogenic disorders, disruption of sperm transport and maturation, failure of sperm–oocyte interactions and coital disorders that limit the exposure of the oocyte to sperm. It is not possible to provide a comprehensive discussion of each of these areas in this chapter, and readers should consult the remaining chapters of this book and other recent publications for further details *(1,2)*. An overview is provided in Table 1. A summary of the causes of male infertility in patients presenting to our reproductive medicine clinic in 1986 provides an indication of the frequency of the differing causes of male infertility (Table 2). It is evident that the etiology of their spermatogenic disorder was unknown in about 40% of the men. Further, 40% of men had a varicocele identified, and given the current controversy of the relationship between varicoceles and infertility and spermatogenic disruption *(3,4)*, it could be argued that in about 80% of these men, the cause of their spermatogenic disturbance was unknown.

Twenty years later, the situation has not changed greatly. In many countries where vasectomy is popular, requests for reversal or the achievement of pregnancies by sperm retrieval from the epididymis or testis now represent a new cause of male infertility. The major advance in the area of genetics is the accepted view that in about 3–5% of men with sperm counts of less than 5 million/mL, a Y-chromosome deletion can be identified as the cause of infertility *(5–7)*. In addition, in a small number of men, mutations in other genes have been causally related to spermatogenic

Table 3
Genes in Which Mutations May Cause an Impairment
in Hormonal Stimulation of Spermatogenesis

- *Gonadotrophin-releasing hormone (GnRH)*
  - Kalig 1 gene
  - Fibroblast growth factor receptor
  - GnRH receptor
- *Follicle-stimulating hormone (FSH)*
  - β-subunit
  - α-subunit common to luteinizing hormone (LH) and thyroid-stimulating hormone (TSH)
  - FSH receptor
- *LH*
  - β-subunit
  - α-subunit common to FSH and TSH
  - LH receptor
- *Testosterone*
  - Steroid biosynthetic enzymes, some common to adrenal
  - Steroid acute regulatory protein gene
  - Androgen receptor gene including CAG repeat length

defects or duct abnormalities. Some examples of these include androgen receptor defects *(8)*, mutations in the cystic fibrosis transmembrane regulator gene *(9)*, genes related to primary ciliary dyskinesia *(10,11)*, the *SYCP3* gene that encodes a component of the synaptonemal complex *(12)*, and genes related to disturbed hormonal control of spermatogenesis (Table 3; refs. *13–22*). Unfortunately, in these genetic defects the pathophysiology involved is still poorly understood, preventing therapeutic developments. Consequently, spermatogenic disorders classified as idiopathic still represent between 30 and 35% of the infertile men.

In view of the dearth of therapeutic options, the last 20 yr has seen the development of assisted reproductive techniques to assist the infertile male, and in many clinics the use of intracytoplasmic sperm injection (ICSI) represents between 40 and 50% of all treatment cycles. The success of ICSI has raised the inevitability that we are transmitting genetic defects that cause infertility to the next generation. Indeed, several papers have reported the transmission of Y-chromosomal deletions to children conceived by the use of ICSI *(23,24)*. The unanswered question is whether there are other genetic causes of infertility that when transmitted to the next generation may cause diseases other than infertility. Data from Lamb's work suggests that some infertile men may carry and transmit mutations that may increase the risk not only of infertility, but also neurodegenerative diseases such as the cerebellar ataxias *(25)*.

There is now an emerging and reasonably well developed body of evidence that genetic defects are causally related to a major portion of the spermatogenic defects that are currently classified as "idiopathic spermatogenic disorders" *(26,27)*. There are several reports and reviews that have established that targeted disruption of genes can result in spermatogenic damage and infertility as the sole phenotype or accompanied by other pathology in mice *(28)*. In this chapter, the known and postulated genetic mechanisms are assembled into a framework that can assist the clinician in the application of these developments to patient management and facilitate clinical research into genetic mechanisms of male infertility.

2. PHYSIOLOGICAL FRAMEWORK

There are multiple control points in the physiology of spermatogenesis that could be disrupted by mutations in specific genes. The resultant defects are divisible into two major groups: those that are reproductive tract-specific and result in infertility as the only phenotype and others that involve alterations in many organ systems. A clear example of the latter are the mutations in the cystic fibrosis transmembrane regulator, which cause cystic fibrosis and congenital absence of the vas deferens. In some instances, however, the same mutation can cause absence of the vas without cystic fibrosis *(9)*.

Key processes in male reproduction that can be disrupted may be classified as follows:

1. Hormonal mechanisms.
2. Mechanisms controlling spermatogenic output.
   a. Migration of germ cells into developing gonad.
   b. Spermatogonial proliferation and survival.
   c. Meiosis.
   d. Spermiogenesis.
   e. Multiple checkpoints.
3. Leydig cell defects.
4. Sperm-transporting system.
5. Sperm–oocyte interactions.

3. THE APPROACH TO THE IDENTIFICATION OF GENETIC DEFECTS

The approaches that have been undertaken to identify genetic defects causing infertility have varied. Frequently, these have arisen from the identification of a crucial control mechanism with a subsequent targeted disruption of a key gene or genes leading to the phenotype in mice (*see* reviews in refs. *28–30*). This has been followed by a search for the equivalent human phenotype. For all of the key processes listed previously, it would be possible to list functional sets of genes that should be examined in men exhibiting the phenotype that might be expected if the control system was disrupted. To date, examples of the successful transition from mouse mutations to human mutations are rare but will hopefully increase rapidly in the future. One example relates to our understanding of the need for Sertoli cells to produce stem cell factor that acts, through its receptor c-kit on spermatogonia, to stimulate spermatogonial mitosis and survival. This knowledge has been gained by studying naturally occurring mutations in the c-kit and stem cell factor genes *(31,32)*. A mutation in the c-kit gene in mice results in the white-spotted mutant where failure of normal melanocyte migration (creating the white spots), anaemia, and infertility coexist, indicating crucial actions in several systems. A similar mutation in the *c-kit* gene in certain families results in the condition of human piebaldism, resulting from failure of normal melanocyte migration, but did not result in infertility or anaemia *(32)*. A further example is the mutation in the *SYCP3* gene where mutations in the mouse and human cause disruption of the meiosis *(12)*.

To date, most of the specific gene defects causing infertility have arisen from identification of a disorder with a clear familial transmission with a subsequent search for the specific gene defect. The elucidation of the genetic mechanism of androgen insensitivity syndrome arose from the identification of the hormonal mechanism of androgen insensitivity and the identification of the X-chromosomal location of the androgen receptor gene. Subsequent identification of mutations in this gene demonstrated the genotype–phenotype linkage. Although defective spermatogenesis was not the issue that gained clinical attention in the early reports of patients who were dominated by the male genotype with female external genitalia, there was no doubt that spermatogenesis was disrupted. More recent studies have identified specific mutations in the androgen receptor gene that cause defective spermatogenesis and infertility without altering the male external genitalia *(8,33)*.

Further, expanded CAG repeat length (polyglutamine tract) in exon 1 of the androgen receptor has also been associated with low sperm counts. Several studies have linked a high risk of azoospermia/severe oligospermia to expansions of the CAG repeat beyond 26 (mean for populations 20.7 [United States], 22.4 [Singapore], 21.8 [Australia], 21.8 [Denmark]). These and other observations suggest that the androgen receptor gene with an expanded CAG repeat has low intrinsic androgen receptor activity *(18–22)*. Others have argued against this linkage *(34)*, but often these studies aggregated all infertile men in their populations, thereby potentially obscuring the specific mechanism. The majority of those studies that identified a linkage were done on infertile men in whom other known causes of infertility, including Y-chromosome deletions, were excluded. There is also the possibility that the size of the CAG repeat influences the response to spermatogenic suppression by androgen–gestation combinations *(22)*. Additionally, targeted disruption of the gene encoding the steroid acute regulatory protein established a phenotype in mice that affected all steroid-producing glands, such as the adrenal, testis, and ovary, producing a complex phenotype *(17)*. Mutations in the human gene have largely replicated the findings in mice.

A second approach arose from observations of chromosomal abnormalities in karyotypic studies. The association of small Y chromosomes observed in karyotypes of azoospermic men led to the identification of Y-chromosome deletions as a cause of severe spermatogenic disruption *(5)*. Subsequent studies have defined the nature and mechanisms of Y-chromosome deletions and these are considered in detail in other chapters in this book *(6,7)*. The frequency of Y deletions in reports has varied significantly, ranging from as high as 37% to as low as 2% *(35,36)*. This variation most likely arises from the selection of patients and may also arise from technical issues, such as the poor quality of DNA leading to failure of polymerase chain reactions. Improvements in our ability to localize defects has culminated in the identification of the nature of the deletions and their frequency, which is conservatively estimated to be 6–10% of men with idiopathic seminiferous tubule failure and about 2% of all men with sperm counts less than 10 million/mL.

In a further example of such an approach, Olesen et al. *(37)*, used digital differential display to identify testis-expressed transcripts, and compared their chromosomal mapping position with the breakpoints found in men with balanced reciprocal translocations found in 265 infertile men. They identified several "hot spots" at 1p31-33, 6p21, 6p22.1, Xq28, 7q 31, and 3p21.1-9. Some of these foci represent regions where known testis-expressed genes are located and others may represent the sites of novel genes with respect to testicular function.

A third area demonstrates the extraordinary power of modern genomics. It has been recognized for decades that the immotile cilia syndrome (now termed primary ciliary dyskinesia) was an inherited disorder. The phenotype of immotile cilia causing infertility and respiratory disorders such as bronchiectasis and dextrocardia (Kartagener's syndrome) is associated with abnormalities of the axoneme, where either the dynein arms (a protein complex with adenosine triphosphatase activity), radial spoxes, or nexin linkages were usually absent on electron microscopy *(38)*. Recognizing that the structure of cilia was highly conserved, even to algal organisms such as chlamydomonas, recent studies have used mutant algal forms to identify some of the key genes. Subsequent examination of the human genome identified two genes, *DNAI1* and *DNAH5* with very high sequence homology (~90%) to the orthologs in chlamydomonas *(10,11)*, both of which show point mutations in patients with primary ciliary dyskinesia lacking outer dynein arms.

It is surprising that more examples of this approach leading to the elucidation of mechanisms are not available given the ever-increasing number of targets that arise from gene knockout experiments in mice. In part, this is no doubt a result of the relatively small number of academic institutions focusing on andrology that can collect detailed clinical information and DNA samples. It is also complicated by the fact that many men are now progressing to ICSI without a detailed clinical evaluation, underscoring the need for the training of more andrologists and the education of gynecologists in andrology. Third, family sizes have decreased in developed countries, limiting opportunities for the identification of family histories of infertility. Finally, there is a crucial need for adequate numbers of DNA samples from men who are fertile to ensure that an identified mutation is not found in the control populations. Further studies have identified the need for controls from the same population as those in whom the mutation had been identified especially with regard to Y haplotypes *(39–41)*.

Our own approach has been to develop a DNA collection with accurate clinical information and quality data, such as semen analysis, testicular histology, and electron microscopic imaging of sperm (from men with motility disorders). This has led to a collection of more than 2000 samples of DNA. Accurate histological reporting on testis biopsies when performed is crucial to defining the type of spermatogenic disruption. The latter requires fixation of biopsies in fluids such as Bouin's and not formalin, which causes cell shrinkage and the loss of chromatin patterns essential for identification of germ cell type. In addition, we have also collected DNA from the cord blood of infants born by ICSI and DNA from their fathers and latterly from their mothers, enabling us to trace the transmission of genetic defects by the use of assisted reproduction technology *(23,24,42)*.

The utility of our DNA repositories in helping define the clinical place of a potential genetic test is evident from our studies of the small Y-chromosome deletion termed gr/gr *(42)*. In a collection of 1387 infertile men, we showed that the prevalence of gr/gr deletions was 3.96% compared with 0.4% in 234 controls. This study also showed that the frequency of the gr/gr deletion was 3.6% in 504 men with sperm counts of less than 5 million/mL, 3.3% in 122 men with sperm counts of 5–20 million/mL, and 2.46% in 162 infertile men with sperm counts of more than 20 million/mL; all these frequencies were significantly greater than the control population of 0.4%. These frequencies are similar to the original study describing this deletion *(43)*.

The failure of a specific association of the gr/gr deletion with sperm density raises the possibility that the deletion causes sperm functional abnormalities that have not been recognized previously. The definition of the control groups has been critical in determining the significance of the gr/gr deletion. Some studies have failed to ensure that they have a control group in which all the parameters of the semen analysis are normal *(39)*. The availability of large numbers of men with normal semen parameters combined with demonstrated fertility is crucial for such studies and even more important in the search for rarer genetic defects that cause infertility, such as the immotile cilia syndrome with a frequency of 1 in 10,000 men.

4. MUTAGENESIS MODELS

As indicated in Table 3, it is possible to construct a logical screening program of genes for mutations causing infertility on the basis of known physiological control mechanisms. However, there are many other unknown mechanisms involved in the control of spermatogenesis. Identification of these pathways may well open up new avenues for therapeutic and diagnostic approaches. The use of random mutagenesis in inbred mouse strains using *N*-ethly-*N*-nitrosourea for example, when combined with phenotypic screening for infertility, can establish cohorts of infertile mice *(44,45)*. By the use of these breeding strategies and linkage analysis, the genetic mutation causing the infertility phenotype can be identified and, by inference key, point to key genes for the establishment of fertility *(45)*. (An example of lines arising from such a repository can be seen in refs. *44* and *45* and the Jackson Lab website [http://reprogenomics.jax.org].)

4.1. Can a Greater Understanding Be Gained From Gene Knockout Models?

In the current quest to publish in high-impact-factor journals with constraints on space, many papers concerning gene knockout phenotypes have limited data concerning specific details of testicular phenotypes.

This is especially true if there are abnormalities in multiple organ systems. Some excellent examples that illustrate a thorough characterization of a phenotype can be seen in the studies by Baarends et al. *(46–48)*, who have explored the function of the XY body in primary spermatocytes and its role in the silencing of unpaired DNA during male meiosis. They showed that the XY body forms a transcriptionally silenced chromatin domain and that targeted inactivation of genes encoding several DNA repair-related proteins that localize to the XY body interrupts meiosis *(46–48)*. Unfortunately, detailed cytological analysis is often not performed because of the lack of specific expertise, time taken, and number of animals needed, particularly if developmental studies are required.

For instance, the phenotype in the Bcl-w knockout mice would have been inadequately characterized if quantitative studies had not been performed demonstrating increased apoptosis before the profound "collapse" of spermatogenesis at 6 wk and thereafter *(49,50)*. Follow-up studies identified that Bcl-w and the other prosurvival molecules, Bcl_2 and $Bcl-x_L$, were present in spermatogonia and Sertoli cells but their expression declined in the adult testis and only Bcl-w persisted *(51)*. Thus, in the Bcl-w knockout mice, there are no prosurvival molecules left in the adult, hence the profound germ cell and Sertoli cell depletion.

It was noted that targeted disruption of the β-subunit of follicle-stimulating hormone (FSH) led to disruption of folliculogenesis but maintenance of some fertility in males, albeit with lower testicular volumes *(52)*. More detailed morphometric studies determined that the lower testis volume and decreased sperm output were in part to the result of a decrease in Sertoli cell number as a consequence of the absence of the proliferative action of FSH. However, these studies also showed that the number of germ cells that could be supported by an individual Sertoli cell decreased, indicating a metabolic requirement for FSH to maintain the "carrying capacity" of the Sertoli cells *(53)*.

5. CONCLUSION

A number of other chapters have explored some of the approaches used to identify genes causing infertility in men. A detailed consideration of them in this chapter is unwarranted within the space allocated. Rather, this chapter has assembled many of the genetic defects disrupting fertility into a format that allows a clinical approach to the identification of known genetic defects in patients and facilitates confirmation of genetically determined spermatogenic defects in mice relevant to man. Tables 4–6 use the physiological framework identified earlier to categorize the knowledge to date in some logical arrangement.

Table 4
Examples of Some Genes Involved in Mechanisms Controlling
Spermatogenic Output

- *Migration of germ cells into developing gonad*
  - C-kit (stem cell factor receptor) mutations
  - Stem cell factor mutations
  - RNA-binding protein TIAR knock-out
- *Spermatogonial proliferation and survival*
  - Bax (proapoptotic)
  - Apoptosis protease-activating factor (Apat-1)
  - DFFRY
  - AZFa deletions
  - DNMT-3L: spermatogonial loss; Sertoli cell-only phenotype
- *Defects in meiosis*
  - Bcl 16 (antiapoptotic): ↑ apoptosis in M1 (meiosis 1)
  - Ataxia telangiectasia mutant (ATM): chromosome fragmentation
  - Cyclin A1: desynapsis abnormalities at M1
  - Deleted in azoospermia-like (Dazl): loss in M1
  - Dmc1-meiosis-specific RecA: zygotene arrest
  - HSP70.2: synaptonemal complex desynapsis failure
  - MLH1-DNA mismatch repair enzyme: meiosis arrest
  - RAD6b (hr6b)-ubiquitin conjugating enzyme: postmeiotic
  - Chromatin condensation
  - Synaptonemal complex protein 3 (SCP3): chromosome synapse failure
  - Translocated in liposarcoma (TLS): failure of synapsis
  - Microorchidia (morc): zygotene-leptotene arrest
  - Siah 1a: failure of M1 metaphase to anaphase transition
  - Mouse vasa homolog gene (Mvh): zygotene arrest
  - AZFb deletions: meiosis arrest
- *Specific defects in spermiogenesis*
  - Casein kinase II catalytic subunit (CK2): globozoospermia
  - Cyclic AMP-responsive element modulator (CREM): early spermatid arrest
  - Ca^{++}/calmodulin dependent protein kinase IV (Camk4): elongating spermatid defect
  - Transition nuclear protein1 (TP1): decreased sperm motility
  - Apolipoprotein B (apo B): decreased sperm motility and survival
  - DNAI1: loss of outer dynein arms in primary ciliary dyskinesia
  - DNAI2: candidate for primary ciliary dyskinesia
  - MDHC7 (mouse dynein heavy chain): KO → ciliary dyskinesia
  - DNAH5: absence of outer dynein arms, primary ciliary dyskinesia
  - Sperm calcium ion channel; involvement with hyperactivation of sperm

Table 5
Hypospermatogenesis

- *Generalized germ cell loss (oligospermia)*
  - Bclw (antiapoptotic): progressive germ cell loss
  - Aromatase (cyp19): progressive germ cell loss
  - Complementation group A: age-dependent decrease
  - AZFc deletions: severe oligospermia
  - Hormone sensitive lipase (HSL): oligospermia
  - Leydig insulin-like hormone (Ins 13): cryptorchidism
  - Occludin: progressive germ cell loss
  - Type 1 protein phosphatase Cγ2 (PP1 c γ2): spermatocyte and spermatid loss
- *Generalized germ cell loss (low normal/oligospermia)*
  - Decreased Sertoli cell numbers and "carrying capacity"
  - Follicle-stimulating hormone β-subunit knockout
  - Activin type IIA receptor knockout

Table 6
Other Defects Genetic Mechanisms With the Potential to Cause Infertility

- *Leydig cell agenesis, loss or dysfunction*
  - Desert hedgehog (Dhh): Leydig cell agenesis, peritubular cell defects
  - Macrophage colony-stimulating factor (M-CSF): knockout $\rightarrow$ absent testis macrophages and absent Leydig cells
  - Steroid acute regulatory protein mutations
- *Sperm transport defects*
  - Estrogen receptor α knockout: efferent duct back pressure
  - Cystic fibrosis transmembrane regulator: vas agenesis
  - PEA3 (ets-transcription factor): ejaculatory dysfunction

The large number of potential genetic targets and the costs associated with screening will cause the clinician problems in trying to identify the most appropriate tests that should be ordered in any clinical investigation. Until clear genotype–phenotype associations are defined, the clinician must still rely on careful analysis of the clinical features of the patient and information from routine tests such as semen analyses, FSH, luteinizing hormone, and testosterone and testicular histology to assist in the choice of the emerging genetic investigations. It is also clear that a karyotype should be undertaken in men with sperm counts of less than 10 million/mL. Further, given the frequency of Y deletions in men with sperm counts of less than

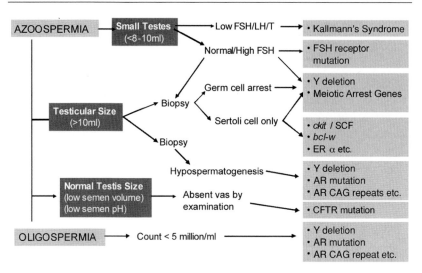

Fig. 1. Schematic approach to identifying groups of patients with a potential genetic basis of infertility.

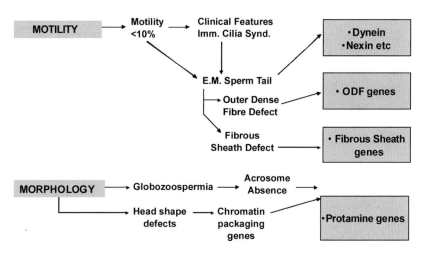

Fig. 2. Schematic approach to identifying groups of patients with a potential genetic basis of infertility for motility or morphology disturbances.

5 million/mL, karyotype should be a routine investigation. Given the data that gr/gr deletions are found in infertile men with a wide variety of spermatogenic abnormalities, the availability of a simple and cheap test could make such an investigation routine for most infertile men.

An outline of an approach to the choice of genetic evaluations for the common phenotypic presentations in infertile men is provided in

Figs. 1 and 2. However, the list of potential genetic targets cannot be listed exhaustively and these figures should be read with reference to Tables 3–6 and recent reviews *(28,30)*.

REFERENCES

1. Baker HWG. Clinical management of male infertility. In: de Groot LJ, Jameson JL, eds. Endocrinology, 5th ed. Elsevier Saunders, Philadelphia; 2006:3199–3225.
2. Irvine DS. Epidemiology and aetiology of male infertility. Hum Reprod 1998;13: 33–44.
3. Evers JL, Collins JA. Assessment of efficacy of varicocele repair for male subfertility: A systematic review. Lancet 2003;361:1849–1852.
4. Hargreave TB. Varicocele: overview and commentary on the results of the World Health Organization varicocele trial. In: Waites GMH, Frick J, Baker HWG, eds. Current Advances in Andrology. Monduzzi Editore, Bologna, 1997;31–44.
5. Tiepolo I, Zuffardi O. Localization of factors controlling spermatogenesis in the nonfluorescent portion of the human Y chromosome long arm. Hum Genet 1976;34:119–124.
6. Reijo R, Lee TY, Salo P, et al. Diverse spermatogenic defects in humans caused by Y chromosome deletions encompassing a novel RNA-binding protein gene. Nat Genet 1995;10:383–393.
7. Najmabadi H, Huang V, Yen P, et al. Substantial prevalence of microdeletions of the Y chromosome in infertile men detected using a sequence tagged site (STS)-based strategy. J Clin Endocrinol Metab 1996;81:1347–1352.
8. Wang QI, Ghadessy FJ, Trounson AO, et al. Azoospermia associated with a mutation in the ligand-binding domain of the androgen receptor displaying normal ligand binding but defective transactivation. J Clin Endocrinol Metab 1998;83: 4303–4309.
9. Chillon M, Casals T, Mercier B, et al. Mutations in the cystic fibrosis gene in patients with congenital absence of the vas deferens. New Engl J Med 1995;332: 1475–1480.
10. Pennarun G, Escudier E, Chapelin C, et al. Loss-of-function mutations in a human gene related to Chlamydomonas reinharditii dynein IC78 result in primary ciliary dyskinesia. Am J Hum Genet 1999;65:1508–1519.
11. Olbrich H, Haffner K, Kispert A, et al. Mutations in DNAH5 cause primary ciliary dyskinesia and randomisation of left-right asymmetry. Nat Genet 2002;30:143–144.
12. Miyamoto T, Hasuike S, Yogev L, et al. Azoospermia in patients heterozygous for a mutation in SYCP3. Lancet 2003;362:1714–1719.
13. Dode C, Levilliers J, Dupont JM, et al. Loss-of-function mutations in FGFR1 cause autosomal dominant Kallmann syndrome. Nat Genet 2003;33:463–465.
14. Achermann JC, Jameson JL. Fertility and infertility: genetic contributions from the hypothalamic–pituitary–gonadal axis. Mol Endocrinol 1999;13:812–818.
15. Huhtaniemi I. Mutations of gonadotrophin and gonadotrophin receptor genes: what do they teach us about reproductive physiology. J Reprod Fert 2000;119:173–186.
16. Martens JWM, Verhoef-Post M, Abelin N, et al. A homozygous Mutation in the luteinizing hormone receptor causes partial Leydig cell hypoplasia: correlation between receptor activity and phenotype. Mol Endocrinol 1998;12:775–784.
17. Hasegawa T, Zhao L, Caron KM, et al. Developmental roles of the steroidogenic acute regulatory protein (StAR) as revealed by StAR knockout mice. Mol Endocrinol 2000;14:1462–1671.

18. Tut TG, Ghadessy F, Trifiro MA, Pinsky L, Yong EL. Long polyglutamine tracts in the androgen receptor are associated with reduced trans-activation, impaired sperm production, and male infertility. J Clin Endocrinol Metab 1997;82:3777–3782.

19. Dowsing AT, Yong EL, McLachlan RI, de Kretser DM, Trounson AO. Linkage between male infertility and trinucleotide expansion in the androgen receptor gene. Lancet 1999;354:640–643.

20. Mifsud A, Sim CKS, Boettger-Tong H, et al. Trinucleotide (CAG) repeat polymorphisms in the androgen receptor gene: molecular markers of risk for male infertility. Fertil Steril 2001;75:275–281.

21. Rajpert-De Meyts E, Leffers H, Petersen JH, et al. CAG repeat length in androgen-receptor gene and reproductive variables in fertile and infertile men. Lancet 2002;359:44–46.

22. Eckardstein SV, Schmidt A, Kamischke A, Simoni M, Gromoll J, Nieschlag E. CAG repeat length in the androgen receptor gene and gonadotrophin suppression influence the effectiveness of hormonal male contraception. Clin Endocrinol 2002;57:647–655.

23. Kent-First MG, Kol S, Muallem A, et al. The incidence and possible relevance of Y-linked microdeletions in babies born after intracytoplasmic sperm injection and their infertile fathers. Mol Hum Reprod 1996;2:943–950.

24. Cram DS, Ma K, Bhasin S, et al. Y chromosome analysis of infertile men and their sons conceived through intracytoplasmic sperm injection: vertical transmission of deletions and rarity of de novo deletions. Fertil Steril 2000;74:909–915.

25. Gordon F, Maduro MR, Murthy L, et al. Neurodegenerative disease microsatellite expansions in infertile men undertaking assisted reproductive treatment. Abstracts of the Endocrine Society 2005;OR:51–52.

26. Lilford R, Jones AM, Bishop DT, Thornton J, Mueller R. Case–control study of whether subfertility in men is familial. BMJ 1994;309:570–573.

27. Bhasin S, de Kretser DM, Baker HWG. Pathophysiology and natural history of male infertility. J Clin Endocrinol Metab 1994;79:1525–1529.

28. Matzuk MM, Lamb DJ. Genetic dissection of mammalian fertility pathways. Nat Cell Biol 2002;8:S41–S49.

29. Cram DS, O'Bryan MK, de Kretser DM. Male infertility genetics—the future. J Androl 2001;22:739–745.

30. O'Bryan MK, de Kretser DM. Mouse models for genes involved in impaired spermatogenesis. Int J Androl 2005;29:76–89.

31. Loveland KL, Schlatt S. Stem cell factor and c-kit in the mammalian testis: lessons from Mother Nature's gene knock-outs. J Endocrinol 1997;153:337–344.

32. Giebel LB, Spritz RA. Mutation of the KIT (mast/stem cell growth factor receptor) protooncogene in human piebaldism. Proc Natl Acad Sci USA 1991;88: 8696–8699.

33. Gottlieb B, Lombroso, Beital LK, Trifiro MA. Molecular pathology of the androgen receptor in male (in)fertility. Reprod Biomed Online 2005;10:42–48.

34. Ruhayel Y, Lundin K, Giwercman Y, Hallden C, Willen M, Giwercman A. Androgen receptor gene GGN and CAG polymorphisms among severely oligozoospermic and azoospermic Swedish men. Hum Reprod 2004;19:2076–2083.

35. Foresta C, Moro E, Ferlin A. Y chromosome microdeletions and alterations of spermatogenesis. Endocr Rev 2001;22:226–239.

36. Cram DS, Lynch M, O'Bryan MK, Salvado C, McLachlan R, de Kretser DM. Genetic screening of infertile men. Reprod Fertil Dev 2004;16:573–580.

37. Olesen C, Hansen C, Bendsen E, et al. Identification of human candidate genes for male infertility by digital differential display. Mol Hum Reprod 2001;7:11–20.

38. Chodhari R, Mitchison HM, Meeks M. Cilia, primary ciliary dyskinesia and molecular genetics. Paediatric Respir Rev 2004;5:69–76.
39. Machev N, Saut N, Longepied P, et al. Sequence family variant loss from the AZFc interval of the human Y chromosome, but not gene copy loss, is strongly associated with male infertility. J Med Genet 2004;41:814–825.
40. Repping S, van Daalen SK, Korver CM, et al. A family of human Y chromosomes has dispersed throughout northern Eurasia despite a 1.8 MB deletion in the azoospermia factor c region. Genomics 2004;83:1046–1052.
41. Repping S, Korver CM, Oates RD, et al. Are sequence family variants useful for identifying deletions in the human Y chromosome? Am J Hum Genet 2004;75:514–517.
42. Lynch M, Cram DS, Reilly A, et al. The Y chromosome gr/gr subdeletion is associated with male infertility. Mol Hum Reprod 2005;11:507–512.
43. Repping S, Skaletsky H, Brown L, et al. Polymorphism for a 1.6Mb deletion of the human Y chromosome persists through a balance between recurrent mutation and haploid selection. Nat Genet 2003;35:247–251.
44. Ward JO, Reinholdt LG, Hartford SA, et al. Toward the genetics of mammalian reproduction: induction and mapping of gametogenesis mutants in mice. Biol Reprod 2003;69:1615–1625.
45. Kennedy CL, O'Connor AE, Sanchez-Partida LG, et al. A repository of ENU mutant mouse lines and their potential for male fertility research. Mol Hum Reprod 2005;11:871–880.
46. Baarends WM, Wassenaar E, Hoogerbrugge JW, et al. Loss of HR6B ubiquitin-conjugating activity results in damaged synaptonemal complex structure and increasing crossing-over frequency during male meiotic prophase. Mol Cell Biol 2003;23:1151–1162.
47. Van der Laan R, Uringa EJ, Wassenaar E, et al. Ubiquitin ligase RAD 18Sc localizes to the XY body and to other chromosomal regions that are unpaired and transcriptionally silenced during male meiotic prophase. J Cell Sci 2004;117:5023–5033.
48. Baarends WM, Wassenaar E, van der Laan R, et al. Silencing of unpaired chromatin and histone H2A ubiquination in mammalian meiosis Mol Cell Biol 2005;25:1041–1053.
49. Print CG, Loveland KL, Gibson L, et al. Apoptosis regulator Bcl-w is essential for spermatogenesis but is otherwise dispensable. Proc Natl Acad Sci USA 1998;95:12,423–12,431.
50. Russell LD, Warren J, Debeljuk L, et al. Spermatogenesis in Bclw-deficient mice. Biol Reprod 2001;65:318–332.
51. Meehan T, Loveland KL, de Kretser D, Cory S, Print CG. Developmental regulation of the bcl-2 family during spermatogenesis: insights into the sterility of bcl-w-/- male mice. Cell Death Differ 2001;8:225–233.
52. Kumar TR, Wang Y, Lu N, Matzuk M. Follicle stimulating hormone is required for ovarian follicle maturation but not for male fertility. Nat Genet 1997;15:201–204.
53. Wreford NG, Kumar TR, Matzuk MM, de Kretser DM. Analysis of the testicular phenotype of the follicle-stimulating hormone beta-subunit knockout and the activin type II receptor knockout mice by stereological analysis. Endocrinology 2001;142:2916–2920.

17 The Future of the Diagnosis of Male (In)Fertility

Christopher De Jonge, *PhD, HCLD*

Summary

Traditionally, the diagnosis of male (in)fertility has relied on the results from clinical evaluation and semen analysis. Although these approaches have undeniable merit, often times causes for subfertility are more covert and are not readily identified by these traditional approaches. In these instances, the diagnosis is simply written as idiopathic or undiagnosed. The genomic and proteomic eras have promised great potential to remedy those cases defined as undiagnosed and further advance our understanding of the complex processes that combine and contribute to the so-called fertile and infertile male.

Key Words: Male infertility; semen analysis; diagnosis; genetics; clinical prognosis.

1. INTRODUCTION

In the absence of clinical pathology, accurate diagnosis of male infertility is further complicated if one must rely solely on results from semen analysis. Although there are strong correlates between abnormalities in one or more semen parameters and subfertility, there remains a substantial gray or indeterminate range for which diagnostic ability is at best equivocal.

The genomic and proteomic eras have promised great potential to offer remedy for those cases defined as undiagnosed and further advance our understanding of the complex processes that combine and contribute to the so-called fertile and infertile male (*see* accompanying chapters in this book).

This chapter briefly reviews some of the traditional approaches to male infertility diagnosis, what the new molecular technologies offer in the way of diagnostic promise and, finally, what the future clinical realities might be for diagnosing male (in)fertility.

From: *The Genetics of Male Infertility*
Edited by: D.T. Carrell © Humana Press Inc., Totowa, NJ

2. DIAGNOSIS AND MALE INFERTILITY

Before delving into the practical aspects of infertility diagnosis, perhaps it would be instructive to define what is meant by "diagnosis." Essentially three levels of complexity can be identified in defining the term diagnosis. The simplest definition is the *identification* of the nature or cause of some phenomenon. A more complex definition for diagnosis is the *process of identifying* a disease by its signs, symptoms, and results of various diagnostic procedures. Last, the most complex definition of diagnosis is the *comparison of the condition* of the patient to patterns from diseases sharing similarities, based on the examination of the specific clinical condition and on results from additional assays.

The clinician and clinical andrology laboratory collaborate in an attempt to offer the male patient answers as to why they are unable to conceive with their presumably fertile partner. The clinician relies on typical history and physical evaluations to determine whether follow-up investigation, such as sonography, radiography, endocrine, and chromosome testing, is warranted. Often, through one of these investigations, a specific diagnosis (cause) can be identified. For example, based on simple physical examination, bilateral cryptorchidism identifies the cause for the infertility (first definition presented earlier). However, although identification is made for infertility, it does not identify the cause for the undescended testes. That process of identification may result after implementing other diagnostic procedures.

The preceding analysis may appear to be arbitrary, yet it weighs significantly on exactly what is meant, perhaps semantically, by "diagnosis of male infertility." For instance, is the identification of one or more variances in semen parameters from established reference values diagnostic, or merely the manifestation of an etiology yet to be uncovered?

3. SEMEN ANALYSIS AND DIAGNOSIS

It can safely be asserted that the ability of semen parameters to distinguish between the subfertile and fertile male in the general population is suspect *(1–5)*. Indeed, investigators *(6)* performed a structured review of the literature focusing on articles published in English between 1983 and 2002 and using semen parameters (i.e., concentration, motility, and morphology) to establish thresholds that would distinguish between fertile and subfertile populations. For this study, the investigators were able to identify only 4 out of 265 articles that fit their structured review criteria. This small portion of directly comparable clinical research publications, in terms of design and methods, seems rather astounding when considered on balance with the heightened awareness and practice of global standardization for semen analysis in the andrology laboratory (e.g., ref. *7*). The purpose of this example is to point out the overwhelming heterogeneity that exists in the clinical research database regarding semen parameter attributes that character-ize the fertile and/or infertile male, thereby making it difficult to formu-late diagnostic thresholds.

In the face of the aforementioned rather dire situation, there exists a plethora of publications in which semen analysis is demonstrated to have irrefutable merit. For example, there are those situations in which the number of countable or motile or normal spermatozoa is so small that a conclusion regarding fertility potential can be made with relative confi-dence (e.g., severe oligozoospermia, necrozoospermia, globozoosper-mia). Results from semen analysis such as these provide clear indication that therapeutic intervention is required for fertility, albeit no cause of the abnormality has been diagnosed. These results may also provide indica-tion for additional diagnostic testing, such as Y-chromosome microdele-tion analysis. Thus, perhaps the truer merit of semen analysis lies more squarely not so much with strict diagnostic ability but rather as a "signal" assay for stimulating further diagnostic investigation (e.g., refs. *8–10*).

Recent advances in the andrology research laboratory have shed light on the importance of sperm chromatin and DNA packaging as an additional attribute of fertile spermatozoa (*see* Chapter 20). Several dif-ferent assays to evaluate DNA fragmentation have been developed, all of which have been purported to have clinical diagnostic merit *(11,12)*. Indeed, numerous reports, mostly from the in vitro fertilization labora-tory, have detailed that if sperm DNA is fragmented and/or if protamine deficiency is evident, then the likelihood for term birth is decreased (e.g., ref. *13*). These DNA assays have not, however, made the transi-tion into the clinical andrology laboratory for routine global applica-tion, primarily because of assay complexity and data diversity *(14)*.

It serves well to mention the World Health Organization (WHO) manual for semen analysis *(7)*. The WHO manual is the only text glob-ally accepted to be the standard on which procedures and rationale for conducting examination of semen is performed. The manual has under-gone several revisions since its first appearance in 1980. Perhaps the most conspicuous change that is evident today is the content dedicated to quality control. Sections pertaining to improvements in actual diag-nostic ability have improved only marginally. Morphology assessment and its potential implications stand out as perhaps the only parameter that has gained in relative clinical significance. That said, morphology assessment (and all other semen parameters for that matter) is only as reliable as the technician, their training, and persistent proficiency training *(15)*. Standardized training and methods for proficiency testing still remain somewhat enigmatic worldwide.

The aforementioned statements are in no means meant to slight the tremendous significance of the WHO manual, for without it we would be lost on the foggy mountaintop without a map and compass. I believe the content and relative stasis of the manual is reflective more of the disparate nature of the clinical research reports, as discussed earlier, rather than a failing by the editors who have written the manual over the years. The forthcoming version (5th edition in preparation) will prove to be the most transitional and reflective of the current global clinical pulse.

4. CLINICAL REALITIES

What then is the current global clinical pulse? Regrettably, the answer to this question involves far greater discourse than is reasonable for present purposes. Suffice to say that consumer demand, cost, health care systems, and insurance weigh considerably on how much effort will be placed on diagnosis vs that expended on treatment. Although it is inarguable that a patient expects a diagnosis for their malady, that desire is balanced keenly against their desire for a result, and for present context that means a healthy baby, and the sooner the better.

In the WHO manual for the standardized investigation, diagnosis, and management of the infertile male *(16)*, it is written that with the exception of azoospermia and congenital bilateral absence of the vas deferens there should be a second semen analysis to serve as comparison for the first. So, a diagnosis is made for congenital bilateral absence of the vas deferens, not from semen analysis *per se*, but what about for the azoospermic male? The manual recommends genetic testing for these and severe oligozoospermic males. That leaves a majority of men who might have one or more abnormal semen parameters and for whom the only diagnostic test recommended is a repeat semen analysis. But what is being diagnosed in a third or fourth repeat semen analysis—perhaps nothing! No infection, no varicocele...only the symptoms of low sperm count, motility, or morphology have been revealed. No clear reason (diagnosis) can be determined yet. This is what proteomics and or genomics might offer—the diagnosis.

However, the subfertile male that has a moderately diminished total sperm number, for example, 30×10^6, 40% of which are motile and whose strict morphology criteria score is 6%. What is his diagnosis? In fact, can one even be made? So, let's return to global pulse and finances.

The advent of intracytoplasmic sperm injection (ICSI) largely negated strong impetus to advance diagnostic ability in the clinical andrology laboratory, with exception made to genetic testing. The perfect assisted reproductive technology universe now exists in the unity of one sperm and one egg. Who now cares whether there is 10 or 20 million sperm? The patients want a baby, so let us try a couple rounds of superovulation with intrauterine insemination and if that fails we will go straight to ICSI. The patient (couple) will likely get their baby, but is this the most cost-effective approach? The answer is not straightforward, nor is it likely to be globally unanimous. Cost-effectiveness is regionally dependent on whether the health care is government-sponsored, self-paid, state-mandated, or variations in between.

Cost also includes the emotional expense for the patients. It is well described that infertility is emotionally expensive. A more protracted diagnostics in lieu of expedited therapy might not be the option of choice for most patients. Applying the example of the oligozoospermic male with a presumed fertile female partner, would this infertile couple, by definition, be willing to go home and have timed intercourse for yet 1 yr more because the odds favor that they will conceive—at some point? No, at least probably not in the majority, these consumers will demand and likely their insurance or their own finances will urge a more rapid route straight to therapy rather than diagnosis. So, once again, superovulation with intrauterine insemination will likely be attempted and, if unsuccessful after several tries, then in vitro fertilization, with or without ICSI, will be the therapy of choice (therapy is a very loose term in this situation because no therapy is actually applied to remedy the oligozoospermia).

5. THE MOLECULAR GENETIC REVOLUTION

Without question, the unraveling and deciphering of the human genome has opened a treasure trove of potential diagnostic and therapeutic possibilities for both male and female factor infertility. The cause for a man's hypospermatogenesis may be determined using DNA microarray analysis, proteomics, and other technologies (e.g., refs. *17* and *18*). However, will a better ability to diagnosis male infertility lead to better therapeutic strategies? This is the million dollar question. Because, to reiterate, there is therapeutic ICSI and for male factor infertility this is the *panacea du jour*, and is not likely to be replaced any time soon.

6. CONCLUSION

It is important to heavily underscore that because of ICSI, and assisted reproductive technology in general, the importance of molecular genetic diagnostics in the field will likely blossom as greater understanding of these technologies in association with epigenetics is gained *(19)*. Whether or not these technologies become routinely applied in the clinical andrology laboratory as diagnostic tools for unraveling the cause of a man's infertility remains to be seen.

REFERENCES

1. Ayala C, Steinberger E, Smith DP. The influence of semen analysis parameters on the fertility potential of infertile couples. J Androl 1996;17:718–725.
2. Barratt CL, Naeeni M, Clements S, Cooke ID. Clinical value of sperm morphology for in-vivo fertility: comparison between World Health Organization criteria of 1987 and 1992. Hum Reprod 1995;10:587–593.
3. Bonde JP, Ernst E, Jensen TK, et al. Relation between semen quality and fertility: a population-based study of 430 first-pregnancy planners. Lancet 1998;352: 1172–1177.
4. Chia SE, Tay SK, Lim ST. What constitutes a normal seminal analysis? Semen parameters of 243 fertile men. Hum Reprod 1998;13:3394–3398.
5. Chia SE, Lim ST, Tay SK, Lim ST. Factors associated with male fertility: a case–control study of 218 infertile and 240 fertile men. BJOG 2000;107:55–61.
6. van der Merwe FH, Kruger TF, Oehninger SC, Lombard CJ. The use of semen parameters to identify the subfertile male in the general population. Gynecol Obstet Invest 2005;59:86–91.
7. World Health Organization. WHO laboratory manual for the examination of human semen and sperm–cervical mucus interaction. Cambridge University Press, Cambridge; 1999.
8. Oehninger S, Franken D. Testing sperm manufacturing quality: the sperm-zona binding assay. In: De Jonge C, Barratt C, eds. The Sperm Cell. Production, Maturation, Fertilization, Regeneration. Cambridge University Press, Cambridge; 2006;194–216.
9. Shefi S, Turek PJ. Sex chromosome abnormalities and male infertility: a clinical perspective. In: De Jonge C, Barratt C, eds. The Sperm Cell. Production, Maturation, Fertilization, Regeneration. Cambridge University Press, Cambridge; 2006; 261–278.
10. Vogt PH. Genetics: a basic science perspective. In: De Jonge C, Barratt C, eds. The Sperm Cell. Production, Maturation, Fertilization, Regeneration. Cambridge University Press, Cambridge; 2006;217–260.
11. Evenson DP, Larson KJ, Jost LK. Sperm chromatin structure assay: its clinical use for detecting sperm DNA fragmentation in male infertility and comparisons with other techniques. J Androl 2002;23:25–43.
12. Chohan KR, Griffin JT, LaFromboise M, De Jonge CJ, Carrell DT. Comparison of chromatin assays for DNA fragmentation evaluation in human sperm. J Androl 2006;27:53–59.
13. Henkel R, Hajimohammad M, Stalf T, et al. Influence of deoxyribonucleic acid damage on fertilization and pregnancy. Fertil Steril 2004;81:965–972.
14. De Jonge C. The clinical value of sperm nuclear DNA assessment. Hum Fertil (Camb) 2002;5:51–53.
15. Riddell D, Pacey A, Whittington K. Lack of compliance by UK andrology laboratories with World Health Organization recommendations for sperm morphology assessment. Hum Reprod 2005;20:3441–3445.
16. World Health Organization. WHO manual for the standardized investigation, diagnosis and management of the infertile male. Cambridge University Press, Cambridge; 2000.

17. Gianotten J, Lombardi MP, Zwinderman AH, Lilford RJ, van der Veen F. Idiopathic impaired spermatogenesis: genetic epidemiology is unlikely to provide a short-cut to better understanding. Hum Reprod Update 2004;10:533–539.
18. Moldenhauer JS, Ostermeier GC, Johnson A, Diamond MP, Krawetz SA. Diagnosing male factor infertility using microarrays. J Androl 2003;24:783–789.
19. La Salle S, Trasler JM. Epigenetic patterning in male germ cells: importance of DNA methylation to progeny outcome. In: De Jonge C, Barratt C, eds. The Sperm Cell. Production, Maturation, Fertilization, Regeneration. Cambridge University Press, Cambridge; 2006;279–322.

18 Polymorphisms and Male Infertility

Csilla Krausz, MD, PhD

Summary

The analysis of polymorphisms in genes involved in spermatogenesis represents one of the most exciting areas of research in the genetics of male infertility. These studies are not only important for identifying genetic risk factors for male infertility, but they may also represent an important starting point for searching for genes involved in spermatogenesis through linkage analysis. Despite many efforts, we often face frustrating situations in which initial promising data are not confirmed in later studies. Discrepancies between association studies are rather frequent and can be related to different factors, such as inadequate sample size, the pathogenetic heterogeneity of infertility, inappropriate control subjects, positive publication bias, and ethnic and geographic differences.

It is likely that some polymorphisms only lead to testicular dysfunction when associated with a specific genetic background or with environmental factors. The role of genetic background seems to be especially relevant for one of the most promising genetic risk factors, the gr-gr deletions of the Y chromosome. Certain gene variants may cause specific phenotypes and consequently only the analysis of a specific subgroup of patients is able to identify their clinical significance. To obtain reliable and clinically useful data, much more attention should be focused on the correct study design, which is still the major weakness of association studies.

Key Words: Polymorphism; spermatogenesis; gr-gr deletion; infertility genetics; Y chromosome.

1. INTRODUCTION

Despite our increasing knowledge of the physiology of male reproduction and the availability of new diagnostic tools, the pathogenesis of testicular failure remains undefined in about 50% of cases and is referred to as "idiopathic infertility" *(1)*. Idiopathic testicular failure is likely to be of genetic origin because the number of genes involved in human spermatogenesis is possibly thousands or more and only a small proportion of them has been identified and screened in infertile men.

From: *The Genetics of Male Infertility*
Edited by: D.T. Carrell © Humana Press Inc., Totowa, NJ

Table 1
Polymorphisms and Male Infertility

Polymorphisms	More than one study	Single study
in GENES involved in:		
Endocrine regulation	Androgen receptor[a,b]	Estrogen receptor β
of spermatogenesis	Follicle-stimulating	Combined single-
	hormone receptor	nucleotide
	Estrogen receptor α	polymorphisms°
Specific spermatogenic	DAZL[a,b]	USP26
functions	PRM1[a]	GRTH
		CREM
Different cell functions	POLG[a,b]	GSTM1
(metabolism, cell	MTHFR[a]	PHGPx
cycle, mutation repair)		BRCA2
in DNA sequences:	Y-chromosome	Mitochondial DNA
	haplogroups[a]	haplogroups
	gr/gr deletions[a]	

[a]Data in the literature are contradictory.
[b]Polymorphisms that are not considered risk factors in the Caucasian populations.

Several reports have focused on the role of certain haplogroups, allele variants, and single-nucleotide polymorphisms (SNPs) in male infertility (Table 1). In many cases, only sporadic data are available, or alternatively, when more studies are published on the same polymorphism, the results are often contradictory. Inadequate sample size, pathogenetic heterogeneity of infertility, inappropriate control subjects, and ethnic and geographic differences (probably also related to environmental factors) may be responsible for discrepancies among case–control studies. On the other hand, these studies are not only important for identifying genetic risk factors, but they may also represent an important starting point in searching for genes involved in spermatogenesis through linkage analysis. In this regard, association studies dealing with human leukocyte antigen haplotypes are relevant for the identification of candidate major histocompatibility complex genes *(2,3)*, and mitochondrial DNA (mtDNA) haplogroups for genes involved in mithocondrial functions *(4,5)*. Similarly, Y-chromosome-related factors (other than azoospermia factor [AZF] deletions) can be determined indirectly by the definition of Y-chromosome haplogroups predisposing to male infertility *(6,7)*. In this chapter, recent findings concerning polymorphisms and male infertility are discussed.

2. POLYMORPHISMS IN GENES INVOLVED IN THE ENDOCRINE REGULATION OF SPREMATOGENESIS

The crucial role of androgens, gonadotropins, and estrogens in the endocrine regulation of spermatogenesis is well known, thus genes of their receptors represent a logical target for mutational analysis in the infertile male.

2.1. The Androgen Receptor

The androgen receptor (AR) is a ligand-activated transcription factor that is encoded by the *AR* gene located on the long arm of the X chromosome (Xq11-q12). The *AR* gene has been the object of a large quantity of studies, and both mutation screenings of the entire coding sequence and the promoter region have been reported (for review, *see* ref. 8). The first exon of the *AR* codes for the transactivation-regulating domain and contains two polymorphic tracts: a CAG and a GGC repeat sequence. The polymorphic (CAG)n codes for a polyglutamine, whereas the (GGC)n repeat for a polyglycine stretch. It has been demonstrated in vitro that the length of the polyglutamine tract, while remaining within the polymorphic range, is inversely correlated with the transactivation activity of the receptor *(9)*. According to this observation, the first association studies dealing with CAG repeat length and male infertility have shown a significant association between relatively long CAG repeats and impaired sperm production. However, subsequent studies gave rather contradictory results, which in part can be the consequence of ethnic differences (the association seems to be more consistent in the Asiatic populations), although the heterogeneity of the control (unselected men or proven fertile men or normospermic men) and of the infertile (different inclusion criteria) groups (for review, *see* ref. *8* and references therein) may play also an important role. A repeat number more than 23 has been reported as significant risk factor only in 5 out of 11 studies, mainly involving Singaporean, Australian, North American, and Japanese subjects, whereas this association is not evident in the European studies *(10)*.

Two groups from Europe attempted to evaluate the joint effect of both exon 1 and polymorphic microsatellites on male infertility *(11,12)*. Although the two populations were both Caucasian, the "protective" and "at risk" CAG/GGC haplotypes were different. In the Swedish study, the <21CAG and GGN = 23, whereas in the Italian study the >23CAG and <16GGC combined haplotype confers a lower risk of infertility to the carriers. Because of these discordant association data and the lack of in vitro expression studies on the effect of varying GGC length in combination with different CAG repeats, the clinical utility of the CAG/GGC haplotype definition remains unclear.

In summary, if only data based on large study populations are considered, the CAG repeat length polymorphism is an unlikely risk factor for male infertility. However, its role in modulating androgen action is evident in patients affected by Klinefelter syndrome *(13)*, in hypogonadal men undergoing T-replacement therapy *(14)*, and in hypoandrogenic males *(15)*. It is therefore possible that the mild functional effect of a long polyglutamine strech can be compensated by a relatively high serum testosterone level, ergo the polymorphism should not be evaluated in isolation but always in the context of environmental factors.

2.2. The Follicle-Stimulating Hormone Receptor

Besides testosterone, follicle-stimulating hormone (FSH) is another fundamental hormone for normal gametogenesis. FSH stimulates spermatogenesis through its specific receptor (FSHR) that is a member of the G protein-coupled receptor family. The receptor consists of 10 exons, located on chromosome 2 (2p21-p16). Mutation screening of the FSHR gene revealed various SNPs, among them the SNP in the core promoter at position -29 and two others situated in exon 10 (for review, *see* ref. *16*). Exon 10 codes for the C-terminal part of the extracellular, transmembrane, and intracellular domains. The two SNPs in exon 10 correspond to amino acid positions 307 and 680 of the mature protein. The two SNPs result in two major, almost equally common allelic variants in the Caucasian population: Thr^{307}-Asn^{680} and Ala^{307}-Ser^{680}. Studies comparing the distribution of the two SNPs in normal and infertile men did not show significant differences *(17)*, whereas the combination of the exon 10 SNPs with the -29 SNP evidenced specific allelic combinations, which can be considered as a new genetic factor for severe spermatogenic impairment *(18)*. Further confirmation of these promising data is awaited in other populations.

2.3. Genes Involved in the Estrogenic Pathway

Although the physiological role of estrogens in spermatogenesis is not clearly defined, human and animal models evidenced an association between estrogen insufficiency and abnormal spermatogenesis. Although recent studies suggest a role as a survival factor *(19)*, the excess of this hormone during the neonatal period or adulthood can impair sperm production in rats *(20)*. The physiological responses to estrogens are known to be mediated by at least two functional isoforms of estrogen receptors (ERs), namely ERα and ERβ, encoded by two different genes in different chromosomes (6q25 and 14q23-24, respectively). Apart from estradiol, other compounds with estrogen-like activity (xenoestrogens) may bind to ERs and may account for the reported decline in sperm count as well as for the increased incidence of other components of the testicular dysgenesis syndrome (hypospadias, cryptorchidism, and testicular cancer) observed in the last 50 yr *(21)*.

Genetic screening of the ERα and ERβ genes has revealed the existence of several polymorphic sites in both genes and some of them have been the object of association studies dealing with male infertility. In the ERα gene, the most widely studied are the PvuII (T397C) and XbaI restriction fragment length polymorphisms (RFLPs) in intron I and the $(TA)_n$ variable number of tandem repeats within the promoter region. To date, four studies have been published in four different populations: Greek *(22)*, Japanese *(23)*, Spanish *(24)*, and Italian *(25)*. A significant association between male infertility and the XbaI RFLP *(22)* or the exon 4 codon 325C-G *(23)* polymorphisms was reported, however, the interpretation of these results is difficult because of the small sample size, especially in the Japanese study (only 31 patients). The Spanish *(24)* and our own study *(25)* on the Italian population aimed to define the role of TA repeats in the promoter region. Both investigations reached the conclusion that the distribution of TA genotype is not different between controls and patients; therefore, this polymorphism cannot be considered a risk factor for male infertility. However, further analysis in the Italian population showed a significant effect of this polymorphism on sperm output in both the control and the infertile groups. The number of TA repeats showed a significant inverse correlation with sperm count and the subdivision of the allelic combinations into two major genotypes (genotype A and B) revealed that men with higher TA repeat number on both alleles (genotype A) have significantly lower sperm production. Because previous studies on lumbar bone mineral density observed that allelic combinations with higher TA repeats are functionally more active *(26)*, our finding indicates that allelic combinations, which confer a stronger estrogen effect, may negatively influence human spermatogenesis. A plausible explanation would be that not only a deficit of estrogens, but also an exaggerated estrogen action related to this genetic variant (eventually combined with environmental factors), can be deleterious. Whether the observed negative effect reflects the expression of a disturbance in the early testis development or in the adult testis, and whether it is related to xenoestrogens, remains to be established. In the Spanish study, besides ERα, other estrogen-related genes have also been analyzed for polymorphic markers (ERβ, FSHR, CYP19A1, and NRIPI). The results support a relevant role for the estrogenic pathway, especially for SNPs in the ERα gene, but also indicate that the combination of different allelic variants in the five genes may protect or predispose to male infertility. However, again because of the limited sample size, these data need to be confirmed in a larger study population.

Thus far, only one association study has been performed for ERβ gene SNPs (RsaI [G1082A] and AluI [G1730A]) and male infertility. The frequency of the heterozygous RsaI AG-genotype was three times higher in infertile men than in controls, indicating that this polymorphism may have modulating effects on spermatogenesis (27).

In summary, preliminary data suggest that ERα and ERβ polymorphisms may influence male fertility and spermatogenic efficiency. It will be of interest to verify the effect of the aforementioned ER polymorphisms on spermatogenic potential in a selected group of subjects with different levels of exposure to xenoestrogens.

3. TWO EXAMPLES OF POLYMORPHISMS IN CANDIDATE AUTOSOMAL SPERMATOGENESIS GENES: PROTAMINE 1, PROTAMINE 2, AND DAZL

A number of spermatogenesis, autosomal, candidate genes have been identified and represent the most obvious targets for mutation analysis. Among them the Protamine (PRM) 1 and PRM2 and deleted azoospermia-like (DAZL) genes were the object of several studies, finally leading to the conclusion that PRM1 polymorphism is relevant in a specific subset of patients, whereas the DAZL gene polymorphism is relevant only in a specific ethnic group.

After the completion of meiosis, in the late phases of spermatogenesis, the haploid genome is compacted within the sperm head by two DNA-binding proteins, PRM1 and PRM2. This remarkable repackaging event is related to the requirement for a unique chromatin architecture that would enable a specific transcription schedule after fertilization. Premature translation of PRM1 messenger RNA causes precocious nuclear condensation and arrests spermatid differentiation in mice (28) and the disruption of either the *Prm1* or *Prm2* gene in mice leads to haploinsufficieny, abnormal cromatin compaction, sperm DNA damage, and male infertility.

Although reduction of PRM2 has been reported in infertile men, mutations in the PRM2 gene have not been reported in association with reduced PRM2 content (29). Nishimune et al. (29) identified a number of SNPs in both the PRM1 and PRM2 genes in a large number of infertile men presenting mainly with azoospermia and proven fertile controls. No association between any of the SNPs and infertility was observed. However, one mutation in the PRM2 gene induced a nonsense codon C248T and was present in heterozygosity in one azoospermic patient. Unfortunately, the testis histology of the patient is unknown and this makes difficult to interpret the consequences of this mutation. In a recent study, a highly selected group of infertile male patients were screened for PRM1 gene mutations *(30)*. A novel SNP, G197T, in a highly conserved region of the gene was identified in 3 out of 30 patients. Based on the absence of this SNP in more than 700 individuals, it appears to be a promising new genetic risk factor for a specific subgroup of infertile patients with normal sperm count associated with abnormal sperm DNA fragmentation and/or teratozoospermia.

The *DAZL* gene is an autosomal homolog of the Y-chromosomal *DAZ* gene cluster and is mapping to chromosome 3p24 *(31)*. *DAZ*, *DAZL*, and *BOULE* are members of the same family and encode RNA-binding proteins with important role in spermatogenesis *(32)*. No clinically relevant mutations for the *BOULE (33,34)* and the *DAZL* genes have been reported so far, except one SNP in the *DAZL* gene sequence in exon 3 (T54A), which was reported as a susceptibility factor to oligospermia/azoospermia in the Chinese population *(35)*. This SNP is situated within the highly conserved RNA-recognition motif domain of the DAZL protein and it may lead to functional consequences such as reduced RNA binding. Despite this promising finding, subsequent studies in Caucasian populations *(36–38)* and in the Japanese population *(39)* failed to detect the T54A mutation in more than 900 men tested, strongly contrasting with the relatively high frequency of this mutation (7.4%) in the Chinese patients. This remarkable difference represents an example of how ethnic background is also important for polymorphisms involved in spermatogenesis.

4. THE POLG GENE POLYMORPHISM

Normal function of sperm mitochondria is a prerequisite for normal spermatogenesis and motility. The mtDNA polymerase γ (POLG) is the sole polymerase for mtDNA and an impaired activity of this protein leads to mitochondrial dysfunction through accumulation of mtDNA mutations. The gene maps to 15q24-15q26 and its first exon contains a polyglutamine tract encoded by a motif $(CAG)_{10}$ CAACAGCAG *(40)*. The length of the CAG repeat is polymorphic with a major allele at 10 repeats.

Rovio and colleagues *(41)* proposed an association between the absence of the common 10 CAG allele and male infertility in a relatively small group of infertile (*n* = 99) and fertile (*n* = 98) men. This finding has been extensively debated by subsequent larger studies. One study on the Danish population observed a significantly higher frequency of homozygous not10 CAG repeat allele in a subgroup of men affected by unexplained infertility (i.e., normal sperm count, motility, and morphology; ref. *42*). However, this conclusion was based on an interpretation bias (i.e., the seven unexplained infertile men with the homozygous not10/not10 CAG genotype were not normospermic, with the exception of one subject). The recalculated real frequency, 1 of 42 (2.38%) instead of 7 of 49 (14.3%), shows no significant difference in respect to the control fertile group (0.8%). In the same year, based on our own study on the Italian population (*n* = 385), we concluded that there is no relationship between the polymorphic CAG repeat in the POLG gene and idiopathic male infertility *(43)*. The same conclusion was achieved later in another large study on the French population *(44)*.

It is therefore clear that the POLG CAG polymorphism has no clinical significance, neither for idiopathic, nor for unexplained male infertility. Considering the importance of mitochondria for sperm motility, the question of whether pure asthenozoospermia (with the sole symptom of reduced sperm motility) can be the consequence of the not10/not10 CAG genotype, remains to be addressed. However, before performing such a study, it would be important to clarify if the length of the CAG tract has any functional effect on the polymerase activity (for review, *see* ref. *45)*.

5. Y-CHROMOSOME POLYMORPHISMS: THE GR/GR DELETIONS

Apart from the classical AZF deletions, a new type of Yq deletion has recently attracted the attention of geneticists and andrologists. A partial deletion in the AZFc region, termed gr/gr has been described specifically in infertile men with varying degrees of spermatogenic failure *(46)*. This deletion removes half the AZFc gene content, including two copies of the major AZFc candidate gene called DAZ *(47)*. In the last 2 yr, an intensive search for gr/gr deletions in infertile and control normospermic men has started to define their frequency and clinical significance *(48–53)*. From the first studies, it was clear that in contrast to the classical AZF deletions, gr/gr deletions can be found also in normospermic men *(49,51,52)*, although at a significantly lower frequency. Therefore, rather than a specific cause, this genetic anomaly represents a risk factor for spermatogenic failure. Among a number of plausible explanations for the heterogeneous phenotype, we hypothesized the presence of polymorphisms or mutations in the autosomal homolog of

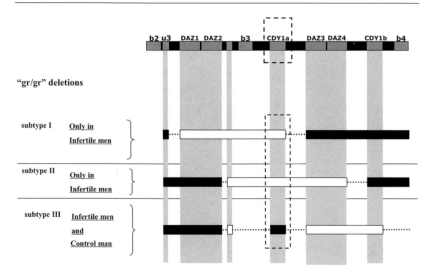

Fig. 1. Following molecular characterization of the gr/gr deletions (gene copy dosage and type of DAZ and CDY1 gene deletion), three subtypes of gr/gr deletions were identified in a large group of infertile and control men of Italian origin *(52)*. CDY1b copy seems to be specifically deleted in infertile men, suggesting that different deletion patterns may have different phenotypic effects.

the DAZ gene, *DAZL (36)*. However, similar to the AZFc-deleted patients, we found no new mutations in the entire coding region of the DAZL gene except the polymorphic Thr12-Ala change (T12A), which, because of its relatively high frequency in the normospermic group, does not seem to have any modulating effect *(36,52)*. The currently used method for the detection of gr/gr deletions is based on STS plus/minus type of analysis, which alone does not provide information about the type of missing gene copies. This analysis may also detect false deletions as a result of rearrangements of the STS-containing sequence, and is also unable to rule out a duplication of the nondeleted part of the AZFc region. The majority of gr/gr studies lack a detailed molecular analysis (i.e., the reduced gene dosage is not confirmed and the type of deleted gene copies is also unknown; refs. *49–51* and *53*). Mitchell et al. *(48)* developed a method able to detect the type of the missing CDY and DAZ copies, whereas Vogt et al. *(54)* developed an RFLP-based DAZ copy analysis. Using the first method, our preliminary data indicate that gr/gr deletions associated with the loss of CDY1a copy are found only in infertile men and not in normospermic controls (Fig. 1; ref. *52*). However, the number of controls is low and further combined studies are needed.

Aside from the gr/gr deletions, the AZFc region predisposes to a number of other possible partial deletions *(55,56)*. The Y-chromosome background seems to play an important role in the pathogenic consequence of these deletions. For example, another deletion named b2/b3 *(57)* or u3-gr/gr *(48)* or g1/g3 *(58)*, which removes a similar quantity of AZFc genes compared with the gr/gr deletion, seems to have no effect on fertility status in association with a certain Y-chromosome background commonly present in Northern Eurasian populations (Y haplogroup N; refs. *57* and *58*). A similar conclusion can also be drawn for the gr/gr deletion found in association with Hgr D2b, which is present in 20% of Japanese subjects *(7)*. Consequently, a combined molecular characterization (haplogroup, gene dosage, and gene copy type definition) of the gr/gr deleted patients and controls will probably allow the distinction between pathogenic and neutral deletions. In the meantime, the screening for gr/gr deletions can be advised for patients undergoing assisted reproductive techniques, because this test is able to provide the identification of a transmissible genetic risk factor (odds ratio = 10.2, confidence interval 1.28–80.3) for reduced sperm count *(52)*.

6. VARIOUS OTHER POLYMORPHISMS

A number of other association studies dealing with different polymorphisms (SNPs or microsatellites) in autosomal and X-linked genes have been published in the recent years. Among them are genes that encode for proteins involved in protection against oxidative stress, such as glutathione S-transferase M1 (GST M1) and Phospholipid hydroperoxide glutathione peroxidase (PHGPx; refs. *59* and *60*). Polymorhisms in these genes are not associated with idiopathic infertility, however, they may have a role in specific conditions associated with oxidative stress (e.g., varicoceles; ref. *60*). Similarly, another gene polymorphism C677T in the methylenetetrahydrofolate reductase gene seems to have clinical relevance only in specific environmental conditions characterized by low dietary intake of folates, which is more common in Indian, African, and Southeast Asian populations *(61–64)*.

New variants in a number of genes with proven or potential role in human spermatogenesis were recently identified and are of interest for future case–control association studies. The common variant N372 in *BRCA2* gene *(65)*, polymorphisms in the *USP26 (66)*, and the gonadotropin-regulated testicular helicase *(GRTH*; ref. *67)* genes have been recently proposed as potential risk factors for severe spermatogenic failure. Among the most relevant spermiogenesis candidate genes, the cyclic adenosine monophosphate-responsive element modulator *(CREM)* gene has been the object of mutation screening in a specific group of men with round spermatid arrest *(68,69)*. In this pilot study, a number of genetic changes have been identified and it seems that certain patterns of homozygous and heterozygous alterations could exert pathological effects *(69)*.

7. CONCLUSIONS

The analysis of polymorphisms in genes involved in spermatogenesis represents one of the most exciting areas of research in the study of the genetics of male infertility. However, we are often facing frustrating situations in which initial promising data are not confirmed in later studies. Discrepancies between association studies are rather frequent and can be related to different factors. Low sample size represents one of the most frequent causes for lack of replication and there are many evidences in the literature showing the critical value of the sample size. According to a meta-analysis by Joannidis et al., a minimum of 150 subjects (controls and cases) should be required for association studies *(70)*. This problem is especially important when subjects are further divided into subgroups according to different allelic combinations.

Apart from the sample size bias, genuine ethnic and geographic differences can also contribute to the lack of confirmation of results in different populations. The recently described DAZL gene polymorphism represents a remarkable example of ethnic differences *(36)*. Finally, control group bias is also a common weakness of many association studies. It is important to distinguish between normal spermatogenesis and fertility because a control group selected on the basis of fertility status may contain up to 10% of men with severe spermatogenic failure *(71)*. If the expected effect of a polymorphism is spermatogenic failure, the correct control group should be normospermic men, whereas if the polymorphism is predicted to influence the sperm fertilization capacity, the most appropriate controls should be proven fertile men.

Polymorphisms should be considered as risk factors rather than direct etiological causes for spermatogenic disturbances or male infertility. Although data are controversial for the majority of polymorphisms, some of them, such as POLG, AR, and the DAZL gene, clearly cannot be considered as genetic risk factors for male infertility.

It is likely that some polymorphisms lead to testicular dysfunction only in association with a specific genetic background or with specific environmental factors. The role of genetic background seems to be especially relevant for one of the most promising genetic risk factors, the gr-gr deletions. Environmental factors may be relevant for ER polymorphisms, MTHR, and genes involved in oxidative stress. Certain gene variants may cause specific phenotypes (e.g., PRM1 and CREM) and consequently only the analysis of a specific subgroup of patients is able to identify their clinical significance. To obtain reliable and clinically useful data, much more attention should be focused on the correct study design, which is still the major weakness of association studies.

REFERENCES

1. Forti G, Krausz C. Clinical review 100: evaluation and treatment of the infertile couple. J Clin Endocrinol Metab 1998;83:4177–4188.
2. van der Ven K, Fimmers R, Engels G, van der Ven H, Krebs D. Evidence for major histocompatibility complex-mediated effects on spermatogenesis in humans. Hum Reprod 2000;15:189–196.
3. Matsuzaka Y, Makino S, Okamoto K, et al. Susceptibility locus for non-obstructive azoospermia is localized within the HLA-DR/DQ subregion: primary role of DQB1*0604. Tissue Antigens 2002;60:53–63.
4. Ruiz-Pesini E, Lapena AC, Diez-Sanchez C, et al. Human mtDNA haplogroups associated with high or reduced spermatozoa motility. Am J Hum Genet 2000;67:682–696.
5. St John JC, Jokhi RP, Barratt CL. The impact of mitochondrial genetics on male infertility. Int J Androl 2005;28:65–73.
6. Krausz C, Quintana-Murci L, Rajpert-De Meyts E, et al. Identification of a Y chromosome haplogroup associated with reduced sperm counts. Hum Mol Genet 2001;10:1873–1877.
7. Krausz C, Quintana-Murci L, Forti G. Y chromosome polymorphisms in medicine. Ann Med 2004;36:573–583.
8. Yong EL, Loy CJ, Sim KS. Androgen receptor gene and male infertility. Hum Reprod Update 2003;9:1–7.
9. Tut TG, Ghadessy FJ, Trifiro MA, Pinsky L, Yong EL. Long polyglutamine tracts in the androgen receptor are associated with reduced trans-activation, impaired sperm production, and male infertility. J Clin Endocrinol Metab 1997;82: 3777–3782.
10. Asatiani K, von Eckardstein S, Simoni M, Gromoll J, Nieschlag E. CAG repeat length in the androgen receptor gene affects the risk of male infertility. Int J Androl 2003;26:255–261.
11. Ferlin A, Bartoloni L, Rizzo G, Roverato A, Garolla A, Foresta C. Androgen receptor gene CAG and GGC repeat lengths in idiopathic male infertility. Mol Hum Reprod 2004;10:417–421.
12. Ruhayel Y, Lundin K, Giwercman Y, Hallden C, Willen M, Giwercman A. Androgen receptor gene GGN and CAG polymorphisms among severely oligozoospermic and azoospermic Swedish men. Hum Reprod 2004;19:2076–2083.
13. Lanfranco F, Kamischke A, Zitzmann M, Nieschlag E. Klinefelter's syndrome. Lancet 2004;364:273–283.
14. Zitzmann M, Depenbusch M, Gromoll J, Nieschlag E. X-chromosome inactivation patterns and androgen receptor functionality influence phenotype and social characteristics as well as pharmacogenetics of testosterone therapy in Klinefelter patients. J Clin Endocrinol Metab 2004;89:6208–6217.
15. Canale D, Caglieresi C, Moschini C, et al. Androgen receptor polymorphism (CAG repeats) and androgenicity. Clin Endocrinol 2005;63:356–361.
16. Gromoll J, Simoni M. Genetic complexity of FSH receptor function. Trends Endocrinol Metab 2005;16:368–373.

17. Simoni M, Weinbauer GF, Gromoll J, Nieschlag E. Role of FSH in male gonadal function. Ann Endocrinol 1999;60:102–106.
18. Ahda Y, Gromoll J, Wunsch A, et al. Follicle-stimulating hormone receptor gene haplotype distribution in normozoospermic and azoospermic men. J Androl 2005;26:494–499.
19. Pentikainen V, Erkkila K, Suomalainen L, Parvinen M, Dunkel L. Estradiol acts as a germ cell survival factor in the human testis in vitro. J Clin Endocrinol Metab 2000;85:2057–2067.
20. Atanassova N, McKinnell C, Turner KJ, et al. Comparative effects of neonatal exposure of male rats to potent and weak (environmental) estrogens on spermatogenesis at puberty and the relationship to adult testis size and fertility: evidence for stimulatory effects of low estrogen levels. Endocrinology 2000;141:3898–3907.
21. Sharpe RM, Skakkebaek NE. Are oestrogens involved in falling sperm counts and disorders of the male reproductive tract? Lancet 1993;341:1392–1395.
22. Kukuvitis A, Georgiou I, Bouba I, et al. Association of oestrogen receptor alpha polymorphisms and androgen receptor CAG trinucleotide repeats with male infertility: a study in 109 Greek infertile men. Int J Androl 2002;25:149–152.
23. Suzuki Y, Sasagawa I, Itoh K, Ashida J, Muroya K, Ogata T. Estrogen receptor alpha gene polymorphism is associated with idiopathic azoospermia. Fertil Steril 2002;78:1341–1343.
24. Galan JJ, Buch B, Cruz N, et al. Multilocus analyses of estrogen-related genes reveal involvement of the ESR1 gene in male infertility and the polygenic nature of the pathology. Fertil Steril 2005;84:910–918.
25. Guarducci E, Nuti F, Becherini L, Rotondi M, Balercia G, Forti G, Krausz C. Estrogen receptor-α promoter polymorphism: stronger estrogen action is coupled with lower sperm count. Hum Reprod 2006;21:994–1001.
26. Becherini L, Gennari L, Masi L, et al. Evidence of a linkage disequilibrium between polymorphisms in the human estrogen receptor alpha gene and their relationship to bone mass variation in postmenopausal Italian women. Hum Mol Genet 2000;9:2043–2050.
27. Aschim EL, Giwercman A, Stahl O, et al. The RsaI polymorphism in the estrogen receptor-beta gene is associated with male infertility. J Clin Endocrinol Metab 2005;90:5343–5348.
28. Lee K, Haugen HS, Clegg CH, Braun RE. Premature translation of protamine 1 mRNA causes precocious nuclear condensation and arrests spermatid differentiation in mice. Proc Natl Acad Sci USA 1995;92:12,451–12,455.
29. Tanaka H, Miyagawa Y, Tsujimura A, Matsumiya K, Okuyama A, Nishimune Y. Single nucleotide polymorphisms in the protamine-1 and -2 genes of fertile and infertile human male populations. Mol Hum Reprod 2003;9:69–73.
30. Iguchi N, Yang S, Lamb DJ, Hecht NB. An SNP in protamine 1: a possible genetic cause of male infertility? J Med Genet 2006;43:382–384.
31. Yen PH, Chai NN, Salido EC. The human autosomal gene DAZLA: testis specificity and a candidate for male infertility. Hum Mol Genet 1996;5:2013–2017.
32. Yen PH. Putative biological functions of the DAZ family. Int J Androl 2004;27: 125–129.
33. Lepretre AC, Patrat C, Jouannet P, Bienvenu T. Mutation analysis of the BOULE gene in men with non-obstructive azoospermia: identification of a novel polymorphic variant in the black population. Int J Androl 2004;27:301–303.
34. Westerveld GH, Repping S, Leschot NJ, van der Veen F, Lombardi MP. Mutations in the human BOULE gene are not a major cause of impaired spermatogenesis. Fertil Steril 2005;83:513–515.

35. Teng YN, Lin YM, Lin YH, et al. Association of a single-nucleotide polymorphism of the deleted-in-azoospermia-like gene with susceptibility to spermatogenic failure. J Clin Endocrinol Metab 2002;87:5258–5264.

36. Becherini L, Guarducci E, Degl'Innocenti S, Rotondi M, Forti G, Krausz C. DAZL polymorphisms and susceptibility to spermatogenic failure: an example of remarkable ethnic differences. Int J Androl 2004;27:375–381.

37. Tschanter P, Kostova E, Luetjens CM, Cooper TG, Nieschlag E, Gromoll J. No association of the A260G and A386G DAZL single nucleotide polymorphisms with male infertility in a Caucasian population. Hum Reprod 2004;19:2771–2776.

38. Bartoloni L, Cazzadore C, Ferlin A, Garolla A, Foresta C. Lack of the T54A polymorphism of the DAZL gene in infertile Italian patients. Mol Hum Reprod 2004;10:613–615.

39. Yang XJ, Shinka T, Nozawa S, et al. Survey of the two polymorphisms in DAZL, an autosomal candidate for the azoospermic factor, in Japanese infertile men and implications for male infertility. Mol Hum Reprod 2005;11:513–515.

40. Ropp PA, Copeland WC. Cloning and characterization of the human mitochondrial DNA polymerase, DNA polymerase gamma. Genomics 1996;36:449–458.

41. Rovio AT, Marchington DR, Donat S, et al. Mutations at the mitochondrial DNA polymerase (POLG) locus associated with male infertility. Nat Genet 2001;29: 261–262.

42. Jensen M, Leffers H, Petersen JH, et al. Frequent polymorphism of the mitochondrial DNA polymerase gamma gene (POLG) in patients with normal spermiograms and unexplained subfertility. Hum Reprod 2004;19:65–70.

43. Krausz C, Guarducci E, Becherini L, et al. The clinical significance of the POLG gene polymorphism in male infertility. J Clin Endocrinol Metab 2004;89:4292–4297.

44. Aknin-Seifer IE, Touraine RL, Lejeune H, et al. Is the CAG repeat of mitochondrial DNA polymerase gamma (POLG) associated with male infertility? A multicentre French study. Hum Reprod 2005;20:736–740.

45. Longley MJ, Graziewicz MA, Bienstock RJ, Copeland WC. Consequences of mutations in human DNA polymerase gamma. Gene 2005;354:125–131.

46. Repping S, Skaletsky H, Brown L, et al. Polymorphism for a 1.6-Mb deletion of the human Y chromosome persists through balance between recurrent mutation and haploid selection. Nat Genet 2003;35:247–251.

47. Reijo R, Lee TY, Salo P, et al. Diverse spermatogenic defects in humans caused by Y chromosome deletions encompassing a novel RNA-binding protein gene. Nat Genet 1995;10:383–393.

48. Machev N, Saut N, Longepied G, et al. Sequence family variant loss from the AZFc interval of the human Y chromosome, but not gene copy loss, is strongly associated with male infertility. J Med Genet 2004;41:814–825.

49. Ferlin A, Tessari A, Ganz F, et al. Association of partial AZFc region deletions with spermatogenic impairment and male infertility. J Med Genet 2005;42:209–213.

50. Llanos M, Ballesca JL, Gazquez C, Margarit E, Oliva R. High frequency of gr/gr chromosome Y deletions in consecutive oligospermic ICS candidates. Hum Reprod 2005;20:216–220.

51. Hucklenbroich K, Gromoll J, Heinrich M, Hohoff C, Nieschlag E, Simoni M. Partial deletions in the AZFc region of the Y chromosome occur in men with impaired as well as normal spermatogenesis. Hum Reprod 2005;20:191–197.

52. Giachini C, Guarducci E, Longepied G, et al. The gr/gr deletion(s): a new genetic test in male infertility? J Med Genet 2005;42:497–502.

53. Lynch M, Cram DS, Reilly A, et al. The Y chromosome gr/gr subdeletion is associated with male infertility. Mol Hum Reprod 2005;11:507–512.

54. Fernandes S, Huellen K, Goncalves J, et al. High frequency of DAZ1/DAZ2 gene deletions in patients with severe oligozoospermia. Mol Hum Reprod 2002; 8:286–298.
55. Yen P. The fragility of fertility. Nat Genet 2001;29:243–244.
56. Vogt PH. Genomic heterogeneity and instability of the AZF locus on the human Y chromosome. Mol Cell Endocrinol 2004;224:1–9.
57. Repping S, Van Daalen SK, Korver CM, et al. A family of human Y chromosomes has dispersed throughout northern Eurasia despite a 1.8-Mb deletion in the azoospermia factor c region. Genomics 2004;83:1046–1052.
58. Fernandes S, Paracchini S, Meyer LH, Floridia G, Tyler-Smith C, Vogt PH. A large AZFc deletion removes DAZ3/DAZ4 and nearby genes from men in Y haplogroup N. Am J Hum Genet 2004;74:180–187.
59. Maiorino M, Bosello V, Ursini F, et al. Genetic variations of gpx-4 and male infertility in humans. Biol Reprod 2003;68:1134–1141.
60. Chen SS, Chang LS, Chen HW, Wei YH. Polymorphisms of glutathione S-transferase M1 and male infertility in Taiwanese patients with varicocele. Hum Reprod 2002;17: 718–725.
61. Bezold G, Lange M, Peter RU. Homozygous methylenetetrahydrofolate reductase C677T mutation and male infertility. N Engl J Med 2001;344:1172–1173.
62. Stuppia L, Gatta V, Scarciolla O, et al. The methylenetethrahydrofolate reductase (MTHFR) C677T polymorphism and male infertility in Italy. J Endocrinol Invest 2003;26:620–622.
63. Singh K, Singh SK, Sah R, Singh I, Raman R. Mutation C677T in the methylenetetrahydrofolate reductase gene is associated with male infertility in an Indian population. Int J Androl 2005;28:115–119.
64. Ebisch IM, van Heerde WL, Thomas CM, van der Put N, Wong WY, Steegers-Theunissen RP. C677T methylenetetrahydrofolate reductase polymorphism interferes with the effects of folic acid and zinc sulfate on sperm concentration. Fertil Steril 2003;80:1190–1194.
65. Zhoucun A, Zhang S, Yang Y, Ma Y, Zhang W, Lin L. The common variant N372H in BRCA2 gene may be associated with idiopathic male infertility with azoospermia or severe oligozoospermia. Eur J Obstet Gynecol Reprod Biol 2006;124:61–64.
66. Stouffs K, Lissens W, Tournaye H, Van Steirteghem A, Liebaers I. Possible role of USP26 in patients with severely impaired spermatogenesis. Eur J Hum Genet 2005;13:336–340.
67. Zhoucun A, Zhang S, Yang Y, Ma Y, Lin L, Zhang W. Single nucleotide polymorphisms of the gonadotrophin-regulated testicular helicase (GRTH) gene may be associated with the human spermatogenesis impairment. Hum Reprod 2006;21:755–759.
68. Krausz C, Sassone-Corsi P. Genetic control of spermiogenesis: insights from the CREM gene and implications for human infertility. Reprod Biomed Online 2005;10:64–71.
69. Vouk K, Hudler P, Strmsnik L, et al. Combinations of genetic changes in the human cAMP-responsive element modulator gene: a clue towards understanding some forms of male infertility? Mol Hum Reprod 2005;11:567–574.
70. Ioannidis JP, Ntzani EE, Trikalinos TA, Contopoulos-Ioannidis DG. Replication validity of genetic association studies. Nat Genet 2001;29:306–309.
71. Almagor M, Dan-Goor M, Hovav Y, Yaffe H. Spontaneous pregnancies in severe oligoasthenozoospermia. Hum Reprod 2001;6:780–781.

19 The Genetics of Abnormal Protamine Expression

Vincent W. Aoki, PhD
and Douglas T. Carrell, PhD

Summary

During spermiogenesis, the sperm chromatin undergoes dramatic remodeling. The testis-specific protamine proteins facilitate these nuclear changes by replacing the somatic cell histones, a process that produces highly condensed, transcriptionally silent chromatin. In humans, there are two forms of sperm protamine: protamine 1 (P1) and protamine 2 (P2), which occur in a strictly regulated 1:1 ratio. Sperm protamine-deficiency and P1:P2 ratio deregulation have been implicated in male infertility. The details of the underlying genetic basis of abnormal protamine expression are just emerging. This chapter summarizes our current knowledge of the sperm protamines, their relationship with male infertility, and what is currently understood regarding the genetic basis of abnormal protamine expression.

Key Words: Chromatin; genetics; expression; protamine; sperm.

1. INTRODUCTION TO THE SPERM PROTAMINE PROTEINS

During spermiogenesis, the haploid sperm chromatin undergoes a dramatic remodeling *(1)*. Two classes of sperm-specific nuclear proteins, the transition proteins and protamines, are responsible for packaging the sperm chromatin into a highly compact transcriptionally silent form *(2)*.

The protamine proteins replace the somatic cell histones in a two-stage process (Fig. 1) *(3)*. The first step occurs in haploid round spermatids and involves replacement of the histones with the transition proteins (TP1 and TP2). Subsequently, in elongating spermatids, the protamine proteins (P1 and P2) replace TP1 and TP2. The resulting chromatin is highly condensed and transcriptionally silent.

From: *The Genetics of Male Infertility*
Edited by: D.T. Carrell © Humana Press Inc., Totowa, NJ

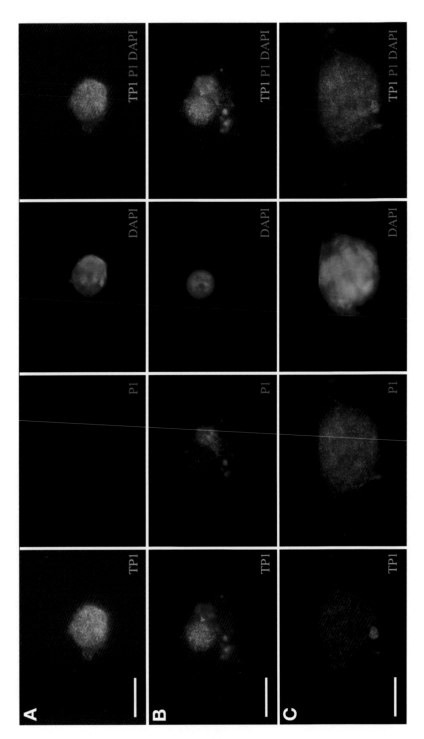

The protamine proteins are ubiquitous in the sperm of all mammals, a testament to their importance during sperm development *(4)*. P1 is present in all mammalian species, whereas P2 has been detected in spermatozoa of mouse hamster, vole, rat, stallion, and man *(4)*. Although the P2 protein is not present in some other mammals, such as the bull and boar, the gene encoding P2 is present and transcribed in these species.

From an evolutionary standpoint, mammals have likely inherited the *P1 gene* from a common ancestor because it is present in all species studied to date *(5)*. There are two possible explanations for the origin of the *P2 gene*. The most plausible is that P2 derived from P1 through a gene duplication event *(6)*. Alternatively, P1 and P2 may have been inherited from a single common ancestor and successive species have subsequently lost the ability to express P2 *(6)*.

The human *P1* and *P2 genes* encode a 50-amino acid protein and a final processed protein of 57 amino acids, respectively *(7,8)*. Overall, there is roughly 50% identity between human P1/P2. In various mammalian species, the P2 content may vary from 0 to 80% *(4)*. However, within a given genus the ratio of P1 to P2 (P1:P2) is strictly regulated and in humans, is approx 1:1 *(4)* (Fig. 2).

From a structural standpoint, the protamines are relatively small proteins but are highly basic in character because of a high level of arginine residues present in their amino acid sequences (~50% of the total amino acid compliment; refs. *7,8*). This aspect of the protamine structure promotes their association with the negatively charged DNA backbone. In addition, P1 and P2 contain copious amounts of cysteine residues (~10%), which foster a highly stable chromatin structure resulting from inter- and intramolecular interactions via disulfide bond formation *(7,8)*.

During the elongating stage of spermatogenesis, P1 is synthesized as a mature protein product, whereas P2 is synthesized as a precursor protein of 103 amino acids and undergoes proteolytic cleavage of its amino-terminus to produce a mature P2 protein *(3)*. Like many other proteins, phosphorylation of the protamines is required for their proper DNA incorporation and subsequent processing. P1 is rapidly phosphorylated

---

Fig. 1. *(Opposite page)* Immunofluorescence micrographs showing protamine 1 (P1) and transition protein 1 (TP1) expression in round and elongating spermatids. **(A)** Early round spermatid displaying TP1 nuclear localization without detectable P1 immunofluorescence. **(B)** Early elongating spermatid showing TP1 nuclear localization in concert with P1 cytoplasmic production. **(C)** Later elongating spermatid showing P1 nuclear localization with minimal residual TP1. Bar = 10 μm for A, B; 25 μm for C.

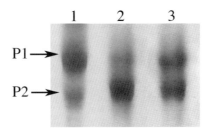

Fig. 2. Protamine detection via gel electrophoresis. Protamine 1 (P1) and P2 bands are located on the top and bottom rows of the gel, respectively. The banding patterns show examples of patients with elevated (lane 1), reduced (lane 2), and normal (lane 3) P1:P2 stoichiometry.

after translation by the serine/arginine protein-specific kinase (SRPK) 1 *(9)*. An intermediate form of P2, one derived by proteolysis of the precursor P2, is also rapidly phosphorylated by another protein, the Ca^{2+}/calmodulin-dependent protein kinase (Camk) 4 *(10)*.

The protamine genes, which contain only a single intron, are highly conserved in the sperm of all mammalian species *(4)*. The haploid genome encodes a single copy of the human P1 and P2 genes mapped to chromosome 16p13.3. In addition, TP2 is mapped to the same locus on chromosome 16p13.3. This *P1–P2–TP2* locus spans a 28.5-kb region and is organized in a linear array, a structural feature affording concurrent expression of the P1, P2, and TP2 genes *(11)*. This multigenic locus, therefore, represents a single coordinately expressed chromatin domain.

2. THE RELATIONSHIP BETWEEN ABNORMAL PROTAMINE EXPRESSION AND MALE INFERTILITY

Numerous reports have emerged in the last decade establishing a relationship between abnormal protamine expression and male infertility. These studies indicate aberrations in the P1:P2 ratio are related to impaired sperm quality and male infertility *(12–19)*. The majority of studies highlight populations of infertile men with abnormally elevated P1:P2 ratios *(12–19)*. Two of these reports document small populations of infertile males with undetectable levels of P2 *(16,17,19)*. Taken together, these data have led to the assumption that abnormal expression of P2 accounts for aberrant P1:P2 ratios in infertile men.

A population of infertile males was also identified with abnormally low P1:P2 ratios *(12,20,21)*. The identification of infertile men with abnormally low P1:P2 ratios raised the possibility that P1 is also abnormally expressed in patients with deregulated protamine stoichiometry. Indeed, protein quantification data strongly suggests P1 underexpression underlies the majority of cases involving abnormally reduced P1:P2 ratios *(12,20)*. Conversely, P2 underexpression appears responsible for the majority of abnormally elevated P1:P2 ratios *(12,20)*. Taken together, these data suggest deregulated expression of both P1 and P2 underlie aberrant sperm P1:P2 ratios. However, it appears that P2 underexpression is more common than P1 underexpression, evidenced by the increased incidence of patients with elevated P1:P2 ratios vs those with reduced P1:P2 ratios.

Sperm functional ability and semen quality parameters, including sperm count, motility, and head morphology, are significantly diminished in patients with abnormal P1:P2 ratios vs patients with normal P1:P2 ratios *(12,13,19,22)*. The ability of these sperm to successfully penetrate oocytes appears to be compromised, evidenced by significantly impaired oocyte penetration abilities *(12,19)*. Furthermore, patients with abnormal protamine expression also display reduced sperm DNA integrity and increased chromatin fragmentation *(21)*. Sperm functional ability, semen quality parameters, and sperm DNA integrity are markedly reduced in patients with abnormally reduced P1:P2 ratios, even vs patients with abnormally elevated P1:P2 ratios *(12,20,21)*. These data suggest P1 deficiency may be particularly detrimental to spermatogenesis in humans.

Animal knockout studies further highlight the importance of the protamines during mouse spermatogenesis and embryogenesis *(23,24)*. Consistent with the human data, mouse P1 and P2 haploinsufficiency results in severely abnormal spermatogenesis and increased DNA damage and sperm cell apoptosis *(23,24)*. Additionally, this induced protamine deficiency directly impairs in vitro embryonic development in mice *(23)*.

It is somewhat surprising that sperm concentration is significantly lower in patients with aberrant P1:P2 ratios, because late spermiogenesis events are not closely linked to events regulating sperm concentration. One possible hypothesis may be that patients lacking P1 or P2 reflect severely abnormal spermatogenesis. Thus, protamine deregulation may occur because of generalized spermatogenetic problems and/or an early aberration in the spermatogenic pathway that results in downstream deregulated protamine expression. Alternatively, the link between semen quality and protamine levels may also be the result of a generalized defect during late spermiogenesis, the point at which stored protamine transcripts undergo translation and posttranslational modifications *(25)*. Coincidentally, this is the stage at which numerous sperm function attributes are acquired, some of which are defective in protamine-deficient sperm.

Another alternative explanation for the link between protamines and semen quality is that protamine transcription and/or translation may act as a "checkpoint" during spermatogenesis, with spermatogenesis directly tied to the relative quantities of P1 and P2. The role of protamines as a checkpoint may seem unlikely, but two facts may indicate that it is not an unreasonable hypothesis. First, protamines are ubiquitous in mammals and critical for normal fertilization ability *(4)*. Second, the mouse knockout studies have shown that protamine haploinsufficiency leads to complete male infertility, including a diminished sperm count *(23,24)*. Although it is possible that the mouse model is not reflective of human spermatogenesis, that study, along with the human data, indicates a strong relationship between protamines and spermatogenesis.

3. THE GENETIC BASIS OF ABNORMAL PROTAMINE EXPRESSION

The etiology of human sperm protamine deficiency has remained elusive. Protamine expression deregulation may occur at multiple points along the expression pathway, including mutations in the protamine genes, aberrant transcription regulation, unfaithful translation repression or activation, and incomplete posttranslational protein processing. A number of studies have emerged in the last decade that have sought to elucidate the genetic basis of abnormal protamine expression.

Genetic sequencing approaches targeting the testis-specific nuclear proteins P1, P2, TP1, and TP2 suggest it is unlikely that aberrations in the coding and intronic regions underlie the majority of cases involving abnormal protamine expression *(16,26–33)*. Initial genetic screens of the protamine genes failed to reveal any pathogenic mutations in the small populations of infertile men *(28,32)*. More recent studies have led to the identification of a number of polymorphisms in the protamine and transition protein genes *(27,29–31,33)*. However, the majority of these studies have failed to correlate direct measures of protamine content with the incidence of these various polymorphisms. In general, there appears to be a very low incidence of these protamine gene polymorphisms. Thus, it does not appear that protamine gene mutations and polymorphisms underlie the majority of abnormal protamine expression cases.

This conclusion appears to be confirmed by a study from our laboratory comparing the identity and frequency of nuclear protein gene polymorphisms in protamine-deficient populations, severely infertile populations, and fertile controls *(42)*. A total of 15 single-nucleotide polymorphisms (SNPs) were identified in the P1, P2, TP1, and TP2 genes. A number of these SNPs resulted in amino acid changes, but occurred in similar frequencies within protamine-deficient patients, severely infertile men, and the fertile control population. Although unlikely, it may be possible that three of the intronic P2 variants may influence aberrant P2 expression, because their presence was limited to only the protamine-deficient population. However, the rare occurrence of these intronic SNPs suggests they do not contribute to the majority of cases involving P2 deficiency.

One of the most exciting discoveries was the elucidation of a potential mechanism of protamine expression deregulation via protamine transcript quantification *(20)*. Semiquantitative real-time RT-PCR revealed abnormally high levels of sperm P1 messenger RNA (mRNA) retention in cases of P1 protein underexpression *(20)*. This abnormal accumulation of P1 transcripts strongly suggests that protamine mRNA, although produced normally, fails to undergo translation. Therefore, defects in translation regulation may underlie the abnormally reduced P1:P2 ratios associated with P1 underexpression.

During spermiogenesis, protamine transcription and translation are temporally uncoupled *(25,34,35)*. Translational regulation is one of the more important aspects of protamine biology and accounts for this delay in protamine protein production *(12)*. If protamine transcription and translation are allowed to occur concurrently, the chromatin undergoes precocious compaction and sperm development is arrested *(36)*.

Under normal circumstances, protamine translation regulation begins immediately with RNA processing via intron splicing and mRNA polyadenylation *(25)*. Polyadenylation serves a dual function to both protect the mRNA from degradation and provide a binding site for translation repressor proteins. As the poly-A mRNA enters the cytoplasm, it is translationally repressed via storage in messenger ribonucleoprotein particles and binding by specific translation repressor proteins, which target the 5′-untanslated region, 3′-untanslated region, and poly-A sequences *(25)*.

Translation repression is removed a few days later, during the elongating spermatid stage, by covalent modification of the messenger ribonucleoprotein particles, release of translatable mRNA, and removal or migration of the translation repressor proteins, leaving the poly-A tail susceptible to degradation. Subsequently, the protamine proteins are translated, phosphorylated, and incorporated into the chromatin. The increased P1 mRNA retention observed in patients underexpressing P1 protein may arise as a result of defects in any of these translation repression/activation steps or abnormalities in the primary mRNA regulatory sequences.

In the case of P2 underexpression, the mRNA data suggests a multi-faceted deregulation pattern *(20)*. Although the majority of cases involving P2 deficiency are associated with decreased mRNA levels, nearly 25% of the P2-deficient patients appear to have an abnormal retention of P2 transcripts, similar to observed scenario for P1-deficient patients *(20)*. This dichotomy in P2 mRNA levels within P2-deficient patients suggests various mechanisms potentially underlie deregulated P2 expression.

Abnormal posttranslational P2 processing may play an important role in P2 underexpression. After translation, P2 is rapidly phosphorylated by Camk4 *(10)*. This phosphorylation step is an absolute requirement for proper binding of P2 to the DNA *(10)*. After the full-length phosphorylated form of P2 is bound to the DNA, it undergoes proteolytic cleavage to produce a mature shortened P2 protein *(37)*. Thus, P2-deficient patients with abnormally elevated P1:P2 ratios may possess defects in the Camk4 protein itself or defective signaling pathways that activate the kinase. Indeed, support for this hypothesis is provided by a study demonstrating an abnormal accumulation of P2 precursors in patients with reduced P2 levels *(17)*.

The decreased P2 levels associated with low P2 mRNA levels may also derive from diminished levels of P2 transcription. Intuitively this scenario does not appear likely, given P1 and P2 are transcribed from a single coordinately expressed gene cluster with similar upstream regulatory elements *(3,5,38,39)*. However, a variable length GA-repeat specific to the P2 promoter has now been identified that may serve to modulate transcription efficiency *(30,38)*.

Finally, there may also be a relationship between disruptions of the hypothalamic–pituitary–gonadal axis and abnormal protamine expression. Two studies in particular highlight a specific relationship between normal endocrine signaling pathways and the normal expression of the sperm nuclear proteins *(40,41)*. The first study evaluated the effects of mouse follicle-stimulating hormone (FSH) receptor disruption on sperm nuclear protein expression patterns *(40)*. A dramatic reduction of TP1, TP2, and P2 expression was observed in 21-d-old mice. Furthermore, in sexually mature mice there was a 50% reduction in total protamine (P1 + P2) levels with an abnormal retention of mono-ubiquitinated histone 2A.

The second study demonstrated cyproterone acetate mediated disruption of testosterone binding to the androgen receptors resulted in a downstream reduction of protamine expression *(41)*. Taken together, these studies indicate endocrine-signaling pathways play an important role in protamine expression. Although the mechanisms are not well understood, FSH is thought to regulate protamine expression through its activation of the cycle adenosine monophosphate response element modulator, which in turn, upregulates protamine transcription. Nevertheless, a generalized malfunction of the hypothalamic–pituitary–gonadal axis, defects in the FSH and androgen receptors, or disruption of the proper signal cascades may also be at the root of abnormal protamine expression.

4. CONCLUSION

The protamine proteins play a critical role during spermatogenesis in the proper remodeling and packaging of the sperm chromatin. Populations of infertile men have now been identified that abnormally express the protamine proteins. In particular, these patients display abnormally protamine stoichiometry, either in the form of reduced or elevated P1:P2 ratios. These abnormal P1:P2 ratios have been shown to arise as a result of deregulated expression of the P1 and P2 proteins, respectively. Aberrations in protamine expression are associated with diminished semen quality, compromised sperm functional ability, and reduced sperm DNA integrity. Deregulated protamine expression does not appear to be a principle result of nuclear protein gene mutations, but instead may arise because of mechanisms of aberrant translation regulation, posttranslational processing defects, or improper endocrine signaling.

REFERENCES

1. Dadoune JP. The nuclear status of human sperm cells. Micron 1995;26: 323–345.
2. Hecht NB. Mammalian protamines and their expression. In: Hnilica LS, Stein JL, Stein GS, eds. Histones and Other Basic Nuclear Proteins. CRC Press, Orlando; 1989:347–373.
3. Oliva R, Dixon GH. Vertebrate protamine genes and the histone-to-protamine replacement reaction. Prog Nucleic Acid Res Mol Biol 1991;40:25–94.
4. Corzett M, Mazrimas J, Balhorn R. Protamine 1: protamine 2 stoichiometry in the sperm of eutherian mammals. Mol Reprod Dev 2002;61:519–527.
5. Domenjoud L, Kremling H, Burfeind P, Maier WM, Engel W. On the expression of protamine genes in the testis of man and other mammals. Andrologia 1991;23: 333–337.
6. Rooney AP, Zhang J. Rapid evolution of a primate sperm protein: relaxation of functional constraint or positive Darwinian selection? Mol Biol Evol 1999;16: 706–710.
7. McKay DJ, Renaux BS, Dixon GH. The amino acid sequence of human sperm protamine P1. Biosci Rep 1985;5:383–391.
8. McKay DJ, Renaux BS, Dixon GH. Human sperm protamines. Amino-acid sequences of two forms of protamine P2. Eur J Biochem 1986;156:5–8.
9. Papoutsopoulou S, Nikolakaki E, Chalepakis G, Kruft V, Chevaillier P, Giannakouros T. SR protein-specific kinase 1 is highly expressed in testis and phosphorylates protamine 1. Nucleic Acids Res 1999;27:2972–2980.

10. Wu JY, Ribar TJ, Cummings DE, Burton KA, McKnight GS, Means AR. Spermiogenesis and exchange of basic nuclear proteins are impaired in male germ cells lacking Camk4. Nat Genet 2000;25:448–452.

11. Nelson JE, Krawetz SA. Linkage of human spermatid-specific basic nuclear protein genes. Definition and evolution of the P1→P2→TP2 locus. J Biol Chem 1993;268:2932–2936.

12. Aoki VW, Liu L, Carrell DT. Identification and evaluation of a novel sperm protamine abnormality in a population of infertile males. Hum Reprod 2005;20: 1298–1306.

13. Balhorn R, Reed S, Tanphaichitr N. Aberrant protamine 1/protamine 2 ratios in sperm of infertile human males. Experientia 1988;44:52–55.

14. Belokopytova IA, Kostyleva EI, Tomilin AN, Vorob'ev VI. Human male infertility may be due to a decrease of the protamine P2 content in sperm chromatin. Mol Reprod Dev 1993;34:53–57.

15. Chevaillier P, Mauro N, Feneux D, Jouannet P, David G. Anomalous protein complement of sperm nuclei in some infertile men. Lancet 1987;2:806–807.

16. de Yebra L, Ballesca JL, Vanrell JA, Bassas L, Oliva R. Complete selective absence of protamine P2 in humans. J Biol Chem 1993;268:10,553–10,557.

17. de Yebra L, Ballesca JL, Vanrell JA, Corzett M, Balhorn R, Oliva R. Detection of P2 precursors in the sperm cells of infertile patients who have reduced protamine P2 levels. Fertil Steril 1998;69:755–759.

18. Khara KK, Vlad M, Griffiths M, Kennedy CR. Human protamines and male infertility. J Assist Reprod Genet 1997;14:282–290.

19. Carrell DT, Liu L. Altered protamine 2 expression is uncommon in donors of known fertility, but common among men with poor fertilizing capacity, and may reflect other abnormalities of spermiogenesis. J Androl 2001;22:604–610.

20. Aoki VW, Liu L, Carrell DT. A novel mechanism of protamine expression deregulation highlighted by abnormal protamine transcript retention in infertile human males with sperm protamine deficiency. Mol Hum Reprod 2006;12:41–50.

21. Aoki VW, Moskovtsev SI, Willis J, Liu L, Mullen JBM, Carrell DT. DNA integrity is compromised in protamine-deficient human sperm. J Androl 2005;26:741–748.

22. Aoki VW, Carrell DT. Human protamines and the developing spermatid: their structure, function, expression and relationship with male infertility. Asian J Androl 2003;5:315–324.

23. Cho C, Jung-Ha H, Willis WD, et al. Protamine 2 deficiency leads to sperm DNA damage and embryo death in mice. Biol Reprod 2003;69:211–217.

24. Cho C, Willis WD, Goulding EH, et al. Haploinsufficiency of protamine-1 or -2 causes infertility in mice. Nat Genet 2001;28:82–86.

25. Steger K. Transcriptional and translational regulation of gene expression in haploid spermatids. Anat Embryol (Berl) 1999;199:471–487.

26. Queralt R, Oliva R. Identification of conserved potential regulatory sequences of the protamine-encoding P1 genes from ten different mammals. Gene 1993;133: 197–204.

27. Schnulle V, Schlicker M, Engel W. A (GA)n repeat polymorphism in the human protamine 2 (PRM 2) gene. Hum Mol Genet 1994;3:1445.

28. Schlicker M, Schnulle V, Schneppel L, Vorob'ev VI, Engel W. Disturbances of nuclear condensation in human spermatozoa: search for mutations in the genes for protamine 1, protamine 2 and transition protein 1. Hum Reprod 1994;9:2313–2317.

29. Kramer JA, Zhang S, Yaron Y, Zhao Y, Krawetz SA. Genetic testing for male infertility: a postulated role for mutations in sperm nuclear matrix attachment regions. Genet Test 1997;1:125–129.

30. Tanaka H, Miyagawa Y, Tsujimura A, Matsumiya K, Okuyama A, Nishimune Y. Single nucleotide polymorphisms in the protamine-1 and -2 genes of fertile and infertile human male populations. Mol Hum Reprod 2003;9:69–73.
31. Iguchi N, Yang S, Lamb DJ, Hecht NB. An SNP in protamine 1: a possible genetic cause of male infertility? J Med Genet 2006;43:382–384.
32. de Yebra L, Oliva R. Rapid analysis of mammalian sperm nuclear proteins. Anal Biochem 1993;209:201–203.
33. Miyagawa Y, Nishimura H, Tsujimura A, et al. Single-nucleotide polymorphisms and mutation analyses of the TNP1 and TNP2 genes of fertile and infertile human male populations. J Androl 2005;26:779–786.
34. Steger K, Klonisch T, Gavenis K, Drabent B, Doenecke D, Bergmann M. Expression of mRNA and protein of nucleoproteins during human spermiogenesis. Mol Hum Reprod 1998;4:939–945.
35. Steger K, Pauls K, Klonisch T, Franke FE, Bergmann M. Expression of protamine-1 and -2 mRNA during human spermiogenesis. Mol Hum Reprod 2000;6:219–225.
36. Lee K, Haugen HS, Clegg CH, Braun RE. Premature translation of protamine 1 mRNA causes precocious nuclear condensation and arrests spermatid differentiation in mice. Proc Natl Acad Sci USA 1995;92:12,451–12,455.
37. Balhorn R, Cosman M, Thornton K. Protamine mediated condensation of DNA in mammalian sperm. In: Gagnon C, ed. The Male Gamete: From Basic Science to Clinical Applications. Cache River Press, Vienna, IL; 1999:55–70.
38. Nelson JE, Krawetz SA. Characterization of a human locus in transition. J Biol Chem 1994;269:31,067–31,073.
39. Domenjoud L, Nussbaum G, Adham IM, Greeske G, Engel W. Genomic sequences of human protamines whose genes, PRM1 and PRM2, are clustered. Genomics 1990;8:127–133.
40. Xing W, Krishnamurthy H, Sairam MR. Role of follitropin receptor signaling in nuclear protein transitions and chromatin condensation during spermatogenesis. Biochem Biophys Res Commun 2003;312:697–701.
41. Aleem M, Padwal V, Choudhari J, Balasinor N, Parte P, Gill-Sharma M. Cyproterone acetate affects protamine gene expression in the testis of adult male rat. Contraception 2005;71:379–391.
42. Aoki VW, Christensen BL, Atkins JF, Carrell DT. Identification of novel polymorphisms in the nuclear protein genes and their relationship with human sperm protamine deficiency and sever male infertility. Fertil Steril, in press.

20 Chromatin Damage and Male Infertility

Denny Sakkas, PhD,
Davide Bizzaro, PhD,
and Gian C. Manicardi, PhD

Summary

There is accumulating evidence linking sperm chromatin damage to poor reproductive outcome. The chromatin damage is associated to sperm anomalies that manifest themselves as breaks in the sperm nuclear DNA, aberrant ratios of protamine and histones in the chromatin, and the presence of apoptotic marker proteins in the ejaculated spermatozoa. This chapter examines the mechanisms involved in generating chromatin damage during spermatogenesis in the human, the techniques used to test sperm chromatin and how they may affect reproductive outcome, and how to reduce the risk of using spermatozoa with chromatin damage.

Key Words: Sperm chromatin; apoptosis; intracytoplasmic sperm injection; DNA damage; spermatogenesis.

1. INTRODUCTION

The classic semen parameters (sperm concentration, motility, and morphology) have long been seen as a true indication of the fertility potential of a man. Although these will always provide a frontline indication of fertility potential, the advent of new assisted reproduction technologies (ARTs) has caused a rethinking of how spermatozoa is assessed. With the use of intracytoplasmic sperm injection (ICSI), in vitro fertilization (IVF), and to a lesser extent intrauterine insemination (IUI), many of the deficiencies revealed in a classic semen analysis (e.g., a low sperm count) can be overcome. Subsequently, the classic semen analysis is now proving less conclusive in some cases and has led us to examine the ejaculated spermatozoa for more subtle characteristics that may affect reproductive outcome.

From: *The Genetics of Male Infertility*
Edited by: D.T. Carrell © Humana Press Inc., Totowa, NJ

One key characteristic has been a more thorough examination of the sperm nucleus. This has led to an abundance of articles being published indicating that chromatin damage in the form of DNA strand breaks and aberrant protamine:histone ratios are clearly detectable in ejaculated spermatozoa and their presence is heightened in the ejaculates of men with poor semen parameters *(1)*.

Damaged chromatin in sperm heightens the risk that the paternal genome is compromised. The impact an abnormal paternal genome may have on reproductive outcome *(2)* is unquestionably less when compared with its female counterpart's role. Egg quality is clearly the major driving force in respect to the chances of a couple achieving a pregnancy. In contrast, the influence of the human sperm on reproductive outcome has been less well characterized, however we recently showed that in 10–15% of IVF cycles a paternal factor may exist *(3)*. The factors present in the paternal genome that impact on poor reproductive outcome are still hypothetical. However, in the last decade the quality of the sperm nuclear chromatin has been more rigorously examined.

2. MECHANISMS INVOLVED IN THE ORIGIN OF CHROMATIN DAMAGE

Spermatogenesis is a complex process of proliferation and differentiation transforming spermatogonia into mature spermatozoa. This unique process involves a series of mitoses and a meiotic division followed by marked changes in cell structure, in addition to proliferation and differentiation. It is clear that spermatozoa can arise in the ejaculate possessing various nuclear anomalies related to chromatin damage. These arise because of the failure of a number of processes that can either cause and/or fail to detect or eliminate the abnormal spermatozoa. Two processes that may fail in their task during spermatogenesis, leading to abnormal sperm in the ejaculate, are apoptosis and chromatin remodeling.

3. APOPTOTIC MARKERS PRESENT ON EJACULATED SPERMATOZA

Apoptosis may play two putative roles during normal spermatogenesis: limitation of the germ cell population to numbers that can be supported by the Sertoli cells and selective depletion of abnormal spermatozoa.

In mouse models, numerous pro- and antiapoptotic proteins have been found to play key roles in spermatogenesis. The Bcl-2 family includes both prosurvival and proapoptotic members, and provides a signaling pathway that appears imperative in maintaining male germ cell homeostasis *(4)*. Bcl-2 and Bcl-x_L are pro-survival members of the

Bcl-2 family. Transgenic overexpression of Bcl-2 and Bcl-x$_L$ results in blockage of cell death at a critical stage, and results in disruption of normal spermatogenesis and infertility in male mice *(5,6)*. Concurrently, knockout models of the pro-apoptotic factor Bax results in germ cell death and testicular atrophy *(7)*. These studies show that an increase in proapoptotic or antiapoptotic proteins can result in disruption of normal spermatogenesis and suggest that apoptosis plays an important role in male gametogenesis by regulating the size of the spermatogenic cell population. Meanwhile, although it seems plausible, the role of apoptosis in selective depletion of abnormal spermatozoa is yet to be proven.

In the human, we originally found that men with abnormal sperm parameters display higher levels of the apoptotic protein Fas on their ejaculated spermatozoa *(8)*. The presence of Fas on ejaculated spermatozoa correlated strongly with a decreased sperm concentration and sperm with abnormal morphology. More recently, we and others also found that other apoptotic markers such as Bcl-x, p53, caspase, and annexin V are also present on ejaculated human spermatozoa and show distinct relationships with abnormal semen parameters *(9–12)*. Double-labeling experiments have shown that ejaculated human sperm expressing apoptotic marker proteins can also display chromatin damage and show signs of immaturity, such as cytoplasmic retention *(10,13)*.

4. CHROMATIN REMODELING DURING SPERMIOGENESIS

A key change in chromatin structure occurs during spemiogenesis when histones are replaced by protamines to confer the compacted chromatin/DNA packaging seen in mature spermatozoa *(14)*. McPherson and Longo demonstrated the presence of endogenous DNA strand breaks in elongating rat spermatids, when chromatin structure and nucleoproteins are modified *(15)*. They proposed that the presence of endogenous nicks in ejaculated spermatozoa might be indicative of incomplete maturation during spermiogenesis. They also postulated that chromatin packaging might involve endogenous nuclease activity to create and ligate nicks during the replacement of histones by protamines, and that an endogenous nuclease, topoisomerase II, may play a role *(16,17)*. Topoisomerase II functions by transiently introducing DNA double-strand breaks, allowing the passage of one double helix through another, and resealing the double-strand break *(18)*. Although the role of topoisomerase II in spermatogenesis is yet to be clarified, it is expressed in the human testis *(19)*. The transient presence of DNA breaks has been reported in both mouse and human *(20,21)*. An abundance of articles have been published indicating that DNA strand breaks are clearly detectable in ejaculated spermatozoa and their presence is heightened in the ejaculates of men with poor semen parameters *(2,22–25)*.

5. GENERATING SPERMATOZOA
WITH DAMAGED CHROMATIN

The presence of spermatozoa with damaged chromatin in the ejaculate is likely influenced by a failure of one or both of the apoptosis and chromatin remodeling mechanisms to function effectively. We have previously hypothesized that the presence of spermatozoa with apoptotic marker proteins in the ejaculate is the result of a process we have termed *abortive apoptosis (8,26–28)*, which is when germ cells are earmarked for apoptosis during spermatogenesis but fail to be cleared and remain in the spermatogenic pool. In addition, failure of the chromatin remodeling process to proceed correctly may allow the production of spermatozoa with DNA breaks. Indeed our own studies have shown that DNA strand breaks are not always present in the same spermatozoa that show apoptotic markers *(10)*. Further failure in other systems to detect abnormal sperm during spermatogenesis, such as DNA repair pathways, will also contribute to this pool of abnormal spermatozoa in the ejaculate. Additionally, we believe that sperm arising from these inadequacies during spermatogenesis will be more susceptible to reactive oxygen species (ROS).

5.1. Reactive Oxygen Species

Further to the events affecting sperm DNA in the testes are posttesticular DNA damage and the possible implication of ROS. Greco et al. recently reported that DNA fragmentation in ejaculated spermatozoa detected by the terminal deoxynucleotidyl transferase [TdT]-mediated dUTP nick end-labeling (TUNEL) assay is significantly higher compared with that in testicular spermatozoa (23 vs 4.5%; ref. *29*). They also found higher pregnancy rates using testicular sperm compared with ejaculated spermatozoa *(29)*. Steele et al. *(30)* found similar results when they compared epididymal sperm with testicular sperm using the Comet assay. One of the theories attempting to explain the differences in DNA damage between testicular and epididymal spermatozoa implicates ROS. Ollero et al. *(31)* suggested that high levels of ROS production and DNA damage observed in immature spermatozoa may be indicative of derangements in the regulation of spermiogenesis and that DNA damage in mature spermatozoa may be the result of oxidative damage harming immature spermatozoa during sperm migration from the seminiferous tubules to the epididymis. Although there are indications that post-testicular events affect sperm DNA integrity, it is still unclear whether it is a testicular failure to generate normal spermatozoa that makes them more susceptible to the effects of ROS.

6. TECHNIQUES USED TO TEST SPERM CHROMATIN AND HOW THEY MAY AFFECT REPRODUCTIVE OUTCOME

6.1. Testing Sperm

A number of tests have been reported in recent years as indicators of sperm nuclear chromatin integrity; however, their effectiveness is increasingly being questioned *(32)*. One of the tests most commonly used to detect DNA strand breaks is TUNEL. The TUNEL technique labels single- or double-stranded DNA breaks, but does not quantify DNA strand breaks in a given cell. Other tests of sperm nuclear DNA integrity include *in situ* nick translation *(33)* and the Comet assay *(34,35)*.

The most widely used test relating to pregnancy data in the human is the sperm chromatin structure assay (SCSA™). This test has its origins in the large animal field where it was clearly shown to have an impact on providing evidence of fertility potential and was proposed as early as 1980 as a test of sperm integrity in the human *(36)*. The SCSA is a flow-cytometric test that measures the susceptibility of sperm nuclear DNA to acid-induced DNA denaturation *in situ*, followed by staining with acridine orange *(37–39)*. Acridine orange is a metachromatic dye that fluoresces red when associated with denatured (fragmented) DNA and green when bound to double-stranded (normal) DNA. Therefore, an increase in the percentage of cells with a high ratio of red to green fluorescence indicates an overall increase in DNA fragmentation in the spermatozoa from that ejaculate. Because the SCSA is a quantitative (on a continuous scale), as opposed to a qualitative measurement, it has the potential to better define thresholds associated with reproductive outcome *(38)*.

6.2. Sperm Chromatin Assessment and Predicting Pregnancy

The SCSA has now been proposed clinically as a service. It provides two main measures: the DNA fragmentation index (DFI; i.e., the sperm fraction with detectable denaturable single-stranded DNA mainly resulting from DNA breaks) and the highly DNA-stainable (HDS) cells (i.e., the sperm fraction showing increased double-stranded DNA accessibility to acridine orange mainly because defects in the histone-to-protamine transition process) *(38,39)*. Because these parameters are not correlated to each other, they represent independent

aberrations of the human mature male gamete in the ejaculate. DFI has
been shown to influence normally initiated pregnancy *(40,41)*: increasing levels of DFI (>30%), independently from World Health
Organization standard semen parameters, were associated with a
decreased probability to father a child. Studies have been set up also to
challenge the SCSA prediction power in the context of ART. In the first
one, a small (24 men) pilot study showed that when DFI was more than
27%, no pregnancies could be obtained after IVF/ICSI *(42)*. Last year,
two other studies reinforced this finding. Larson-Cook et al. *(38)* examined 89 couples undergoing IVF/ICSI. The end point was clinical pregnancy 14 d after embryo transfer as assessed by positive serum human
chorionic gonadotrophin (hCG) and ultrasound detection for a fetal sac.
They showed that all patients who achieved a pregnancy had a DFI less
than 27% (on the other hand, HDS was not correlated to pregnancy).
Saleh et al. *(43)* considered 19 couples undergoing IUI, 10 couples
undergoing IVF, and 4 couples undergoing ICSI. In this study, levels of
DFI (but not of HDS) were negatively correlated with biochemical
pregnancy. The highest DFI value in biological fathers was 28%.
Although quite consistent in their finding, some discrepancies emerged
from these two studies: sperm concentration, % motility, and % morphology were significantly lower in patients who failed to initiate a
clinical pregnancy in the Saleh et al. *(43)* study but not in the Larson-
Cook et al. *(38)* study; the fertilization rate was related to DFI in the
Saleh et al. *(43)* study but not in the Larson-Cook et al. *(38)* study. It is
worthwhile to note that Benchaib et al. *(44)*, who assessed the clinical
pregnancy rate in a cohort of 50 IVF patients and 54 ICSI patients by
positive plasma hCG and ultrasound detection of a fetal heartbeat, also
showed that higher (>10%) sperm DNA fragmentation levels (this time
evaluated by TUNEL assay on the discontinuous gradient centrifugation selected sperm) was a negative factor to obtain pregnancies via
ICSI (but not via IVF) and no pregnancies were started if DNA fragmentation was more than 20%.

The enthusiasm originated by these original studies, on the existence of an upper DNA fragmentation threshold above which no
pregnancy can be obtained after ART, has been cooled down as more
investigations have been published. First, Gandini et al. *(45)*, in a
study involving 34 couples (12 IVF and 22 ICSI) did not note any
difference between patients initiating pregnancies or not and, above
all, they reported healthy full-term pregnancies even with high levels
of DFI (up to 66.3%). Pregnancy rates were 25% for IVF and 40.9%
for ICSI. HDS was not correlated either with pregnancy or delivery.
No association between the SCSA parameters and the fertility rate

was found. Second, Bungum et al. *(46)* investigated 306 consecutive couples undergoing ART (131 IUI, 109 IVF, and 66 ICSI), taking into account biochemical pregnancy (positive plasma hCG), clinical pregnancy (intrauterine gestational sac with a heartbeat 3 wk after a positive hCG test), and delivery. Delivery rate was 15.3% after IUI, 28.4% after IVF, and 37.9% after ICSI. They reported that, for IUI, the chance of pregnancy/delivery was significantly higher in the group with DFI less than 27% (and HDS <10%): only one delivery was obtained in the 23 males having a DFI more than 27%. The combination of DFI and HDS gave a higher predictive value regarding the outcome of IUI. On the other hand, no statistically significant difference in the outcome after IVF/ICSI was noted by dividing patients according to the DFI level of 27%. However, the results of ICSI were significantly better than those of IVF: for example, in the group with DFI more than 27%, the authors reported higher clinical pregnancy (52.9 vs 22.2%), implantation (37.5 vs 19.4%), and delivery (47.1 vs 22.2%) rates when comparing ICSI with IVF performances. In addition, by restricting the analysis to IVF patients only, the group with less than 27% DFI level consistently showed better clinical pregnancy (36.6 vs 22.2%), implantation (33.3 vs 19.4%), and delivery (29.7 vs 22.2%) rates as compared with the group of men with DFI more than 27%. Finally, Virro et al. *(47)* studied 249 couples undergoing IVF/ICSI and noted that men with DFI less than 33% had a significantly greater chance of initiating a clinical pregnancy (positive hCG), lower rate of spontaneous abortions, and an increase of ongoing pregnancies at 12 wk (47 vs 28%). HDS and standard World Health Organization parameters were not related to pregnancy outcomes. Further, Gardner et al. did not find a difference in the implantation and pregnancy rates between two groups that had 16 vs 40% fragmentation rates detected by SCSA *(48)*. All these studies demonstrate that high levels of DNA damage were compatible with pregnancy and delivery after IVF/ICSI.

The increasing number of publications in this field indicates that the relevance of sperm nuclear DNA is not completely black and white. A number of conclusions from the ever-increasing wealth of data collected about the various sperm nuclear DNA integrity tests and their predictive power in ART *(49)* can be made. Briefly, the conclusions can be summarized by the following points:

1. An increased fraction of sperm showing DNA damage is a negative trait that reduces the chances to father a child.
2. An absolute number or percentage of DNA strand breaks not compatible with pregnancy is far from being established.

3. The predictive power of the current sperm DNA integrity tests seem to lose their strength from natural conception to ICSI, passing through IUI and IVF.

7. REDUCING THE RISK OF USING SPERMATOZOA WITH CHROMATIN DAMAGE

Human semen is heterogeneous in quality, not only between males but also within a single ejaculate. Differences in quality are evident, both when examining the classical parameters of sperm number, motility, and morphology and in the integrity of the sperm nucleus. Potentially the greatest risk of using spermatozoa with damaged chromatin is present when using ICSI.

The ability to improve the efficiency of preparation techniques to eliminate spermatozoa with nuclear anomalies, selection of the best spermatozoa prior to ICSI, and/or selection of embryos that may have an abnormal paternal complement may all assist in eliminating the risk of using spermatozoa possessing damaged chromatin and making ICSI a safer technique. A number of studies have shown that spermatozoa prepared using a density gradient centrifugation technique significantly improves the quality of spermatozoa in the preparation *(33,50)*. In our own study, we showed that there was a significant ($p < 0.001$) decrease in both chromomycin A3 positivity and DNA strand breakage in sperm samples from different men after preparation by density gradient centrifugation. Chromomycin A3 indirectly demonstrates a decreased presence of protamines. These results indicated that density gradient centrifugation can enrich the sperm population by separating out those with nicked DNA and with poorly condensed chromatin. Another technique we proposed in 1999 was culturing ICSI embryos post-embryonic genome activation to the blastocyst stage *(51)*. This was based on the idea that the extent of nuclear DNA damage in spermatozoa is related to embryo development to the blastocyst stage, a time when the embryonic genome is activated, transcriptional activity has begun, and the paternal genome plays a significant contributory role in embryo function. Subsequently, we have shown that a significant negative correlation exists between the extent of DNA strand breaks in sperm samples and blastocyst development after IVF or ICSI *(52)*.

A final methodology is to improve the selection of spermatozoa before ICSI. One technique that has been reported is the selection of spermatozoa under high magnification. Bartoov et al. *(53)* reported that they were able to achieve a pregnancy rate of 58% in patients who had previously failed at least five consecutive routine cycles of IVF and

ICSI. They have also reported a follow-up study showing improved pregnancy rates with ICSI and morphologically selected sperm compared with conventional ICSI *(54)*. Aitken's group *(55)* also reported a novel electrophoretic sperm isolation technique for the isolation of functional human spermatozoa free from significant DNA damage. Briefly, the separation system consists of a cassette comprising two chambers. Semen is introduced into one chamber and a current applied that leads to a purified suspension of spermatozoa collecting on one side of the chamber within seconds. Suspensions generated by the electrophoretic separation technique contain motile, viable, morphologically normal spermatozoa that exhibit lower levels of DNA damage. A technique using magnetic cell sorting using annexin V-conjugated microbeads that eliminates apoptotic spermatozoa based on the externalization of phosphatidylserine residues has also been reported as a means of ameliorating sperm samples *(56)*.

Another promising sperm selection technique has recently been reported by Huszar and collaborators. They had previously reported that sperm that are able to bind to hyaluronic acid (HA) are mature and have completed the spermiogenetic process of sperm plasma membrane remodeling, cytoplasmic extrusion, and nuclear histone–protamine replacement *(57)*. Testing of a newly invented ICSI sperm selection method based on the binding ability of spermatozoa to HA has shown that the HA-bound sperm is less likely to show chromatin damage, apoptotic marker proteins, cytoplasmic retention, and aneuploidy compared with unselected sperm *(58)*. A limitation of this technique is that it may not be optimal for use in patients with very low sperm counts and motility.

8. CONCLUSIONS

There is now an abundance of studies showing a range of nuclear anomalies in ejaculated spermatozoa. It is also apparent that they are more likely to be present in men with poor semen parameters. The concern as to the level of this relationship is definitely greater in relation to ICSI, in which there is a higher chance that such a sperm will be chosen to fertilize an egg. The tests currently available only provide an inkling of the impact of sperm chromatin damage on reproductive outcome success. However, novel methods are being developed to limit the chance of using chromatin-damaged sperm in ARTs. More research is needed to improve our current knowledge in relation to how and why the chromatin damage arises in spermatozoa, how to detect and remove them more accurately, and how they may relate to failed reproductive outcomes.

REFERENCES

1. Irvine DS, Twigg JP, Gordon EL, Fulton N, Milne PA, Aitken RJ. DNA integrity in human spermatozoa: relationships with semen quality. J Androl 2000;21: 33–44.
2. Seli E, Sakkas D. Spermatozoal nuclear determinants of reproductive outcome: implications for ART. Hum Reprod Update 2005;11:337–349.
3. Sakkas D, D'Arcy Y, Percival G, Sinclair L, Afnan M, Sharif K. Use of the egg-share model to investigate the paternal influence on fertilization and embryo development after in vitro fertilization and intracytoplasmic sperm injection. Fertil Steril 2004;82:74–79.
4. Huynh T, Mollard R, Trounson A. Selected genetic factors associated with male infertility. Hum Reprod Update 2002;8:183–198.
5. Furuchi T, Masuko K, Nishimune Y, Obinata M, Matsui Y. Inhibition of testicular germ cell apoptosis and differentiation in mice misexpressing Bcl-2 in spermatogonia. Development 1996;122:1703–1709.
6. Rodriguez I, Ody C, Araki K, Garcia I, Vasalli P. An early and massive wave of germ cell apoptosis is required for the development of functional spermatogenesis. EMBO J 1997;16:2262–2270.
7. Russell LD, Chiarini-Garcia H, Korsmeyer SJ, Knudson CM. Bax-dependent spermatogonia apoptosis is required for testicular development and spermatogenesis. Biol Reprod 2002;66:950–958.
8. Sakkas D, Mariethoz E, St John JC. Abnormal sperm parameters in humans are indicative of an abortive apoptotic mechanism linked to the Fas-mediated pathway. Exp Cell Res 1999;251:350–355.
9. Barroso G, Morshedi M, Oehninger S. Analysis of DNA fragmentation, plasma membrane translocation of phosphatidylserine and oxidative stress in human spermatozoa. Hum Reprod 2000;15:1338–1344.
10. Sakkas D, Moffatt O, Manicardi GC, Mariethoz E, Tarozzi N, Bizzaro D. Nature of DNA damage in ejaculated human spermatozoa and the possible involvement of apoptosis. Biol Reprod 2002;66:1061–1067.
11. Grunewald S, Paasch U, Wuendrich K, Glander HJ. Sperm caspases become more activated in infertility patients than in healthy donors during cryopreservation. Arch Androl 2005;51:449–460.
12. Oehninger S, Morshedi M, Weng SL, Taylor S, Duran H, Beebe S. Presence and significance of somatic cell apoptosis markers in human ejaculated spermatozoa. Reprod Biomed Online 2003;7:469–476.
13. Cayli S, Sakkas D, Vigue L, Demir R, Huszar G. Cellular maturity and apoptosis in human sperm: creatine kinase, caspase-3 and Bcl-XL levels in mature and diminished maturity sperm. Mol Hum Reprod 2004;10:365–372.
14. Ward WS, Coffey DS. DNA packaging and organization in mammalian spermatozoa: comparison with somatic cells. Biol Reprod 1991;44:569–574.
15. McPherson S, Longo FJ. Chromatin structure–function alterations during mammalian spermatogenesis: DNA nicking and repair in elongating spermatids. Eur J Histochem 1993;37:109–128.
16. McPherson SM, Longo FJ. Nicking of rat spermatid and spermatozoa DNA: possible involvement of DNA topoisomerase II. Dev Biol 1993;158:122–130.
17. McPherson SM, Longo FJ. Localization of DNase I-hypersensitive regions during rat spermatogenesis: stage-dependent patterns and unique sensitivity of elongating spermatids. Mol Reprod Dev 1992;31:268–279.
18. Wang JC, Caron PR, Kim RA. The role of DNA topoisomerases in recombination and genome stability: a double-edge sword? Cell 1990;62:403–406.

19. Seli E, Bizzaro D, Manicardi GC, et al. The Involvement of DNA Strand Breaks and Topoisomerase II in Condensing Sperm Chromatin During Spermatogenesis in Human. Madrid, Spain: 2003.
20. Sakkas D, Manicardi G, Bianchi PG, Bizzaro D, Bianchi U. Relationship between the presence of endogenous nicks and sperm chromatin packaging in maturing and fertilizing mouse spermatozoa. Biol Reprod 1995;52:1149–1155.
21. Marcon L, Boissonneault G. Transient DNA strand breaks during mouse and human spermiogenesis new insights in stage specificity and link to chromatin remodeling. Biol Reprod 2004;70:910–918.
22. Irvine DS, Twigg JP, Gordon EL, Fulton N, Milne PA, Aitken RJ. DNA integrity in human spermatozoa: relationships with semen quality. J Androl 2000;21:33–44.
23. O'Brien J, Zini A. Sperm DNA integrity and male infertility. Urology 2005;65:16–22.
24. Alvarez JG. DNA fragmentation in human spermatozoa: significance in the diagnosis and treatment of infertility. Minerva Ginecol 2003;55:233–239.
25. Agarwal A, Said TM. Role of sperm chromatin abnormalities and DNA damage in male infertility. Hum Reprod Update 2003;9:331–345.
26. Sakkas D, Seli E, Manicardi GC, Nijs M, Ombelet W, Bizzaro D. The presence of abnormal spermatozoa in the ejaculate: did apoptosis fail? Hum Fertil (Camb) 2004;7:99–103.
27. Sakkas D, Mariethoz E, Manicardi G, Bizzaro D, Bianchi PG, Bianchi U. Origin of DNA damage in ejaculated human spermatozoa. Rev Reprod 1999;4:31–37.
28. Sakkas D, Seli E, Bizzaro D, Tarozzi N, Manicardi GC. Abnormal spermatozoa in the ejaculate: abortive apoptosis and faulty nuclear remodelling during spermatogenesis. Reprod Biomed Online 2003;7:428–432.
29. Greco E, Scarselli F, Iacobelli M, et al. Efficient treatment of infertility due to sperm DNA damage by ICSI with testicular spermatozoa. Hum Reprod 2005;20:226–230.
30. Steele EK, McClure N, Maxwell RJ, Lewis SE. A comparison of DNA damage in testicular and proximal epididymal spermatozoa in obstructive azoospermia. Mol Hum Reprod 1999;5:831–835.
31. Ollero M, Gil-Guzman E, Lopez MC, et al. Characterization of subsets of human spermatozoa at different stages of maturation: implications in the diagnosis and treatment of male infertility. Hum Reprod 2001;16:1912–1921.
32. Schlegel PN, Paduch DA. Yet another test of sperm chromatin structure. Fertil Steril 2005;84:854–859.
33. Tomlinson MJ, Moffatt O, Manicardi GC, Bizzaro D, Afnan M, Sakkas D. Interrelationships between seminal parameters and sperm nuclear DNA damage before and after density gradient centrifugation: implications for assisted conception. Hum Reprod 2001;16:2160–2165.
34. Morris ID, Ilott S, Dixon L, Brison DR. The spectrum of DNA damage in human sperm assessed by single cell electrophoresis (COMET assay) and its relationship to fertilization and embryo development. Hum Reprod 2002;17:990–998.
35. Hughes C, Lewis S, McKelvey-Martin V, Thompson W. A comparison of baseline and induced DNA damage in human spermatozoa from fertile and infertile men, using a modified comet assay. Mol Hum Reprod 1996;2:613–619.
36. Evenson DP, Darzynkiewicz Z, Melamed MR. Relation of mammalian sperm chromatin heterogeneity to fertility. Science 1980;210:1131–1133.
37. Evenson D, Jost L. Sperm chromatin structure assay is useful for fertility assessment. Methods Cell Sci 2000;22:169–189.
38. Larson-Cook KL, Brannian JD, Hansen KA, Kasperson KM, Aamold ET, Evenson DP. Relationship between the outcomes of assisted reproductive techniques and sperm DNA fragmentation as measured by the sperm chromatin structure assay. Fertil Steril 2003;80:895–902.

39. Evenson DP, Larson KL, Jost LK. Sperm chromatin structure assay: its clinical use for detecting sperm DNA fragmentation in male infertility and comparisons with other techniques. J Androl 2002;23:25–43.

40. Evenson DP, Jost LK, Marshall D, et al. Utility of the sperm chromatin structure assay as a diagnostic and prognostic tool in the human fertility clinic. Human Reprod 1999;14:1039–1049.

41. Spano M, Bonde JP, Hjollund HI, Kolstad HA, Cordelli E, Leter G. Sperm chromatin damage impairs human fertility. The Danish First Pregnancy Planner Study Team. Fertil Steril 2000;73:43–50.

42. Larson KL, DeJonge CJ, Barnes AM, Jost LK, Evenson DP. Sperm chromatin structure assay parameters as predictors of failed pregnancy following assisted reproductive techniques. Hum Reprod 2000;15:1717–1722.

43. Saleh RA, Agarwal A, Nada EA, et al. Negative effects of increased sperm DNA damage in relation to seminal oxidative stress in men with idiopathic and male factor infertility. Fertil Steril 2003;79:1597–1605.

44. Benchaib M, Braun V, Lornage J, et al. Sperm DNA fragmentation decreases the pregnancy rate in an assisted reproductive technique. Hum Reprod 2003;18: 1023–1028.

45. Gandini L, Lombardo F, Paoli D, et al. Full-term pregnancies achieved with ICSI despite high levels of sperm chromatin damage. Hum Reprod 2004;19:1409–1417.

46. Bungum M, Humaidan P, Spano M, Jepson K, Bungum L, Giwercman A. The predictive value of sperm chromatin structure assay (SCSA) parameters for the outcome of intrauterine insemination, IVF and ICSI. Hum Reprod 2004;19:1401–1408.

47. Virro MR, Larson-Cook KL, Evenson DP. Sperm chromatin structure assay (SCSA) parameters are related to fertilization, blastocyst development, and ongoing pregnancy in in vitro fertilization and intracytoplasmic sperm injection cycles. Fertil Steril 2004;81:1289–1295.

48. Virro MR, Larson-Cook KL, Evenson DP. Sperm chromatin structure assay (SCSA) parameters are related to fertilization, blastocyst development, and ongoing pregnancy in in vitro fertilization and intracytoplasmic sperm injection cycles. Fertil Steril 2004;81:1289–1295.

49. Spano M, Seli E, Bizzaro D, Manicardi GC, Sakkas D. The significance of sperm nuclear DNA strand breaks on reproductive outcome. Current Opin Obstet Gynecol 2005;17:255–260.

50. Sakkas D, Manicardi GC, Tomlinson M, et al. The use of two density gradient centrifugation techniques and the swim-up method to separate spermatozoa with chromatin and nuclear DNA anomalies. Hum Reprod 2000;15:1112–1116.

51. Sakkas D. The need to detect DNA damage in human spermatozoa: possible consequences on embryo development. In: Gagnon C, editor. The Male Gamete: from basic science to clinical applications. Cache River Press, Vienna, IL; 1999:379–384.

52. Seli E, Gardner DK, Schoolcraft WB, Moffatt O, Sakkas D. Extent of nuclear DNA damage in ejaculated spermatozoa impacts on blastocyst development after in vitro fertilization. Fertil Steril 2004;82:378–383.

53. Bartoov B, Berkovitz A, Eltes F. Selection of spermatozoa with normal nuclei to improve the pregnancy rate with intracytoplasmic sperm injection. N Engl J Med 2001;345:1067–1068.

54. Bartoov B, Berkovitz A, Eltes F, et al. Pregnancy rates are higher with intracytoplasmic morphologically selected sperm injection than with conventional intracytoplasmic injection. Fertil Steril 2003;80:1413–1419.

55. Ainsworth C, Nixon B, Aitken RJ. Development of a novel electrophoretic system for the isolation of human spermatozoa. Hum Reprod 2005;20:2261–2270.

56. Said T, Agarwal A, Grunewald S, et al. Selection of non-apoptotic spermatozoa as a new tool for enhancing assisted reproduction outcomes: an in vitro model. Biol Reprod 2005;74:530–537.

57. Huszar G, Ozenci CC, Cayli S, Zavaczki Z, Hansch E, Vigue L. Hyaluronic acid binding by human sperm indicates cellular maturity, viability, and unreacted acrosomal status. Fertil Steril 2003;79:1616–1624.

58. Jakab A, Sakkas D, Delpiano E, et al. Intracytoplasmic sperm injection: a novel selection method for sperm with normal frequency of chromosomal aneuploidies. Fertil Steril 2005;84:1665–1673.

21 Clinical Evaluation of the Genetics of Male Infertility

Peter N. Schlegel, MD

Summary

Clinical evaluation for genetic abnormalities is at the crossroads of investigational and practical patient management. Whereas scientific investigation begs for further evaluation of the likely genetic anomalies that underlie many cases of male infertility, clinical testing and consultation must, wherever possible, be practical and directed toward optimizing patient outcome. Men with congenital obstructive azoospermia as well as patients with severely defective spermatogenesis will commonly have identifiable genetic abnormalities. Men with bilateral congenital absence of the vas deferens are commonly cystic fibrosis (CF) carriers, and their female partner should be tested for CF gene mutations before conception. Severely defective spermatogenesis may reflect a karyotypic abnormality or partial deletion of the Y chromosome. Detection of Y microdeletions or specific chromosome anomalies may affect the chance of sperm retrieval in azoospermic men, whereas it appears that the use of sperm from men with genetic abnormalities does not affect intracytoplasmic sperm injection outcomes. Specific genetic testing is warranted for certain subsets of infertile men. Other genetic tests (sperm DNA integrity testing, sperm aneuploidy analysis) are being evaluated and may prove to be clinically useful in the future.

Key Words: Azoospermia; Y-chromosome microdeletion; diagnosis; treatment; kayotype; chromatin.

1. INTRODUCTION

For all men with infertility, a complete history and physical examination is recommended to identify potentially correctable causes of male factor infertility. The American Urological Association and American Society for Reproductive Medicine Practice Committees recommend that initial evaluation of the man and woman in an infertile couple proceed in parallel and be initiated at the same time *(1)*. The initial evaluation of the man involves semen analysis and reproductive

From: *The Genetics of Male Infertility*
Edited by: D.T. Carrell © Humana Press Inc., Totowa, NJ

history. If abnormalities are found on initial evaluation, then complete evaluation with additional history, complete physical examination, hormone testing, and genetic analysis may be indicated.

An infertile man is evaluated when the results will influence the treatment for a couple. In most cases, evaluation is aimed toward identification of conditions that may be treated and change the chance of achieving a pregnancy. Preferably, evidence that treatment is effective will have been demonstrated in randomized controlled clinical trials of that treatment. Unfortunately, relatively few treatments for male infertility have such a level of evidence to support treatment. Therefore, evaluation is directed toward identifying conditions that may affect male infertility (such as varicoceles, obstruction of the reproductive tract, and so on) despite the lack of strong evidence to support treatment. Medically important conditions associated with infertility (testis tumors, pituitary lesions) are also sought during this evaluation.

A second indication for evaluation exists where there is evidence that a genetic condition may be present in the infertile man that would affect the prognosis for treatment or a condition present in the infertile man could affect the health of offspring. Genetic testing is recommended because certain genetic conditions are found in subgroups of infertile men. The conditions where genetic testing is clearly indicated are discussed in this chapter. Other genetic testing that is considered investigational but not yet recommended for routine use is also discussed.

2. OBSTRUCTIVE AZOOSPERMIA

Men with obstructive azoospermia (OA) may be candidates for microsurgical reconstruction or sperm retrieval with assisted reproduction. Regardless of the approach for fertility treatment, the potential genetic etiology of congenital OA must be evaluated.

Mesonephric (Wolffian) duct anomalies are commonly associated with mutations in the cystic fibrosis transmembrane conductance regulator (CFTR) gene. CF is the most common fatal autosomal-recessive disorder in the white population, with an incidence of approx 1 in 2500 live births and a carrier frequency of 1 in 25 persons of Northern European descent. The CFTR gene was cloned in 1989, with more than 550 mutations described, 51 of which are commonly tested in a CF genetic screening panel. In most ethnic groups, these 51 mutations will define more than 70–90% of patients with CF. In approx 95% of men with CF, the Wolffian derivatives of the vas deferens and most of the epididymis do not develop, resulting in the condition referred to as congenital bilateral absence of the vas deferens (CBAVD). Conversely, 50–80% men with CBAVD (but no digestive or pulmonary symptoms suggestive of CF) will have CFTR mutations definable. This relationship has been summarized nicely by Oates and Amos *(2)*. Jarvi et al. have also reported that up to 47% of men with idiopathic epididymal obstruction will also have CFTR mutations present *(3)*. Given the high prevalence of the CFTR mutation carrier state in women in North America, it is prudent to consider evaluation of the female partner for CFTR mutations when a man presents with Wolffian duct abnormalities including congenital unilateral absence of the vas deferens or idiopathic epididymal obstruction.

Of interest, men with CBAVD who also have renal anomalies (unilateral agenesis or anomalies of ascent) do not appear to be at any higher risk of carrying CFTR anomalies than men in the general population. For developmental or other genetic reasons, an early defect in mesonephric development may affect both the ureteral bud as well as Wolffian duct development. Therefore, not all men with CBAVD will have CFTR mutations. However, all men with CBAVD should be evaluated for renal anomalies, and the female partners of men with CBAVD should be evaluated for CFTR status, because many CFTR anomalies may not be detected with a standard panel of 51 mutations analyzed. Men with CBAVD and two kidneys should be assumed to be carriers of CFTR mutations and their female partners should be tested for CF gene mutations before treatment with assisted reproduction *(1)*.

3. SPERMATOGENIC FAILURE

Men with spermatogenic failure have decreased numbers and/or quality of spermatozoa in the ejaculate. In its most severe form, these patients will have no sperm in the ejaculate (nonobstructive azoospermia [NOA]). External heat or toxic effects or significant medical pathology may be the underlying cause of spermatogenic failure. In both cases, knowledge and removal/management of these conditions is critical before proceeding with assisted reproduction. In addition, genetic evaluation may provide significant prognostic value that can affect decision making for patients who are to be treated with assisted reproduction. Genetic testing (Y-chromosome microdeletion analysis and karyotype) are recommended for men with oligozoospermia (<5–10 million sperm/cc). CFTR gene mutations have also been associated with NOA or idiopathic infertility in anecdotal reports. Larger studies have not confirmed these assertions. Therefore, CF mutation screening of men with impaired spermatogenesis is not currently recommended.

4. GENETIC ABNORMALITIES AND TESTING

The frequency and clinical significance of certain genetic disorders associated with spermatogenic failure, including NOA are adequate to support screening for specific genetic abnormalities. These abnormalities include both chromosomal abnormalities, detectable with routine karyotype testing, and Y-chromosome microdeletions, so-called azoospermia factor (AZF) defects. Other rare genetic causes of male infertility have been reviewed previously (4). For men with severe male factor infertility, including men with sperm concentrations less than 10×10^6/cc and NOA, karyotype evaluation and Y-chromosome microdeletion analysis is recommended before treatment with assisted reproduction.

4.1. Karyotype Evaluation

The most common karyotypic abnormality in men with severe male factor infertility is Klinefelter syndrome, affecting up to 7–13% of azoospermic men. Almost all men with the pure, classic form (47,XXY) of Klinefelter will be azoospermic, whereas limited sperm production is commonly found in men with a mosaic pattern of Klinefelter syndrome. It was previously felt that only spermatogonia with a 46,XY complement could produce spermatozoa; however, observations indicate that a significant proportion of 24,XY spermatozoa are present in the testes of men with Klinefelter (5). General teaching has suggested that men with Klinefelter syndrome can be readily identified by their typical physical appearance of tall stature, gynecomastia, and small, firm testes. We now routinely detect men with nonmosaic Klinefelter syndrome who are normally masculinized, and between 5'6" and 5'10" in height. Observations reported by Oates et al. also confirm that some men with chromosomal abnormalities will have an otherwise normal phenotypic appearance, except for their infertility (2).

The presence of Klinefelter syndrome provides a favorable prognostic feature for sperm retrieval using microdissection testicular sperm extraction (TESE) in azoospermic men. For these patients, the chance of sperm retrieval is 72%, and once sperm is retrieved, the chance of clinical pregnancy is more than 50% at our institution (6). The rate of development of 47,XXY, or 47,XXX embryos after sperm retrieval for men with Klinefelter syndrome appears to be very low. None of the children born at our institution, and only one fetus reported in published literature, had Klinefelter syndrome, despite the slight increased risk of aneuploidy in sperm obtained from such men.

Other karyotypic abnormalities identified include Robertsonian translocations, chromosomal inversions, and non-Klinefelter sex chromosome abnormalities. Detection of these structural chromosomal anomalies results in an increased risk of aneuploidy or unbalanced chromosomal complements in embryos. Couples with structural abnormalities should have genetic counseling, and the use of genetic pre-implantation diagnosis (PGD) is warranted for these couples.

4.2. Y Chromosome (AZF) Microdeletions

Several genes have been identified in the distal portion of the long arm of Y (Yq) that are frequently deleted in men with NOA. The best described gene has multiple copies, and is referred to as deleted azoospermia (DAZ). Deletions involving DAZ were identified in 13% (12/89) of azoospermic men screened by Reijo et al. in 1995 *(7)*. In addition, Reijo et al. observed that men with severe oligozoospermia had a 6% (2/35) chance of DAZ deletions *(7)*. Other investigators have found longer deletions of the Y chromosome associated with male infertility. Vogt et al. have suggested that three relatively discrete regions of Yq, AZFa, AZFb, and AZFc, are deleted in severely infertile men *(8)*. We have further characterized the clinical significance of AZF deletions and found that the deleted region determines the chance of sperm retrieval *(9)*. The AZF regions have also been mechanistically described based on the pallindromic repeat regions that recombined to allow the deletions along the Y chromosome. In addition, short regions of deletion within AZFc that are commonly deleted in normospermic and azoospermic men have been described (gr/gr). Because there is inadequate evidence that gr/gr deletions occur at a higher rate in men with low sperm production or infertility than for men with normal sperm production and fertility, it is likely that such deletions reflect polymorphisms.

Several investigators have found that 3–18% of men with severe sperm production abnormalities, including azoospermia, have Y-chromosome deletions. However, the literature is difficult to evaluate because the data was generated in multiple laboratories, each looking at different patient populations and examining different regions and sites on Yq. For example, some investigators considered a microdeletion present when only a single sequence-tagged site was absent, whereas others considered a microdeletion present only if sequential sites on the Y chromosome failed to amplify with polymerase chain reaction-based analysis. Nevertheless, all investigators consistently found Y microdeletions of the AZFa, AZFb, or AZFc regions in a measurable proportion of severely subfertile men, with no detectable deletions in normal fertile men, or in the fathers or brothers of men with Y microdeletions.

Y-chromosome deletions affecting fertility usually involve deletion of one or more entire AZFa, AZFb, or AZFc regions. An additional region of the Y chromosome referred to as AZFd has been described, however, AZFd is within AZFc, has no prognostic significance, and is not associated with impaired sperm production. Therefore, such deletions appear not to have any clinical relevance. Approximately two-thirds of men with deletions involving only AZFc have sperm in the ejaculate (severe oligozoospermia). In azoospermic men with AZFc deletions, sperm production is commonly present within the testicle, and TESE is at least as successful as for other men with NOA, who have an overall sperm retrieval rate of 58%. At Cornell, sperm was found by TESE in 75% of men with AZFc deletions and azoospermia (9). Once sperm are found from men with AZFc deletions, either in the ejaculate or by TESE, fertilization and pregnancy results following intracytoplasmic sperm injection (ICSI) are comparable to those obtained for other couples (matched for sperm production level and contemporaneously) treated at our center (10).

For men with deletions involving the AZFb region, the chance of having sperm in the ejaculate or finding sperm with TESE is severely decreased (11). Sperm were found in none of 23 men we evaluated with deletions involving AZFb who had a biopsy or sperm retrieval attempted with TESE (9). Therefore, we do not recommend that men with deletions involving the entire AZFb region undergo TESE.

Overall, approx 9% of men with NOA and Sertoli cell-only pattern on diagnostic testis biopsy will have AZFa deletions. Deletions involving the entire AZFa region are also commonly associated with a Sertoli cell-only pattern on diagnostic biopsy (12). It is important to discriminate between partial and complete deletions of an AZF region, given that at least one patient with a deletion of part of the AZFa region had germ cells on testis biopsy. However, to date, no sperm has been retrieved from men with complete deletions of AZFa or AZFb. Because the documented number of cases in the literature is limited, absolute predictive statements are not possible to make at this time. However, the prognosis for sperm retrieval is clearly different and dramatically worse for men with complete AZFa and AZFb deletions than for other patients with NOA (9).

Because Y chromosome abnormalities, including deletions, will be passed on to any male child who is produced after assisted reproduction, these men must have genetic counseling before treatment. In an important preliminary study of fathers and ICSI-derived sons, Kent-First et al. found that 10% (3/32) of unselected ICSI-derived boys had detectable Y-chromosome microdeletions, however, only one of the three boys had a father with Y-chromosome microdeletions detected on testing of his peripheral blood *(12)*. These results suggest that mosaicism with germline deletions on the short segments of the Y chromosome frequently develop in spermatozoa of men with severe male factor infertility. Because men with these genetic defects have rarely or never fathered children naturally, it is uncertain whether any medical conditions will be present in the offspring with Y-chromosome microdeletions, except for infertility. This knowledge makes genetic counseling difficult. On the other hand, common sense suggests that because the fathers are otherwise healthy and normal, the presence of a Y-chromosome microdeletion does not pose a high risk for major congenital defects in potential offspring. A definitive answer will not be available for many years, when the children born from this process are adults.

5. EFFECT OF GENETIC ANOMALIES ON TREATMENT CHOICE

Evaluation of a sequential series of 170 men with NOA who were candidates for TESE at our institution revealed that 17% of these men had definable genetic defects, be it Y-chromosome microdeletions or karyotype abnormalities *(6)*. We have found that the knowledge of having a genetic defect leads many men to pursue options other than TESE-ICSI and that, regardless of treatment choice, the majority of men find it reassuring to know the cause of their infertility.

6. OTHER GENETIC TESTS NOT CURRENTLY RECOMMENDED FOR CLINICAL APPLICATION

6.1. Androgen Receptor Defects

Defects of the androgen receptor (AR) result in phenotypic females (testicular feminization), whereas very mild mutations have been associated in a limited number of cases with a male phenotype and infertility. A variable-length region of exon 1 of the AR has been identified and characterized that contains multiple glutamine (CAG) sequences. This region, referred to as a polyglutamine or trinucleotide-repeat segment, has been associated with several disease states. Long extensions of the polyglutamine region ($\geq$40 CAG repeats), is associated with Kennedy disease, a severe, degenerative, neuromuscular condition. Shorter numbers of CAG repeats are associated with an increased risk of prostate cancer. Men of African-American descent have shorter CAG sequences than Caucasian men, whereas Asian men have the longest CAG repeats.

Interestingly, black men are at the highest risk of developing prostate cancer, with Asian men having a limited risk.

Different studies of CAG repeats in infertile men have been reported. In an article looking at all types of AR mutations in infertile men, in addition to CAG-repeat length polymorphisms, no mutations were found in 35 patients or 32 controls *(13)*. Azoospermic men had significantly longer CAG repeats than controls (23.2 vs 20.5). The odds of having a CAG repeat length of 20 were sixfold higher for men with a defect in spermatogenesis. It was postulated that assisted reproductive techniques may lead to a trend toward higher CAG-repeat lengths and higher risk of Kennedy disease. Other studies have supported a difference in CAG-repeat length in severe male factor infertility *(14,15)*, whereas others have failed to confirm the association *(16)*. Taken together, CAG-repeat length in the AR may be a risk factor for some men with infertility. Several anecdotal reports have suggested that isolated men with longer CAG-repeat sequences associated with infertility have had increased sperm concentration and pregnancies after treatment with clomiphene citrate or exogenous testosterone. The increased serum testosterone provided by these treatments was postulated to overcome the AR defect. Nevertheless, these are uncontrolled case reports. Indeed, most men treated over prolonged periods with exogenous testosterone will have spermatogenesis suppressed because of decreased endogenous pituitary gonadotropin production and subsequent lowering of intratesticular testosterone levels. Therefore, AR receptor analysis is not currently recommended as a genetic screening test because it does not predict infertility, is not associated with an obvious increased risk of disease in offspring, and treatment has not been demonstrated to be of benefit for "affected" patients.

6.2. Sperm DNA Integrity Testing

Several tests allow assessment of DNA integrity within spermatozoa. The deoxynucleotidyl transferase [TdT]-mediated dUTP nick end-labeling (TUNEL) assay detects the number of DNA breaks within the head of spermatozoa. This test has been used to detect sperm that are undergoing apoptosis. The Comet assay similarly detects DNA fragmentation using an *in situ* detection technique. The sperm chromatin structure assay (SCSA™) is now commonly applied for analysis of DNA integrity in men with infertility. This test evaluates spermatozoa DNA as being single-stranded (abnormal) or double-stranded (normal). Unfortunately, its clinical role has not been clearly defined. Initial studies suggested that abnormal SCSA levels (>27% DNA fragmentation index) were associated with no chance of fertility naturally or with assisted reproduction. Many further studies have been done to evaluate the effect of abnormal DNA integrity on pregnancy rates. Most studies have not controlled for female age or other factors that are known to affect the results of IVF/ICSI. However, most studies have suggested that abnormal DNA integrity has a significant negative effect on the chance of pregnancy after assisted reproduction (17). Although it would be of concern to use spermatozoa with grossly abnormal DNA for IVF or ICSI, based on preliminary data, it appears that abnormalities of sperm DNA integrity rarely exist as an isolated finding. In most cases, sperm from semen samples with poor DNA integrity often have abnormal motility, low concentration, and abnormal morphology. However, 8% of infertile men with normal semen parameters will have abnormal sperm DNA integrity (18). Therefore, the role of these tests of DNA integrity as a clinical tool for male factor infertility is yet to be fully defined (19). It is possible that some couples who have poor embryo development or recurrent pregnancy loss may have abnormal DNA integrity as a cause (20).

A more sophisticated test for DNA adducts allows detection of 8-hydroxydeoxyguanosine (8-OhdG), a measure of oxidative damage to spermatozoa (20). Increased DNA damage is seen in spermatozoa from men with oxidative effects, including men who are smokers, and treatment of these men with antioxidants (e.g., vitamin C 250 mg/d) has been shown to decrease 8-hydroxydeoxyguanosine formation (consistent with decreased oxidation (21,22).

6.3. Sperm Aneuploidy Analysis

Defective sperm production is associated with an increased risk of sperm aneuploidy. Whereas normospermic men have approx 1% sperm aneuploidy, oligozoospermic men have 8% aneuploidy and men with NOA have 15% aneuploidy (23). Morphologically abnormal sperm are also more likely to have sperm aneuploidy, although the frequency of sperm aneuploidy is small even in men with 0% normal forms. Aneuploid sperm may fertilize oocytes, especially during assisted reproduction. Sperm aneuploidy may also play a significant role in recurrent pregnancy loss (24). Sperm aneuploidy occurs at a much lower frequency than oocyte aneuploidy, our observation that limits the clinical value of routine sperm aneuploidy testing of any subgroup of infertile men. The lack of increased birth defect rates after assisted reproduction treatment of men with severe infertility supports the limited value of sperm aneuploidy testing. However, the prognostic role of sperm aneuploidy analysis in treatment of infertile men has yet to be demonstrated, and couples that are appropriate candidates for sperm aneuploidy analysis are still being refined. Therefore, sperm aneuploidy analysis is not yet recognized as a useful clinical tool for management of infertile couples.

7. ROLE OF GENETIC ANALYSIS DURING AND AFTER ASSISTED REPRODCTION

Genetic analysis before ICSI can provide several distinct advantages. First, it may allow PGD of genetic defects in embryos. Second, it may provide important prognostic information before treatment. Third, it reassures men that they were born with their infertile condition and did not cause it through sexual or environmental exposures. PGD can detect chromosomal or specific genetic abnormalities in embryos before intrauterine transfer, but knowledge of the specific genetic abnormality is necessary to direct PGD analysis. Finally, it is evident that approx 20% of men with genetic anomalies detected and confirmed will choose to pursue other options rather than sperm retrieval to become fathers *(6)*.

8. CONCLUSION

Men with NOA or severe oligozoospermia (<5–10×10^6 sperm/cc) should be tested with karyotype analysis and evaluated for Y-chromosome microdeletion. This recommendation reflects the American Society for Reproductive Medicine Practice Committee and American Urological Association Male Infertility Best Practice Policy Guidelines published in 2001. Men with less than 10×10^6 sperm/cc should also be counseled regarding Y-chromosome microdeletion analysis.

Men with OA owing to congenital absence of the vas deferens or idiopathic epididymal obstruction are at high risk to be carriers of CF gene mutations. Therefore, their female partners should be tested before treatment with microsurgical reconstruction of the male or assisted reproduction with retrieved spermatozoa. The men are often commonly evaluated for CF gene mutations, because many couples want to know what caused their fertility problem.

REFERENCES

1. Sharlip ID, Jarow JP, Belker AM, et al. Best practice policies for male infertility. Fertil Steril 2002;77:873–882.
2. Oates RD, Amos JA. The genetic basis of congenital absence of the vas deferens and cystic fibrosis. J Androl 1994;15:1.

3. Jarvi K, Zielinski J, Wilschanski M, et al. Cystic fibrosis transmembrane conductance regulator and obstructive azoospermia. Lancet 1995;345:1578.

4. Mak V, Jarvi KA. The genetics of male infertility. J Urol 1996;156:1245–1257.

5. Chevret E, Rousseaux S, Monteil M, et al. Increased incidence of hyperhaploid 24,XY spermatozoa detected by three-colour FISH in a 46,XY/47,XXY male. Hum Genet 1996;97:171–175.

6. Rucker GB, Mielnik A, King P, Goldstein M, Schlegel PN. Preoperative screening for genetic abnormalities in men with non-obstructive azoospermia prior to testicular sperm extraction. J Urol 1998;160:2068–2071.

7. Reijo R, Lee TY, Salo P, et al. Diverse spermatogenic defects in humans caused by Y chromosome deletions encompassing a novel RNA-binding protein gene. Nat Genet 1995;10:383–393.

8. Vogt PH, Edelmann A, Kirsch S, et al. Human Y chromosome azoospermia factors (AZF) mapped to different subregions in Yq11. Hum Mol Genet 1996;5: 933–943.

9. Hopps CV, Mielnik A, Goldstein M, Palermo GD, Rosenwaks Z, Schlegel PN. Detection of sperm in men with Y chromosome microdeletions of the AZFa, AZFb and AZFc regions. Hum Reprod 2003;18:1660–1665.

10. Choi JM, Chung P, Veeck L, Mielnik A, Palermo GD, Schlegel PN. AZF microdeletions of the Y chromsome and in vitro fertilization outcome. Fertil Steril 2004;81:337–341.

11. Brandell RA, Mielnik A, Liotta D, et al. AZFb deletions predict the absence of sperm with testicular sperm extraction: Preliminary report of a prognostic genetic test. Hum Reprod 1998;13:2812–2815.

12. Kent-First MG, Kol S, Muallem A, et al. Infertility in intracytoplasmic sperm-injection-derived sons. Lancet 1996;348:332–333.

13. Dowsing AT, Yong EL, Clark M, McLachlan RI, deKretser DM, Trounsen AO. Linkage between male infertility and trinucleotide repeat expansion in the androgen-receptor gene. Lancet 1999;354:640–643.

14. Yoshida KI, Yano M, Chiba K, Honda M, Kitahara S. CAG repeat length in the androgen receptor gene is enhanced in patients with idiopathic azoospermia. Urology 1999;54:1078–1081.

15. Yong EL, Lim J, Qi W, Ong V, Mifsud A. Molecular basis of androgen receptor diseases. Ann Med 2000;32:15–22.

16. Dadze S, Wieland C, Jakubiczka S, et al. Mol Hum Reprod 2000;6:207–214.

17. Niederberger C. Redefining the relationship between sperm deoxyribonucleic acid fragmentation as measured by the sperm chromatin structure assay and outcomes of assisted reproductive techniques. J Urol 2006;175:663.

18. Zini A, Fischer MA, Sharir S, Shayegan B, Phang D, Jarvi K. Prevalence of abnormal sperm DNA denaturation in fertile and infertile men. Urology 2002;60: 1069–1072.

19. Carrell DT, Liu L, Peterson CM, et al. Sperm DNA fragmentation is increased in couples with unexplained recurrent pregnancy loss. Arch Androl 2003;49:49–55.

20. Shen HM, Chia SE, Ong CN. Evaluation of oxidative DNA damage in human sperm and its association with male infertility. J Androl 1999;20:718–723.

21. Fraga CG, Motchnik PA, Wyrobek AJ, Rempel DM, Ames BN. Smoking and low antioxidant levels increase oxidative damage to sperm DNA. Mutat Res 1996;351:199–203.

22. Fraga CG, Motchnik PA, Shigenaga MK, Helbock HJ, Jacob RA, Ames BN. Ascorbic acid protects against endogenous oxidative DNA damage in human sperm. Proc Natl Acad Sci USA 1991;88:11,003–11,006.

23. Palermo GD, Colombero LT, Hariprashad JJ, Schlegel PN, Rosenwaks Z. Chromosome analysis of epididymal and testicular sperm in azoospermic patients undergoing ICSI. Hum Reprod 2002;17:570–575.

24. Carrell DT, Wilcox AL, Lowy L, et al. Elevated sperm chromosome aneuploidy and apoptosis in patients with unexplained recurrent pregnancy loss. Obstet Gynecol 2003;101:1229–1235.

Index

A

ADAM2, *see* Fertilinβ
ADAM3, *see* Cyritestin
ADAM24, *see* Testase
Androgen receptor,
  CAG repeat, 254,
    255,275,321,322
  gene polymorphisms, 275, 276
  genetic screening, 322
Andrology,
  genomics relationship, 4, 5
  historical perspective, 4
Aneuploidy analysis,
  chromosomal translocations,
    132, 133
  fluorescence *in situ*
    hybridization, 130–134,
    136, 137, 139
  46,XY karyotype, 134, 137
  indications, 139
  inversions, 133, 134
  nonobstructive azoospermia,
    137, 139
  normal men, 129, 130
  offspring studies,
    prospective studies, 136, 137
    retrospective studies, 135,
      136
  recommendations, 323, 324
  sex chromosome abnormalities,
    131, 132, 134
  sperm selection based on
    chromosome content, 134,
    135
Annexin V, sperm apoptosis
  marker, 303

Apoptosis, sperm markers, 302, 303
Argonaute,
  chromatid body association,
    202, 203
  function, 201, 202
ART, *see* Assisted reproductive
  technology
Assisted reproductive technology
  (ART),
  approaches, 301
  costs, 269
  intracytoplasmic sperm
    injection, 232, 252, 268,
    269, 308, 309
  limitations and alternatives, 79,
    90, 269
  offspring infertility, 252, 320,
    321
  pregnancy prediction with
    sperm chromatin damage
    testing, 305–308
  sperm handling, 308, 309
  trends in use, 79
Ataxia telangiectasia, infertility,
  156, 157
ATM, functions, 156, 157
AZF, *see* Azoospermia factor
Azoospermia factor (AZF),
  infertility defects, 233, 234
  microdeletions,
    evaluation, 319–321
    partial AZFc deletions and
      Y-chromosome
      variants, 240, 241, 243–
      245, 280, 282
    types, 233, 234, 239, 240, 319
Azoospermia, definition, 232

329